PROGRESS IN QUANTITATIVE CORONARY ARTERIOGRAPHY

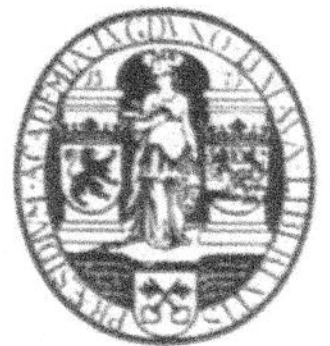

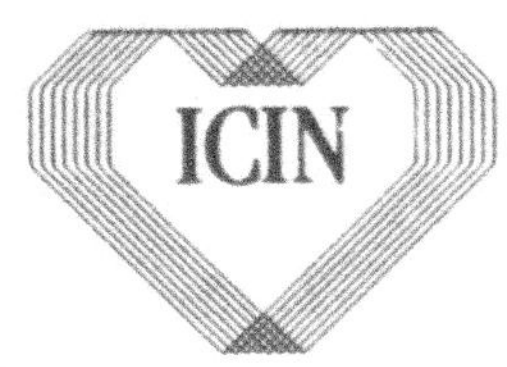

Developments in Cardiovascular Medicine

VOLUME 155

The titles published in this series are listed at the end of this volume.

Progress in quantitative coronary arteriography

Edited by

JOHAN H.C. REIBER
Laboratory for Clinical and Experimental Image Processing, Department of Diagnostic Radiology and Nuclear Medicine, University Hospital Leiden, The Netherlands

and

PATRICK W. SERRUYS
Catheterization Laboratory, Thorax Center, Erasmus University, Rotterdam, The Netherlands

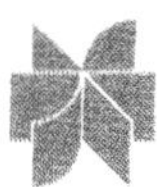

Springer Science+Business Media, B.V.

Library of Congress Cataloging-in-Publication Data

Progress in quantitative coronary arteriography / edited by Johan H.C. Reiber and Patrick W. Serruys.
p. cm. -- (Developments in cardiovascular medicine ; v. 155)
Includes index.
ISBN 978-0-7923-2814-8 ISBN 978-94-011-1172-0 (eBook)
DOI 10.1007/978-94-011-1172-0
1. Angiocardiography. 2. Coronary heart disease--Diagnosis
3. Coronary arteries--Imaging. I. Reiber, J. H. C. (Johan H.C.)
II. Serruys, P. W. III. Series.
[DNLM: 1. Coronary Angiography--methods. 2. Vascular Surgery--methods. W1 DE997VME v. 155 1994 / WG 300 P9647 1994]
RC683.5.A5P77 1994
616.1'2307572--dc20
DNLM/DLC
for Library of Congress 94-13374

ISBN 978-0-7923-2814-8

Printed on acid-free paper

Originally published by Kluwer Academic Publishers in 1994

Table of contents

Part Four: **QCA in progression/regression of atherosclerotic disease**

Part Five: **QCA in recanalization techniques**

Part Six: **'The rivals'**

List of contributors

Andreas Baumbach
Medical Clinic III, Eberhard-Karls-University, Otfried-Müller-Strasse 10, D-72076 Tübingen, Germany
Co-authors: Karl K. Haase & Karl R. Karsch

Glenn J. Beauman
Division of Cardiology, University of Maryland Medical System, Rm N3W77, 22 S. Greene Str, Baltimore, MD 21201, U.S.A.
Co-authors: Johan H.C. Reiber, Gerhard Koning, Roland C.M. van Houdt & Robert A. Vogel

Jack T. Cusma
Cardiac Catheterization Laboratory, Duke University Medical Center, Box 3012, Durham, NC 27710, U.S.A.
Co-author: Thomas M. Bashore

Håkan Emanuelsson
Division of Cardiology, Medical Clinic I, Sahlgrenska Hospital, S-431 45 Göteborg, Sweden
Co-authors: Carl Lamm & Michal Dohnal

Pim J. de Feyter
Thoraxcenter, Bd 432, University Hospital Dijkzigt, P.O. Box 1738, 3000 DR Rotterdam, The Netherlands
Co-authors: Carlo Di Mario, Cees J. Slager, Patrick W. Serruys & Jos R.T.C. Roelandt

Peter Ganz
Cardiovascular Division, Brigham and Women's Hospital, 75 Francis Street, Boston, MA 02115, U.S.A.
Co-authors: François Charbonneau, Ian T. Meredith, Todd J. Anderson, Marie Gerhard, Michael Dyce, Danielle Delagrange & Andrew P. Selwyn

Jürgen Haase
Herzzentrum Frankfurt, Alfred Brehm Platz 5-9, D-60136 Frankfurt, Germany
Co-authors: David Keane, Carlo Di Mario, Javier Escaned, Yukio Ozaki, Cornelis J. Slager, Rob van Bremen, Willem J. van der Giessen & Patrick W. Serruys

Morton J. Kern
Director, J.G. Mudd Cardiac Catheterization Laboratory, St. Louis University Hospital, 3635 Vista Ave at Grand, St. Louis, MO 63110, U.S.A.

John R. Kramer
The Cleveland Clinic Foundation, One Clinic Center, 9500 Euclid Avenue, Cleveland, OH 44195-5066 U.S.A.
Co-authors: Bruce W. Lytle & Michael S. Feld

Jean-Marc Lablanche
Hôpital Cardiologique, Boulevard du Professeur Leclercq, F-59037 Lille, France
Co-authors: (Chapter 22): Eugène P Mc Fadden, Christophe Bauters, Philippe Quandalle & Michel E. Bertrand
Co-authors (Chapter 23): Martial Hamon, Eugène P. Mc Fadden, Christophe Bauters & Michel E. Bertrand

Jacques Lespérance
Montreal Heart Institute, 5000 Bélanger Str. East, Montreal, Quebec, Canada H1T 1C8
Co-authors: Gilles Hudon, Pierre Théroux & David Waters

Thomas Felix Lüscher
Division of Cardiology, University Hospital, Inselspital, Hebelstr. 20, CH-3010 Bern, Switzerland

G.B. John Mancini
Department of Internal Medicine, University Hospital – UBC Site, Room S-169, 2211 Wesbrook Mall, Vancouver, BC, Canada V6T 1Z3

Nico H.J. Pijls
Department of Cardiology, Catharina Hospital, P.O. Box 1350, 5602 ZA Eindhoven, The Netherlands
Co-authors: Bernard De Bruyne, Sherif El Biltagui, Mamdouh El Gamal, Hans J.R.M. Bonnier, Guy R. Heyndrickx, K. Lance Gould, Richard Kirkeeide, G. Jan Willem Bech, Jacques J. Koolen, H. Rolf Michels, Frank A.L.E. Bracke & William Wijns

Jeffrey J. Popma
Director, Angiographic Core Laboratory, Washington Hospital Center, 110 Irving Street, Suite 4 B-1, Washington, DC 20010, U.S.A.
Co-authors: Ya Chien Chuang, Gary S. Mintz, Luella T. Lewis & Martin B. Leon

Johan H.C. Reiber
Department of Diagnostic Radiology, University Hospital Leiden, Building 1, C2-S, P.O. Box 9600, 2300 RC Leiden, The Netherlands
Co-authors (Chapter 3): Gerhard Koning, Craig D. von Land & Pieter M.J. van der Zwet
Co-authors (Chapter 5): Craig D. von Land, Gerhard Koning, Pieter M.J. van der Zwet, Ronald C.M. van Houdt, Martin J. Schalij & Jacques Lespérance

Jos R.T.C. Roelandt
Thoraxcenter, Bd 408, Erasmus University Rotterdam, P.O. Box 1738, 3000 DR Rotterdam, The Netherlands
Co-authors: Andonis G. Violaris, Carlo Di Mario, Patrick W. Serruys & Pim J. de Feyter

Martin T. Rothman
Consultant Cardiologist, The Royal London & Royal Brompton Hospitals, London E1 1BB, U.K.

Martin J. Schalij
Department of Cardiology, University Hospital Leiden, Building 1, P.O. Box 9600, 2300 RC Leiden, The Netherlands
Co-authors: Mariken J.S. Geldof, Pieter M.J. van der Zwet, E.T. van der Velde, Els M. Nagtegaal, Volkert Manger Cats, Johan H.C. Reiber & Albert V.G. Bruschke

Patrick W. Serruys
Thoraxcenter, Ee 2332, Erasmus University Rotterdam, P.O. Box 1738, 3000 DR Rotterdam, The Netherlands
Co-authors: Carlo Di Mario, Rob Krams, Robert Gil & Nicolas Meneveau

Rüdiger Simon
Department of Cardiology, I. Medical Clinic, Christian-Albrechts-University, DW-2300 Kiel, Germany

Jos A.E. Spaan
Department of Medical Physics and Information, Academic Medical Center, Meibergdreef 15, 1105 AZ Amsterdam, The Netherlands

Mark M.J.M. van der Linden
Cardialysis, Westzeedijk 120, 3016 AH Rotterdam, The Netherlands
Co-authors: Jürgen Haase & Patrick W. Serruys

Felix Zijlstra
Department of Cardiology, Hospital De Weezenlanden, Groot Wezenland 20, 8011 JW Zwolle, The Netherlands
Co-authors: P. Widimsky & Harry Suryapranata

Preface

This is the fifth volume in this series on quantitative coronary arteriography (QCA) published over the last nine years. Research and applications in this exciting field are covered in a total of 26 chapters by world renowned experts. This book is subdivided into a total of 6 parts, each emphasizing the latest progress in these respective fields.

In Part One a comprehensive overview is given of the current knowledge and research in endothelial function, which is of eminent importance for the further understanding of the pathophysiology of coronary artery disease in patients.

Fortunately, the use of QCA tools is not limited anymore to leading research institutes; over the last several years these tools have been installed in many cardiology centers world wide. To understand the current possibilities, limitations and future expectations of QCA, several relevant topics are presented in Part Two. First of all, the questions about why and how QCA systems should be validated both at the development site and at the application sites, and whether data from different vendors and core laboratories can be pooled, are discussed. As the X-ray cardiovascular world steadily moves into the digital imaging era, differences and similarities between the conventional cinefilm and the modern digital approaches are presented. Currently, the widespread use of digital imaging is still hindered by the lack of proper archival and exchange media. Requirements and possible solutions for this problem are handled in this section as well.

QCA continues to be an excellent tool for the accurate description of the coronary morphology and the changes therein due to interventions. However, for clinical decision making, data about the functional significance of coronary obstructions and about coronary blood flow and velocity, are of even greater importance. Over the last few years, new imaging and signal developments as well as the necessary clinical applications have gained momentum in attempts to provide such measures. All these topics are extensively described in Part Three.

Part Four focusses among others on regression and progression of coronary artery disease. Until today, QCA was the only available technique to describe quantitatively the changes in vessel morphology over time. However, with the advent of intracoronary ultrasound and intracoronary Doppler, three complementary techniques may soon become available for the complete assessment of progression/regression. Currently no good quantitative descriptors of plaque morphology as assessed from the coronary angiograms exist. However, it is very likely that the diagnosis of coronary artery disease, its prognosis and risk stratification could be improved by a better characterization of this plaque morphology. This is currently limited to an expert qualitative assessment of the angiograms.

In Part Five overviews are presented on the efficacy, limitations and applications of various recanalization approaches, being pulsed excimer laser systems, and three clinically available atherectomy devices (directional, rotational, and extraction atherectomy).

Coronary arteriography is limited by the fact that it produces two-dimensional projection lumenograms. Describing the presence and extent of coronary artery disease is, of course, limited by these same constraints. In attempts to provide better insights in vessel and plaque morphology, other rivaling approaches have arisen, of which intracoronary ultrasound with the potential for three-dimensional reconstruction of the vessel is one of the most exciting ones. Three rivaling approaches (angioscopy, intravascular echo and fluorescence spectroscopy) are finally covered in Part Six. Extensive validation studies are still required to define the applications in which each of these approaches are most suitable.

We sincerely hope that this latest volume provides both the necessary global as well as in depth information about the fundamental and applicatory research and developments in quantitative coronary imaging to the active and interested clinicians and physicists.

Johan H.C. Reiber &
Patrick W. Serruys

PART ONE

Endothelial function

1. Endothelium control of vascular tone and growth: Potential role in coronary artery disease

THOMAS F. LÜSCHER

Summary

The endothelium regulates vascular tone by releasing factors involved in relaxation and contraction, in coagulation and thrombus formation, and in growth inhibition and stimulation. Endothelium-dependent relaxations are elicited by transmitters, hormones, platelet substances, and the coagulation system, and by physical stimuli such as the shear stress from circulating blood. They are mediated by the endothelium-derived relaxing factor, recently identified as nitric oxide, which causes vasodilation and platelet deactivation. Other proposed endothelium-derived relaxing factors include a hyperpolarizing factor and lipooxygenase products. Endothelium-derived contracting factors are produced by the cyclooxygenase pathway. In addition, endothelial cells release the peptide endothelin-1, a potent vasoconstrictor that under normal conditions circulates at low levels. The endothelium also produces growth inhibitors such as heparin-like substances, transforming growth factor ß1 and nitric oxide as well as growth stimulators such as platelet-derived growth factor, basic fibroblast growth factor and connective tissue growth factor. Normally, it appears that the inhibitory signals are more dominant. Denuded or dysfunctional endothelium leads to a proliferative response and intimal hyperplasia in the vessel wall; moreover, platelets adhere to the site and release potent growth factors. Endothelial dysfunction has numerous causes: Aging is associated with increased formation of contraction factor and decreased relaxing factor; denudation, such as by coronary angioplasty, impairs the capacities of regenerated endothelial cells; oxidized low-density lipoproteins and hypercholesterolemia interfere with nitric oxide production; hypertension morphologically and functionally alters the endothelium; and atherosclerosis markedly attenuates endothelium-dependent relaxations. For patients with coronary bypass grafts, differences in endothelium-derived vasoactive factors between the internal mammary artery and the saphenous vein may be important determinants of graft function, with the mammary artery having more pronounced relaxations than the saphenous vein and thus a higher patency rate. Hence, the endothelium is an important regulator of vascular tone, coagulation, platelet function as well as proliferation and migration. Hence, alterations in the production and action of these numerous mediators may contribute to the pathophysiology of coronary artery disease, which is characterized by increased vasoconstriction, augmented platelet-vessel wall interaction and thrombus formation as well as increased migration and proliferation of vascular smooth muscle.

J.H.C. Reiber and P.W. Serruys (eds): Progress in quantitative coronary arteriography. 3–18.

Introduction

Coronary artery disease remains the most important cause of morbidity and mortality in Western countries. Coronary artery disease is characterized by:

1. abnormal vasomotion;
2. increased platelet vessel wall interaction; and
3. increased migration and proliferation of vascular smooth muscle cells in the blood vessel wall.

The endothelium takes part in the regulation of vascular tone, modulates platelet vessel wall interaction and influences vascular smooth muscle cell migration and proliferation [1].

Due to its strategic anatomic position, the endothelium is a target organ for hypertension, diabetes and hyperlipidemia [1]. A reduced release and/or increased breakdown of endothelium-derived relaxing factors and an enhanced liberation of endothelium-derived contracting factors are common under those conditions. Alterations in endothelial function are likely to contribute to the pathogenesis as well as progression and complications of coronary artery disease.

This chapter reviews endothelium-dependent vascular regulation in the coronary circulation as well as in coronary artery bypass grafts, and focuses on the dysfunction of these mechanisms in coronary artery disease.

Endothelium-dependent vascular regulation

Endothelium-derived relaxing factors

Endothelium-derived nitric oxide (EDNO; Figure 1.1)
Endothelium-dependent relaxations are elicited by autocoids, neurotransmitters, hormones, substances derived from platelets and the coagulation system [1–4]. Further, physical stimuli such as shear stress (exerted by the circulating blood) elicit endothelium-dependent vasodilation [5]. The so-called endothelium-derived relaxing factor (EDRF) [2] has recently been identified as nitric oxide (NO) and has a half-life of a few seconds [6–8].

EDNO is formed from L-arginine by oxidation of the guanidine-nitrogen terminal of L-arginine (Figure 1.1) [9]. NO synthase has been cloned [9]; it is a primarily cytosolic enzyme requiring calmodulin, Ca^{+} and NADPH and has similarities with cytochrome P450 enzymes. Isoforms of the enzyme occur in endothelial cells, platelets, macrophages, vascular smooth muscle cells and in the brain [10–13]. In coronary arteries, endothelium-dependent relaxations to serotonin are inhibited by analogues of L-arginine such as L-N^G-monomethyl arginine (L-NMMA) and are restored by L-, but not D-arginine [3, 14], while L-NMMA alone causes endothelium-dependent contractions (Figure

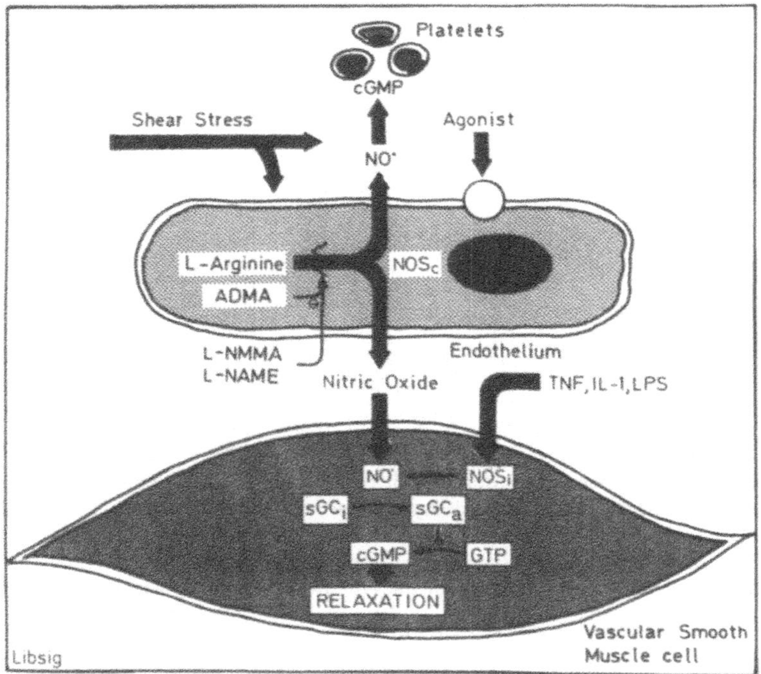

Figure 1.1. The L-arginine pathway in the blood vessel wall: Endothelial cells form nitric oxide (NO) from L-arginine via the activity of the constitutive nitric oxide synthase (NOS_c) specific enzymes which can be inhibited by analogues of the amino acid such as L-N^G-monomethyl arginine (L-NMMA). NO increases soluble guanylyl cyclase (sGC) in vascular smooth muscle and platelets and increases in cyclic 3'5-guanosine monophosphate (cGMP) which mediates relaxation and platelet inhibition, respectively. Shear stress and receptor-operated agonists (not shown) increase the release of NO. In addition, vascular smooth muscle cells can form nitric oxide via the activity of an inducible (by tumor necrosis factor, interleukin 1 and lipopolysaccharide) form of nitric oxide synthase (NOS_I).

1.2; [3]). Furthermore, contractions to norepinephrine and other vasoconstrictors are augmented under these conditions. When infused in rabbits, L-NMMA causes long-lasting increases in blood pressure which are reversed by L-arginine [15]. Hence, the vasculature including the coronary circulation is in a constant state of vasodilation due the continuous release of NO.

Relaxations to EDNO are associated with an increase in cyclic 3'5'-guanosine monophosphate (cGMP) in vascular smooth muscle (Figure 1.1) [14]. Soluble guanylyl cyclase is also present in platelets (Figure 1.1) [17]. Increased levels of cGMP in platelets are associated with a reduced adhesion and aggregation [18]. Thus, EDNO causes both vasodilatation and platelet deactivation and thereby is an antithrombotic feature of the endothelium.

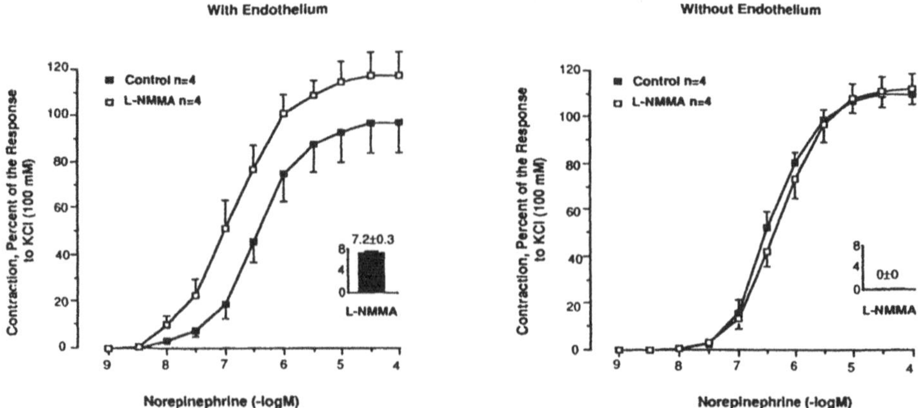

Figure 1.2. Modulation of vasoconstrictor responses to norepinephrine by basal release of nitric oxide in human mammary arteries with or without endothelium. In preparations with endothelium, L-NMMA (L-N^{G}-monomethylarginine, an inhibitor of nitric oxide formation) causes endothelium-dependent contractions (inset) and augments the sensitivity and maximal response to norepinephrine. In contrast, in preparations without endothelium, no effect is appreciable (from Ref. 3, by permission of the American Heart Association).

Nitric oxide derived from vascular smooth muscle

Although the media of the blood vessel wall normally does not produce NO, vascular smooth muscle cells including those obtained from human vessels can do so if stimulated by endotoxin, interleukin-1 or other cytokines (Figure 1.1) [12, 13]. Thus, at least two enzymes for NO production exist, the constitutive endothelial enzyme and the inducible form which is primarily expressed in smooth muscle and monocytes. Activation of the L-arginine pathway in smooth muscle cells by endotoxin, tumor necrosis factor and interleukin-1 may play a role in septic shock and explain, why the cardiovascular system no longer responds to catecholamines under these conditions. Hence, L-NMMA or an analogue may become a therapeutic tool to prevent NO formation in vascular smooth muscle. Preliminary data in patients in septic shock suggest that L-NMMA or a similar pharmacological tool preventing NO formation may be beneficial in these patients [19].

Prostacyclin

Prostacyclin is the major product of vascular cyclooxygenase (see [20]). It is produced in the intima, but also the media and adventitia in response to shear stress, hypoxia and several mediators which also stimulate EDNO. Prostacyclin increases cyclic 3′5′-adenosine monophosphate (cAMP) in smooth muscle and platelets, and thereby inhibits platelet aggregation. In human platelets EDNO and prostacyclin inhibit platelet aggregation synergistically.

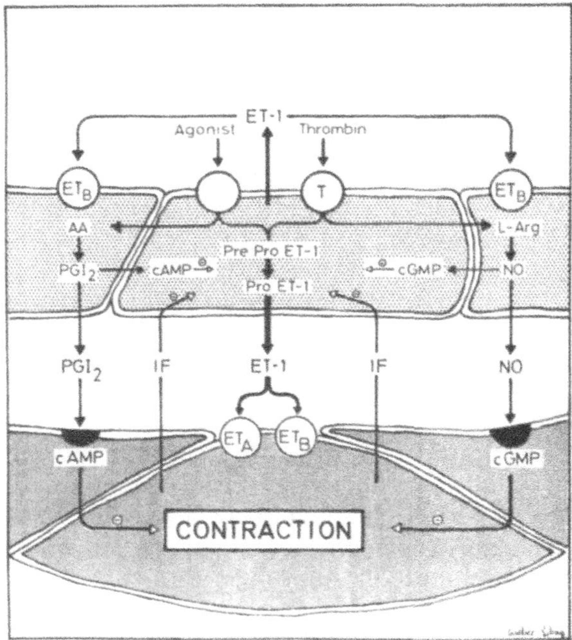

Figure 1.3. Endothelin production and action in the blood vessel wall. Endothelin-1 (ET-1). ET-1 is produced from precursor molecules. The production is inhibited via cyclic AMP-dependent mechanisms, activated by prostacyclin (PGI_2), cyclic GMP-dependent pathway (activated by nitric oxide, NO) formed from L-arginine (L-ARG)) and the putative inhibitory effect (IF) released by vascular smooth muscle. On vascular smooth muscle ET_A- and ET_B-receptors cause contraction, while on endothelial cells ET_B-receptors are linked to the formation of PGI_2 and NO. The contractile effect of ET1 on vascular smooth muscle are modulated by PGI_2 and NO via the activation of cyclic AMP or cyclic GMP respectively (modified from Ref. 29, by permission of the American Heart Association).

Other endothelium-derived relaxing factors

In the porcine coronary circulation, L-NMMA inhibits the relaxations to serotonin, but not to bradykinin [6], suggesting that the endothelium releases relaxing factor(s) other than NO. Since prostacyclin is a weak vasodilator in these arteries and indomethacin does not affect the response, prostacyclin can be excluded. Several candidates for these responses have been proposed, but a hyperpolarizing factor (EDHF) causing hyperpolarization of vascular smooth muscle appears a likely candidate [21].

Endothelium-derived contracting factors (EDCF)

Cyclooxygenase-dependent endothelium-derived contracting factor (EDCF)

Arachidonic acid causes endothelium-dependent contractions which are prevented by indomethacin (an inhibitor of cyclooxygenase) [22]. In the human saphenous vein, acetylcholine and histamine evoke endothelium-dependent contractions; in the presence of indomethacin, however, endothelium-dependent relaxations are unmasked [3]. The products of cyclooxygenase mediating the contractions are thromboxane A_2 and endoperoxides which activate both smooth muscle and platelets [3].

The cyclooxygenase pathway also produces of superoxide anions which induce endothelium-dependent contractions either by the breakdown of NO or direct vascular effects [23].

Endothelin

Endothelial cells produce the 21 amino acid peptide endothelin (Figure 1.3) [1, 24]. In addition, other isoforms such as endothelin-2 and endothelin-3 are produced by non-endothelial cells. Translation of messenger RNA generates preproendothelin, which is processed to big endothelin; its conversion to endothelin-1 by the endothelin converting enzyme (ECE) is necessary for the development of full vascular activity. Expression of messenger RNA and the release of the peptide is stimulated by thrombin, transforming growth factor-beta, interleukin-1, epinephrine, angiotensin II, arginine vasopressin, calcium ionophore and phorbol ester [1, 24, 25].

Endothelin-1 is a potent vasoconstrictor; it causes vasodilation at lower and marked contractions at higher concentrations (Figure 1.3) [24, 26] which in the heart eventually leads to ischemia, arrhythmias and death. Also, in human arterial and venous coronary bypass vessels, endothelin causes marked contractions [27]. However, the circulating levels of endothelin-1 are low. Hence, little peptide is formed under physiological conditions [28] due to the absence of stimuli and the presence of potent inhibitory mechanisms [29]. Importantly, most of the peptide is released abluminally towards smooth muscle [30]. Three inhibitory mechanisms regulating endothelin production have been delineated [29]:

1. cGMP-dependent inhibition [25, 31];
2. cAMP-dependent inhibition [32] and
3. an inhibitor factor produced by vascular smooth muscle (Figure 1.3) [33].

The cGMP-dependent mechanism can be activated by EDNO, nitroglycerine, 3–morpholino sydnonimine (SIN-1) [34] and atrial natriuretic peptide [31]. Thus, after inhibition of the endothelial L-arginine pathway, the thrombin-induced production of endothelin is augmented (Figure 1.3) [25]; on the other hand, SIN-1 prevents the thrombin-induced endothelin release via a cyclic GMP-dependent mechanism [34]. Endothelin also releases NO and prostacyclin from endothelial cells which may represent a negative feedback mechanism [29].

Endothelin does not activate voltage-operated Ca^+ channels on smooth muscles [29]. However, the peptide can indirectly activate voltage-operated Ca^+ channels in certain blood vessels such as the porcine coronary artery where calcium antagonists attenuate endothelin-induced vasoconstriction

[35]. In the human forearm circulation, endothelin-1–induced contractions are inhibited by nifedipine and verapamil [26]. The vasodilator effects of endothelin are mediated by prostacyclin although NO may contribute [36].

Endothelium-dependent regulation of vascular growth
Removal of the endothelium invariably leads to a proliferative response with intimal hyperplasia; this indicates that endothelial cells normally are a source of growth inhibitors (Figure 1.4). This may explain why under normal conditions smooth muscle cells are quiescent, while in the absence of endothelial cells they proliferate in response to pulsatile stretch and platelet-derived growth factor (PDGF; Figure 1.5) [37, 38]. EDNO can act as a growth inhibitor both directly (in vascular smooth muscle) as well as indirectly (together with prostacyclin) by preventing platelet adhesion and aggregation (Figure 1.4) (see [39, 40]). Platelets release large amounts of PDGF once they are activated. Important growth inhibitors produced by the endothelium are heparin and heparin sulphates, EDNO and most likely transforming growth factor $ß_1$ (TGF$ß_1$). Endothelial cells can also produce growth factors such as basic fibroblast growth factor, platelet-derived growth factor (see [39]). Endothelin might also contribute to proliferative responses, at least under certain conditions [41]. Not much is known yet about the regulation of endothelium-dependent mechanisms regulating antiproliferation and proliferation, but it is likely that under normal conditions, inhibitory stimuli are more important (Figure 1.4).

Endothelium dysfunction

Aging and regeneration
Aging is an important determinant of vascular disease. In the rat, ageing leads to an increased formation of the cyclooxygenase-dependent endothelium-derived contracting factor (prostaglandin H_2) [42] as well as a mild decrease in that of EDNO [43]; in contrast, the responsiveness of smooth muscle to NO-forming compounds does not change. In the human coronary microcirculation, the increase in coronary flow induced by intraarterial infusion of acetylcholine declines with ageing [44].

Endothelial regeneration
After mechanical denudation, regenerated endothelial cells have an impaired capacity to release EDNO in response to platelet-derived serotonin, because of a defect G_i-protein linked to the $5HT_1$-serotonergic receptor [45]. In addition, balloon injury induces nitric oxide synthase activity in rat carotid artery [46], while the effects of this procedure on the formation of endothelin are less certain.

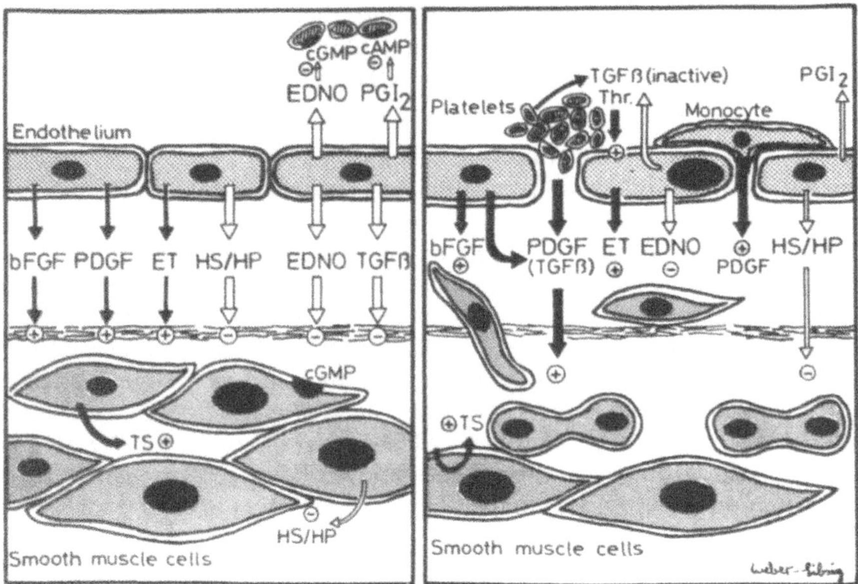

Figure 1.4. Regulation of migration and proliferation in the blood vessel wall. Normally, the endothelium primarily appears to produce inhibitors of vascular migration and proliferation such as heparan-like substances (HS/H), nitric oxide (NO) and transforming growth factor beta-1 (TGF_{beta-1}), while growth promoters released by the endothelium are less important (basic FGF, bFGF; platelet-derived growth factor, PDGF and endothelin, ET) (left panel). The release of EDNO and prostacyclin (PGI_2) also prevent platelet adhesion which importantly contributes to antiproliferative effects as platelets contain PDGF. In contrast, under disease conditions (right panel), platelets and monocytes adhere to the blood vessel wall and release large quantities of PDGF. Endothelial cells now also produce growth factors which leads to migration and proliferation of vascular smooth muscle (modified from Ref. 39).

Lipoproteins and hypercholesteremia

Morphologically, the endothelium remains intact in most stages of atherogenesis, but pronounced functional alterations occur [1]. Oxidized low density lipoproteins (OX-LDL) are present in atherosclerotic lesions which inhibit endothelium-dependent relaxations to platelets, serotonin and thrombin (Figure 1.6) [47]. In contrast, relaxations to the NO-donor SIN-1 are well maintained excluding a reduced responsiveness of smooth muscle to EDNO. The inhibition is specific for OX-LDL and not caused by comparable native LDL. In the rabbit aorta the effect of OX-LDL is mimicked by lysolecithin (a characteristic component of OX-LDL) [48]. OX-LDL appears to activate an endothelial receptor distinct from the LDL receptor (i.e. scavenger receptor; Figure 1.7) [66]. The inhibitor of NO production L-NMMA exerts a similar effect, indicating that OX-LDL interferes with the L-arginine pathway. NO synthetase, however, remains unaffected as L-arginine evokes a full relaxation in vessels treated with OX-LDL. Pretreatment with L-arginine restores

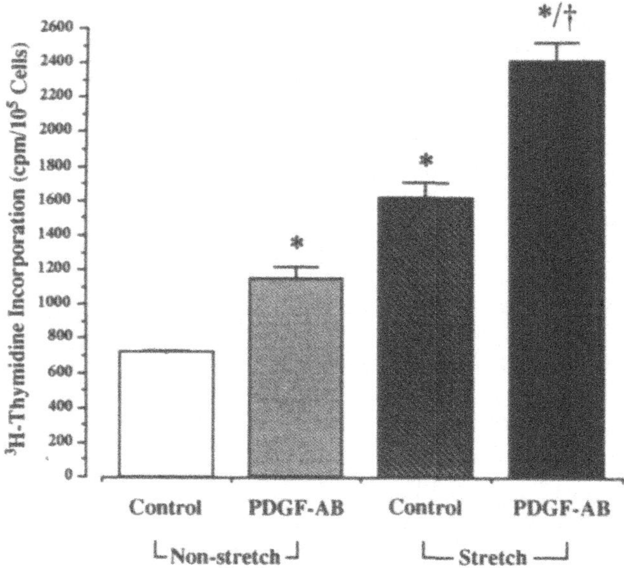

Figure 1.5. Effects of pulsatile stretch and platelet-derived growth factor (PDGF) alone or in combination in cultured human coronary artery smooth muscle cells. Note that each stimulus alone increases thymidine uptake in human vascular smooth muscle cells indicating DNA synthesis or proliferation. The effect of pulsatile stretch and PDGF are additive (from Ref. 38, by permission of the American Heart Association).

the response to serotonin in vessels treated with OX-LDL. Thus, OX-LDL must interact with the intracellular availability of L-arginine or its release mechanisms (for instance G_i-proteins linked to endothelial receptors; Figure 1.7). In hypercholesterolemic pigs, a similar inhibition of endothelium-dependent relaxation is noted as in coronary arteries exposed to OX-LDL *in vitro* [49]. In humans with hypercholesteremia, L-arginine infusion augments the blunted increase in coronary blood flow in response to acetylcholine [50]; in contrast the loss of endothelium-dependent vasodilation to acetylcholine in epicardial coronary arteries in unaffected by the amino acid, possibly because of the presence of fully developed atherosclerosis.

OX-LDL also induce endothelin messenger RNA expression and the release of the peptide from the intact porcine aorta (Figure 1.7) [51]. As thresholds and low concentrations of endothelin potentiate contractions induced by other vasoconstrictors in human arteries, this effect may alter the contractile state of the blood vessel wall (Figure 1.8) [52].

Hypertension

Endothelium-dependent relaxations to acetylcholine are reduced in the aorta, cerebral and peripheral microcirculation of hypertensive rats (see [53]) and

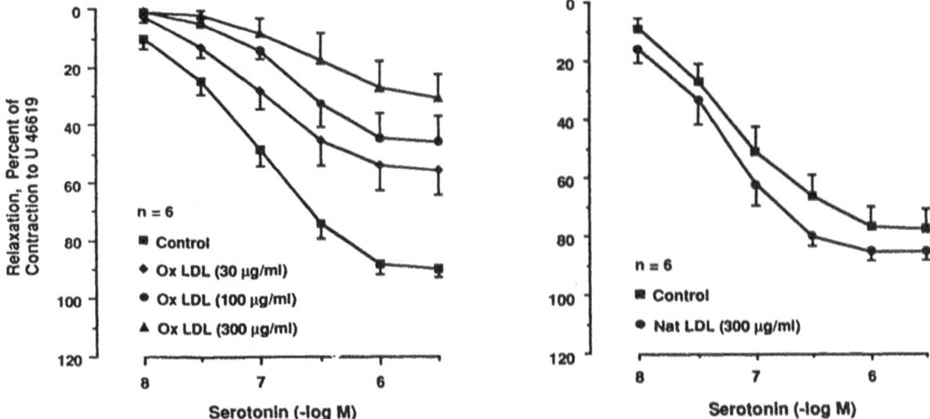

Figure 1.6. Effect of oxidized (left panel) and native low density lipoproteins (right panel) on endothelium-dependent relaxations induced by serotonin in the porcine coronary artery (in the presence of ketanserin). Oxidized but not native LDLs markedly reduce the response to serotonin indicating that oxidation of the lipoproteins is a crucial step for endothelial dysfunction occurring in hyperlipidemia (modified from Ref. 47, by permission of the American Heart Association).

the vasodilator effects of acetylcholine are impaired in the forearm of hypertensive subjects [4]. In the spontaneously hypertensive rat, the reduced response to acetylcholine is related to the production of a cyclooxygenase-dependent endothelium-derived contracting factor (i.e. prostaglandin H_2), while in most other forms of experimental hypertension a reduced formation of EDNO predominates [53]. In the mesenteric microcirculation, intraluminal activation of the endothelium is dysfunctional indicating a predominant alteration of that surface of the endothelium which is most exposed to high blood pressure [54].

Diabetes

Increasing concentrations of glucose and diabetes reduce the release of EDNO [55]. In the aorta of the rabbit, diabetes is associated with an increased formation of endothelium-derived thromboxane A_2 which inhibits the effects of EDNO [1, 56]. In the corpora cavernosa of diabetic patients, the vasodilator effects of acetylcholine are reduced, while those to sodium nitroprusside are maintained [57].

Atherosclerosis

In porcine coronary arteries, established atherosclerosis severely impairs endothelium-dependent relaxations to serotonin and also reduces endothelium-dependent relaxations to bradykinin which are maintained in hypercholesterolemia [49]. However, endothelium-independent relaxations to ni-

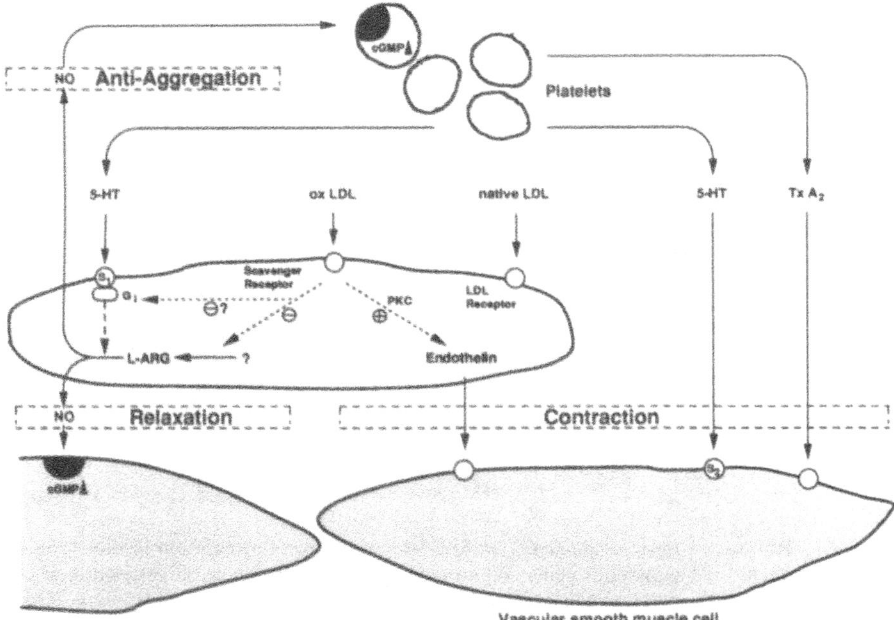

Figure 1.7. Schematic representation of the effects of oxidized low density lipoproteins (OX-LDL) on the endothelial L-arginine pathway in the coronary circulation. OX-LDL activates the scavenger receptor which then interferes with the intracellular availability of L-arginine (L-arg) or receptor-operated mechanisms responsible for its release. This reduces the efficacy of the receptor operated activation of the L-arginine pathway by serotonin (5–HT) and other mediators (modified from Ref. 39, by permission).

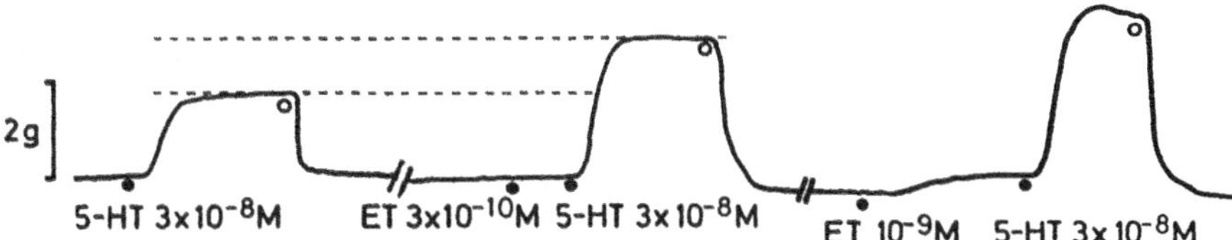

Figure 1.8. Potentiating effects of endothelin on vasoconstrictors responses in the human coronary artery. In an isolated ring of the left anterior descending coronary artery serotonin (5–hydroxytryptamine; 5HT) induces a contraction which is reversed after washout (0). Threshold concentrations of endothelin (ET) which by themselves do no exert a contraction potentiate the vascular response to readded serotonin (5HT). Similar observations can be made with slightly higher concentrations of ET (10^{-9} M; right) (from Ref. 52, by permission of the American Heart Association).

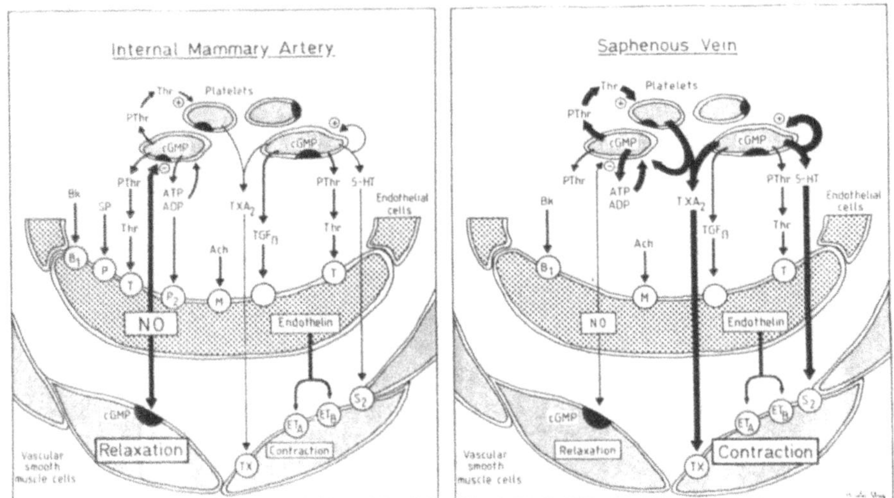

Figure 1.9. Release of nitric oxide (NO) and platelet vessel wall interaction in human internal mammary arteries and saphenous veins. While in the artery (left panel), large quantities of NO are produced leading to relaxation and inhibition of platelet function, this effect is less pronounced in the vein (right panel) leading to preactivation of platelets and vasoconstrictor responses induced by thromboxane A_2 (TXA_2) and serotonin (5HT; 5-hydroxytryptamine). ACH = acetylcholine; ATP/ADP = adenosine trisphosphate and diphosphate; Bk = bradykinin; circles = receptors; PTHR = prothrombin; SP = substance P; THR = thrombin. (modified from Ref. 39).

trovasodilators remain preserved except in severely atherosclerotic arteries [1]. In atherosclerotic human coronary arteries, endothelium-dependent relaxations to substance P, bradykinin, aggregating platelets and calcium ionophore are attenuated [58] and *in vivo* acetylcholine as well as serotonin cause paradoxical vasoconstriction [59].

The exact mechanism responsible for the marked impairment or loss of endothelium-dependent relaxations in atherosclerosis remains controversial. The bioassayable EDRF release in porcine coronary artery with hypercholesteremia and atherosclerosis is reduced [49]. Direct measurements of nitric oxide in the rabbit aorta, however, revealed increased levels of the breakdown products of NO (i.e. NO_2^-, NO_3^-; [60]). The latter observation would suggest an increased formation of superoxide radicals and other products inactivating NO and/or decreased activity of superoxide dismutase. However, it is unknown whether similar alterations occur in human coronary arteries as in the rabbit aorta.

Ischemia, myocardial infarction and reperfusion

Hypoxia can evoke endothelium-dependent contractions due to withdrawal of EDNO [61]. In addition, endothelin is released and its receptors are externalized during hypoxia [62]. After coronary ligation and reperfusion, endothelium-dependent relaxations to thrombin and other agonists are impaired [63]. Myocardial infarction also is associated with marked elevations in the circulating levels of endothelin [64] indicating that a decreased release of EDNO and an increased formation of this potent vasoconstrictor contributes to ischemia occurring in myocardial infarction.

Coronary bypass graft function and patency
Endothelium-derived vasoactive factors may contribute to graft function as they determine the antithrombotic properties and the regulation of blood flow. In addition, the factors may have antiproliferative and proliferative properties determining in late changes occurring in coronary bypass grafts.

The mammary artery exhibits much more pronounced endothelium-dependent relaxations as compared to the saphenous vein, because the release of EDNO to receptor-operated agonists and in particular by aggregating platelets is more efficient in the artery than in the vein (Figure 1.9) [65, 66]. Particularly the release of EDNO to platelet-derived adenosine diphosphate represents an important antithrombotic property. The gastroepiploic artery releases comparable amounts of EDNO as the mammary artery, but exhibits more pronounced contractions (presumably because it represent a muscular rather than elastic artery) [67]. These differences in endothelial and vascular smooth muscle function of various bypass graft vessels may play an important role in graft function and patency and in turn for the survival of patients undergoing coronary bypass surgery.

Acknowledgment

The author is indebted to Amanda de Sola Pinto and to Bernadette Weber-Libsig for their help in the preparation of the manuscript. Original research reported in the manuscript was supported by grants of the Swiss National Research Foundation (No. 32–32541.91), the Karl Mayer Foundation, Vaduz, Liechtenstein, the Swiss Cardiology Foundation and the Swiss Mobiliar Insurance, Bern, Switzerland.

References

1. Lüscher TF, Vanhoutte PM. The Endothelium: Modulator of Cardiovascular Function. Boca Raton, Fl.: CRC Press, 1990.
2. Furchgott RF, Zawadzki JV. The obligatory role of endothelial cells in the relaxation of arterial smooth muscle by acetylcholine. Nature 1980; 299: 373–6.
3. Yang ZH, von Segesser L, Bauer E, Stulz P, Turina M, Lüscher TF. Different activation of endothelial L-arginine and cyclooxygenase pathway in the human internal mammary artery and saphenous vein. Circ Res 1991; 68: 52–60.
4. Linder L, Kiowski W, Bühler FR, Lüscher TF. Indirect evidence for release of endothelium-

derived relaxing factor in human forearm circulation *in vivo*. Blunted response in essential hypertension. Circulation 1990; 81: 1762–7.
5. Rubanyi GM, Romero JC, Vanhoutte PM. Flow-induced release of endothelium-derived relaxing factor. Am J Physiol 1986; 250: H1145–9.
6. Rubanyi GM, Vanhoutte PM. Superoxide anions and hyperoxia inactivate endothelium-derived relaxing factor. Am J Physiol 1986; 250: H822–7.
7. Palmer RMJ, Ferrige AG, Moncada S. Nitric oxide release accounts for the biological activity of endothelium-derived relaxing factor. Nature 1987; 327: 524–6.
8. Palmer RMJ, Ashton DS, Moncada S. Vascular endothelial cells synthesize nitric oxide from L-arginine. Nature 1988; 333: 664–6.
9. Bredt DS, Hwang PM, Glatt CE, Lowenstein C, Reed RR, Snyder SH. Cloned and expressed nitric oxide synthase structurally resembles cytochrome P-450 reductase. Nature 1991; 351: 714–8.
10. Radomski MW, Palmer RMJ, Moncada S. An L-arginine/nitric oxide pathway present in human platelets regulates aggregation. Proc Natl Acad Sci USA 1990; 87: 5193–7.
11. Hibbs JB Jr, Traintor RR, Vavrin Z, Rachlin EM. Nitric oxide: a cytotoxic activated macrophage effector molecule. Biochem Biophys Res Comm 1988; 157: 87–9.
12. Fleming I, Gray GA, Julou-Schaeffer G, Parratt JR, Stoclet JC. Incubation with endotoxin activates the L-arginine pathway in vascular tissue. Biochem Biophys Res Commun 1990; 171 (2): 562–8.
13. Bernhardt J, Tschudi MR, Dohi Z *et al*. Release of nitric oxide from human vascular smooth muscle cells. Biochem Biophys Res Commun 1991; 180(2): 907–12.
14. Knowles RG, Palacios M, Palmer RMJ, Moncada S. Formation of nitric oxide from L-arginine in the central nervous system: a transduction mechanism for stimulation of the soluble guanylate cyclase. Proc Natl Acad Sci USA 1989; 86: 5159–62.
15. Richard V, Tanner FC, Tschudi M, Lüscher TF. Different activation of L-arginine pathway by bradykinin, serotonin, and clonidine in coronary arteries. Am J Physiol 1990; 259: H1433–9.
16. Rees DD, Palmer RMJ, Moncada S. Role of endothelium-derived nitric oxide in the regulation of blood pressure. Proc Natl Acad Sci USA 1989; 86: 3375–8.
17. Rapoport RM, Murad F. Agonist-induced endothelium-dependent relaxation in rat thoracic aorta may be mediated through cGMP. Circ Res 1983; 52: 352–7.
18. Busse R, Lückhoff A, Bassenge E. Endothelium-derived relaxant factor inhibits platelet activation. Naunyn Schmiedeberg's Arch Pharmacol 1987; 336: 566–71.
19. Petros A, Bennett D, Vallance P. Effect of nitric oxide synthase inhibitors on hypotension in patients with septic shock. Lancet 1991; 338: 1557–8.
20. Moncada S, Vane JR. Pharmacology and endogenous roles of prostaglandin endoperoxides, thromboxane A_2 and prostacyclin. Pharmacol Rev 1978; 30: 293–331.
21. Komori K, Lorenz RR, Vanhoutte PM. Nitric oxide, acetylcholine, and electrical and mechanical properties of canine arterial smooth muscle. Am J Physiol 1988; 255: H207–12.
22. Miller VM, Vanhoutte PM. Endothelium-dependent contractions to arachidonic acid are mediated by products of cyclooxygenase in canine veins. Am J Physiol 1985; 248: H432–7.
23. Katusic ZS, Vanhoutte PM. Superoxide anion is an endothelium-derived contracting factor. Am J Physiol 1989; 357: H33–7.
24. Yanagisawa M, Kurihara H, Kimura S *et al*. A novel potent vasoconstrictor peptide produced by vascular endothelial cells. Nature 1988; 332: 411–5.
25. Boulanger C, Lüscher TF. Release of endothelin from the porcine aorta. Inhibition by endothelium-derived nitric oxide. J Clin Invest 1990; 85: 587–90.
26. Kiowski W, Lüscher TF, Linder L, Bühler FR. Endothelin-1 induced vasoconstriction in humans: reversal by calcium channel blockade but not by nitrovasodilators or endothelium-derived relaxing factor. Circulation 1991; 83: 469–75.
27. Lüscher TF, Yang Z, Tschudi M *et al*. Interaction between endothelin-1 and endothelium-derived relaxing factor in human arteries and veins. Circ Res 1990; 66 (4): 1088–94.
28. Suzuki N, Matsumoto H, Kitada C *et al*. Immunoreactive endothelin-1 in plasma detected

by a sandwich-type enzyme immunoassay. J Cardiovasc Pharmacol 1989; 13 (Suppl. 5): S151–2.
29. Lüscher TF, Boulanger CM, Dohi Y, Yang ZH. Endothelium-derived contracting factors. Hypertension 1992; 19: 117–30.
30. Wagner OF, Christ G, Wojta J *et al.* Polar secretion of endothelin-1 by cultured endothelial cells. J Biol Chem 1992; 267: 16066–8.
31. Saijonmaa O, Ristimäki A, Fyhrquist F. Atrial natriuretic peptide, nitroglycerine, and nitroprusside reduce basal and stimulated endothelin production from cultured endothelial cells. Biochem Biophys Res Commun 1990; 173: 514–20.
32. Yokokawa K, Kohno M, Yasunari K, Murakawa K, Takedo T. Endothelin-3 regulates endothelin-1 production in cultured human endothelial cells. Hypertension 1991; 18: 304–15.
33. Stewart DJ, Langleben D, Cernacek P, Cianflone K. Endothelin release is inhibited by coculture of endothelial cells with cells of vascular media. Am J Physiol 1990; 259: H1928–32.
34. Boulanger CM, Lüscher TF. Hirudin and nitrates inhibit the thrombin-induced release of endothelin from the intact porcine aorta. Circ Res 1991; 68: 1768–72.
35. Goto K, Kasuya Y, Matsuki N *et al.* Endothelin activates the dihydropiridine-sensitive, voltage-dependent Ca^+ channel in vascular smooth muscle. Proc Natl Acad Sci USA 1989; 86: 3915–8.
36. Dohi Y, Lüscher TF. Endothelin in hypertensive resistance arteries. Intraluminal and extraluminal dysfunction. Hypertension 1991; 18: 543–9.
37. Predel HG, Yang Z, von Segesser L, Turina M, Bühler FR, Lüscher TF. Implications of pulsatile stretch on growth of saphenous vein and mammary artery smooth muscle. Lancet 1992; 340: 878–9.
38. Yang Y, Noll G, Lüscher TF. Calcium antagonists differently inhibit proliferation of human coronary smooth muscle cells in response to pulsatile stretch and platelet-derived growth factor. Circulation 1993; 88: 832–6.
39. Lüscher TF, Tanner FC. Endothelial regulation of vascular tone and growth. Am J Hypertens 1993; 6: 283s–93s.
40. Garg UC, Hassid A. Nitric oxide-generating vasodilators and 8-bromo-cyclic guanosine monophosphate inhibit mitogenesis and proliferation of cultured rat vascular smooth muscle cells. J Clin Invest 1989; 83: 1774–7.
41. Dubin D, Pratt RE, Cooke JP, Dzau VJ. Endothelin, a potent vasoconstrictor, is a vascular smooth muscle mitogen. J Vasc Med Biol 1989; 1: 13–7.
42. Koga T, Takata Y, Kobayashi K, Takishita S, Yawashita Y. Fujishima M. Age and hypertension promote endothelium-dependent contractions to acetylcholine in the aorta of the rat. Hypertension 1989; 14: 542–8.
43. Dohi Y, Lüscher TF. Aging differentially affects direct and indirect actions of endothelin-1 in perfused mesenteric arteries of the rat. Br J Pharmacol 1990; 100: 889–93.
44. Vita JA, Treasure CB, Nabel EG *et al.* Coronary vasomotor response to acetylcholine relates to risk factors for coronary artery disease. Circulation 1990; 81: 491–7.
45. Shimokawa H, Flavahan NA, Vanhoutte PM. Natural course of the impairment of endothelium-dependent relaxations after balloon endothelium-removal in porcine coronary arteries. Circ Res 1989; 63: 740.
46. Joly GA, Schini VB, Vanhoutte PM. Balloon injury and interleukin-1 beta induce nitric oxide synthase activity in rat carotid arteries. Circ Res 1992; 71: 331–8.
47. Tanner FC, Noll G, Boulanger CM, Lüscher TF. Oxidized native low density lipoproteins inhibit relaxations of porcine coronary arteries. Role of scavenger receptor and endothelium-derived nitric oxide. Circulation 1991; 83: 2012–20.
48. Kugiyama K, Kerns SA, Morrisett JD, Roberts R, Henry PD. Impairment of endothelium-dependent arterial relaxation by lysolecithin in modified low-density lipoproteins. Nature 1990; 344: 160–2.
49. Shimokawa H, Vanhoutte PM. Impaired endothelium-dependent relaxation to aggregating

platelets and related vasoactive substances in porcine coronary arteries in hypercholesterolemia and in atherosclerosis. Circ Res 1989; 64: 900–14.
50. Drexler H, Zeiher AM, Meinzer K, Just H. Correction of endothelial dysfunction in coronary microcirculation of hypercholesterolemic patients by L-arginine. Lancet 1991; 338: 1546–50.
51. Boulanger CM, Tanner FC, Bea ML, Hahn AWA, Werner A, Lüscher TF. Oxidized low density lipoproteins induce mRNA expression and release of endothelin from human and porcine endothelium. Circ Res 1992; 70: 1191–7.
52. Yang ZH, Richard V, von Segesser L *et al.* Threshold concentrations of endothelin-1 potentiate contractions to norepinephrine and serotonin in human arteries. A new mechanism of vasospasm? Circulation 1990; 82: 188–95.
53. Lüscher TF. Imbalance of endothelium-derived relaxing and contracting factors. A new concept in hypertension? Am J Hypertens 1990; 3: 317–30.
54. Dohi Y, Thiel MA, Bühler FR, Lüscher TF. Activation of endothelial L-arginine pathway in resistance arteries. Effect of age and hypertension. Hypertension 1990; 15: 170–9.
55. Bucala R, Tracey KJ, Cerami A. Advanced glycosylation products quench nitric oxide and mediate defective endothelium-dependent vasodilatation in experimental diabetes. J Clin Invest 1991; 87 (2): 432–8.
56. Tesfamariam B, Jakubowski JA, Cohen RA. Contraction of diabetic rabbit aorta caused by endothelium-derived PGH_2/TXA_2. Am J Physiol 1989; 257: H1327–33.
57. Saenz De Tejada I, Goldstein I, Azadzoi K, Krane RJ, Cohen RA. Impaired neurogenic and endothelium-mediated relaxation of penile smooth muscle from diabetic men with impotence. N Engl J Med 1989; 320: 1025–30.
58. Förstermann U, Mügge A, Alheid U, Haverich A, Frölich JC. Selective attenuation of endothelium-mediated vasodilation in atherosclerotic human coronary arteries. Circ Res 1988; 62: 185–90.
59. Ludmer PL, Selwyn AP, Shook TL *et al.* Paradoxical vasoconstriction induced by acetylcholine in atherosclerotic coronary arteries. N Engl J Med 1986; 315: 1046–51.
60. Minor RL Jr, Myers PR, Guerra RJr, Bates JN, Harrison DG. Diet-induced atherosclerosis increases the release of nitrogen oxides from rabbit aorta. J Clin Invest 1990; 86: 2109–16.
61. Rubanyi GM, Vanhoutte PM. Hypoxia releases a vasoconstrictor substance from the canine vascular endothelium. J Physiol (Lond) 1985; 364: 45–56.
62. Rakugi H, Tabuchi Y, Nakamaru M *et al.* Evidence for endothelin-1 release from resistance vessels of rats in response to hypoxia. Biochem Biophys Res Commun 1990; 169: 973–7.
63. Ku DD. Coronary vascular reactivity after acute myocardial ischemia. Science 1982; 218: 576–8.
64. Stewart DJ, Kubac G, Costello KB, Cernacek P. Increased plasma endothelin-1 in the early hours of acute myocardial infarction. J Am Coll Cardiol 1991; 18: 38–43.
65. Lüscher TF, Diederich D, Siebenmann R *et al.* Difference between endothelium-dependent relaxation in arterial and in venous coronary bypass grafts. N Engl J Med 1988; 319: 462–7.
66. Yang ZH, Stulz P, von Segesser L, Bauer E, Turina M, Lüscher TF. Different interactions of platelets with arterial and venous coronary bypass vessels. Lancet 1991; 337: 939–43.
67. Yang Z, Siebenmann R, Studer M, Egloff L, Lüscher TF. Similar endothelium-dependent relaxation, but enhanced contractility of the right gastroepiploic artery as compared to the internal mammary artery. J Thorac Cardiovasc Surg 1992; 104: 459–64.

2. Endothelial function in atherosclerosis

FRANÇOIS CHARBONNEAU, IAN T. MEREDITH, TODD J. ANDERSON, MARIE GERHARD, MICHAEL DYCE, DANIELLE DELAGRANGE, ANDREW P. SELWYN & PETER GANZ

Summary

Traditionally, evaluation and treatment of patients with coronary artery disease (CAD) have mainly focused on the severity of luminal narrowings as assessed by angiography. In the last decade however, several limitations of this approach have emerged, stimulating interest in the composition and function of the arterial wall, rather then the remaining lumen. Located at the interface of blood-borne elements and arterial wall, the endothelium is a major regulator of several critical functions involved in ischemia. Recently, there has been accumulating evidences that endothelium-dependent vasodilator function is impaired not only in patients with symptomatic CAD, but also in healthy subjects with one or more of the traditional cardiac risk factors. This impairment, which equally affects the epicardial arteries and the coronary resistance vessels, may contribute to the genesis of ischemia. Interestingly, endothelial dysfunction can also be detected in peripheral vessels rarely affected by structural atherosclerosis. This suggests that endothelial dysfunction is an early and systemic manifestation of atherosclerosis. Because of its likely involvement in progression of CAD, ischemic syndromes and other cardiovascular diseases, many studies are examining strategies aimed at restoring endothelium-dependent dilation and its effect on clinical outcome.

Introduction

The introduction of cardiac catheterization by Forssmann and the subsequent development of modern angiography in the 1950's, has led to important progress in our understanding of coronary pathophysiology and to new treatments of coronary artery disease (CAD). Unfortunately this success, in conjunction with the purely anatomic nature of the information provided, has focused the attention and therapeutic efforts mainly on the structural modifications of coronary atherosclerosis, as if the severity of stenoses could predict the clinical outcome. Several limitations to this approach have become apparent. First, angiography fails to account for the functional alterations associated with atherosclerosis, which may be responsible for variability in the ischemic threshold of a great number of patients. Second, it

J.H.C. Reiber and P.W. Serruys (eds): Progress in quantitative coronary arteriography, 19–30.

has become clear that luminal size obtained does not necessarily correlate with the clinical outcome. In fact, most myocardial infarctions are associated with stenoses less than 70% in severity, typically considered 'non significant' [1]. This discordance between structure, function and outcome is also highlighted in the results of the recent cholesterol lowering trials where lowering cholesterol was associated with a disproportionately large reduction in cardiovascular events compared to the modest degree of anatomical regression [2]. Third, ischemia may result from impaired function of the microvasculature, which can hardly be studied or diagnosed with angiography.

In view of these limitations, attention has shifted from measuring the residual lumen (arteriography) to examination of the arterial wall architecture (intra-coronary ultrasound, angioscopy) and function. Among the different components of the arterial wall, the endothelial cell has been the focus of intense interest since the discovery by Furchgott of endothelium dependent vasodilation, more than ten years ago [3]. Long considered a passive barrier, the endothelium occupies a key location throughout the vascular system, at the interface of blood-borne elements such as platelets, leukocytes, coagulation factors and lipoproteins and the arterial wall. It plays a major role in:

a) Modulation of hemostasis through interaction with platelets and coagulation factors.
b) Regulation of leukocyte migration from the circulation into the vessel wall.
c) Inhibition of proliferative responses, and
d) Regulation of arterial tone.

Although often studied separately, these functions are interdependent and all affected by the development of atherosclerosis. In this chapter, we will focus on the control of arterial tone by the endothelium, in health and disease states.

Mechanisms of ischemia

Myocardial ischemia can result from an increase in oxygen demand which outstrips a limited capacity to increase supply. Clinicians are familiar with this concept, since the exercise test was designed to increase myocardial oxygen demand through increases in heart rate and blood pressure. Despite its clinical utility, this view is incomplete. With the introduction of continuous Holter monitoring, it has become apparent that in many patients with 'classic' exertional angina, episodes of ischemia occur at variable and lower levels of activity and heart rate, suggesting a decrease in the ischemic threshold. Ischemic episodes occur more frequently in the morning and can be triggered by normal daily events, such as mental or emotional stress. Also, ischemia can be detected at lower heart rate/blood pressure products during a more gradual exercise protocol, compared to the Bruce protocol. These results indicate that in many stable angina patients, a dynamic reduction in oxygen supply may occur in conjunction with increases in myocardial oxygen demand to create ischemia [4].

Abnormal constriction of atherosclerotic arteries may well be involved in this reduction in oxygen supply, both at the conductance and resistance levels. In support of this, the introduction of quantitative angiographic methods has shown abnormal constriction of atherosclerotic coronary arteries to a variety of stimuli including isometric and dynamic exercise, mental stress, cold pressor test and spontaneously at rest [5]. This abnormal vasoconstriction can now be understood in the context of the biology of atherosclerosis.

Endothelium and arterial vasomotion

Locally, arterial tone is determined by the balance of two opposing forces, acting to either expand or constrict the lumen, through contraction or relaxation of the smooth muscle cells in the media. Although abnormal increase in constrictive signals could potentially be involved in the genesis of ischemia, present evidence suggests that a lack of vasodilation is the principal factor resulting in unopposed vasoconstriction. Locally, arterial dilation is largely under the control of the endothelium. Furchgott and Zawadzki first showed that in the presence of intact endothelium, acetylcholine (ACh) produced a dose-dependent relaxation of isolated arterial rings while causing contraction when endothelial cells were removed [3]. Thus acetylcholine has a dual action: a direct constrictor effect on smooth muscle and indirect dilator effect, through an 'endothelium-derived relaxing factor' (EDRF), the net result being the sum of the two. At lower concentrations and in the presence of intact endothelium, vasodilation predominates. In the presence of dysfunctional endothelium or once the maximum effect of EDRF is exceeded, further increase in ACh concentration only promotes constriction.

ACh is not the only substance to evoke 'endothelium-dependent' vasomotor responses. Bradykinin, histamine, ADP, ATP, thrombin, serotonin, and substance P [6], as well as physical factors such as blood flow, pulse pressure and sheer stress [7] are known to release EDRF. Other factors however, have a direct relaxing effect on the smooth muscle either at the conductance or resistance level and are said to be 'endothelium-independent', such as nitrates, papaverine, calcium antagonists and dipyridamole.

There is now good evidence that EDRF is a nitric oxide radical (NO) or a complex containing NO (e.g. nitrosothiol), derived from the guanidino moiety of L-arginine [8]. NO acts on smooth muscle through activation of a soluble guanylate cyclase, phosphorylation of key proteins which eventually leads to *de*phosphorilation of the light chain of myosin and inhibition of Ca^+ release from intracellular stores and its entry through receptor-operated Ca^+ channels [9]. Exogenous sources of NO, such as nitroglycerin, require bioconversion through different enzymatic pathways before they can release nitric oxide. This transformation occurs at different levels along the vascular system according to the compound used, which explains the differences in the vascular bed affected and in the hemodynamic effects [10].

Endothelial Dysfunction in Ischemia

Evidence that abnormal vasoconstriction in humans with CAD is associated with endothelial vasodilator dysfunction was described by Ludmer *et al.*, in 1986. Infusion of ACh into coronary arteries of patients undergoing cardiac catheterization, resulted in vasodilation of angiographically normal vessels. In the presence of atherosclerosis however, constriction was induced by the same concentrations of ACh used to produce dilation of the normal vessels. Because diseased vessels retained the ability to respond adequately to the endothelium-independent vasodilator nitroglycerin, the paradoxical response to ACh was attributed to dysfunctional endothelium [11] (Figure 2.1). Additional support for this conclusion was obtained from studies using inhibitors of NO. Coronary infusions of free hemoglobin (which inactivates NO by direct biding), methylene blue (thought to act predominantly by inactivation of NO via the generation of superoxide free radicals) and the use of a specific inhibitor of NO synthesis, N^G-monomethyl-L-arginine (L-NMMA) all abolished the dilation of normal human coronary arteries to ACh without altering endothelium-independent dilator responses [12–14] (Figure 2.2).

Experimental studies have suggested endothelial injury or dysfunction to be the earliest step in the atherosclerotic process [15]. In support of this at the clinical level, abnormal vasoconstriction to ACh has been observed in vessels with minimal CAD (less than 30% angiographic stenosis) and in angiographically normal coronary arteries of patients with stenosis in the another coronary artery [11]. Abnormal endothelial vasodilator function has also been observed in patients with angiographically normal coronaries but with one or more of the following atherogenic risk factors: hypertension, hypercholesterolemia, male gender, family history or advanced age. Furthermore, the degree of the dysfunction appears to be proportional to risk factor severity (e.g. for cholesterol level and age), as well as to the total number of factors present in a single individual [16]. These results suggest that endothelial dysfunction may not only be an early marker of CAD but that it may be induced by risk factors and precede structural disease. In these patients with multiple risk factors however, the presence of abnormal vasomotion in response to ACh could have been associated with occult atherosclerosis not detected by angiography. To clarify these relationships, Hodgson *et al.* examine vasomotor response to ACh in patients with risk factors and normal coronary arteries by both angiography and intra-vascular ultrasound (IVUS). Endothelial dysfunction was related to the presence of risk factors and appeared to precede the development of intimal thickening [17].

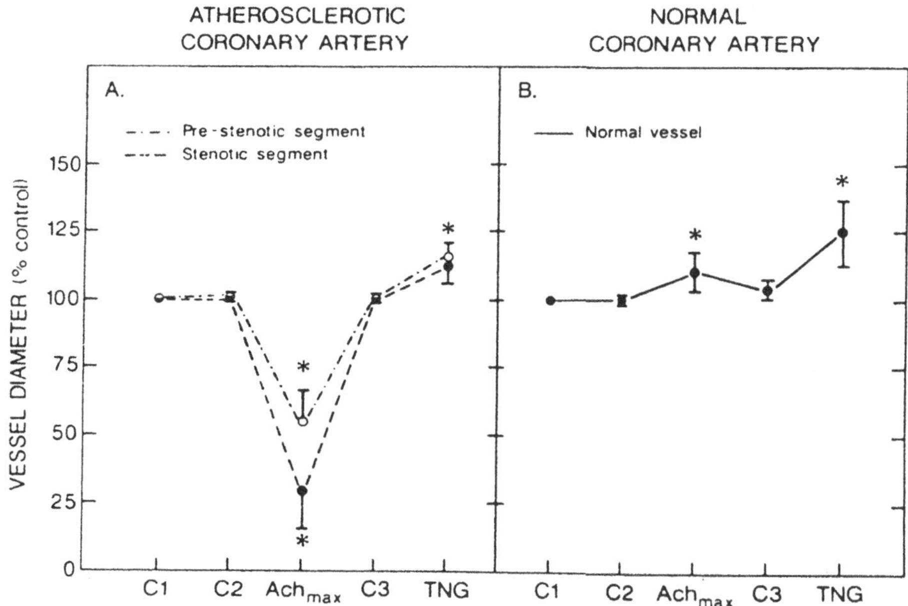

Figure 2.1. Responses of coronary arteries to intracoronary administration of an endothelium-dependent vasodilator (Acetylcholine) and a direct smooth- muscle vasodilator (Nitroglycerin) in eight atherosclerotic coronary arteries (Panel A) and four normal coronary arteries (Panel B). Cl denotes control, C2 vehicle control, Ach max response to maximal dose of acetylcholine, C3 repeated control, and TNG nitroglycerin. Asterisks indicate that P < O.Ol for the comparison with Cl. Reprinted, by permission of The New England Journal of Medicine, (vol. 315; p.1048, 1986).

Endothelial dysfunction: A systemic disease?

If endothelial dysfunction were related to circulating (lipids) or other systemic risk factors (hypertension, smoking, diabetes, genetic factors) as well as other diseases (Table 1), endothelial cells in vascular segments not overtly involved by atherosclerosis might also be affected. Consistent with this view, evidence has accumulated that indeed these insults also affect the endothelium of coronary and peripheral resistance arterioles and conduits arteries rarely involved in obstructive atherosclerosis such as the brachial artery.

Coronary microvascular bed

Coronary resistance vessels, although spared from the structural effects of atherosclerosis, are nevertheless functionally affected by the process. Sellke *et al.* have demonstrated abnormal vasomotion in coronary microvessels

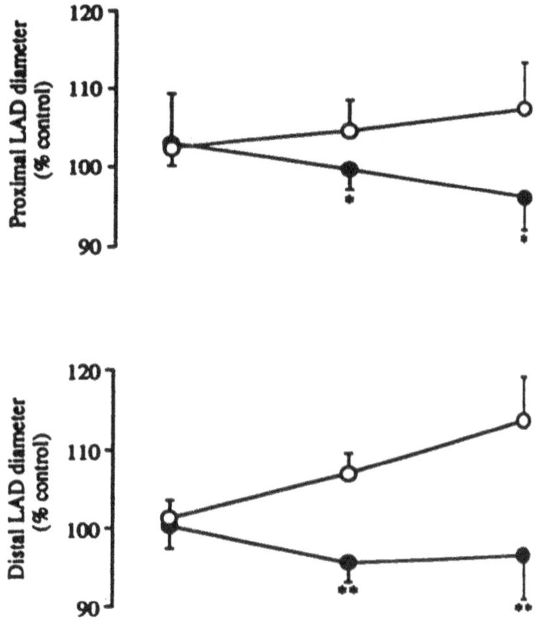

Figure 2.2. Graphs showing effects of the intracoronary infusion of acetylcholine on proximal and distal left anterior descending (LAD) coronary artery diameters before (O) and after (-) the N^G-monomethyl-L-arginine (L- NMMA) infusion. Results are mean ±SEM in six patients. * P < 0.05, **P < O.Ol compared with before L-NMMA infusion. Reproduced with permission. Circulation 88; p. 50, 1993. American Heart Association.

Table 2.1. Human diseases associated with impaired endothelium-dependent dilation.

Atherosclerosis
Transplant arteriosclerosis
Hypercholesterolemia
Post-menopausal state
Hypertension
Diabetes mellitus
Smoking
Homocysteinuria
Idiopathic dilated cardiomyopathy
Chagas' disease cardiomyopathy
Congestive heart failure

(122–220 μm) of hypercholesterolemic cynomolgus monkeys in response to ACh, bradykinin and A23187(a calcium ionophore and endothelium-dependent vasodilator). Responses to adenosine and sodium nitroprusside on the other hand were comparable to those observed in control animals, suggesting a defect at the level of the endothelium [18]. Blood flow studies using Doppler catheters have also documented absent or minimal dilation of coronary resistance vessels in response to ACh and substance P in patients with either minimal atherosclerosis or normal arteries and risk factors, including advanced age, hypercholesterolemia and hypertension. Responses to adenosine or papaverine, used as endothelium-independent dilators, were also blunted but to much lesser extent [19]. Although first demonstrated using pharmacological stimuli, endothelial dysfunction at the resistance level, is probably responsible for limiting blood flow and O_2 delivery during common, everyday events such as cold exposure, exercise or simple increases in heart rate [20, 21] (Figure 2.3).

Peripheral vascular bed

Conduit and resistance peripheral vessels may also be affected by endothelial dysfunction. High resolution ultrasound methods have revealed impaired flow mediated vasodilation in the brachial and/or femoral arteries, not only of patients with established CAD, but also of smokers, diabetics and even children with familial hypercholesterolemia, when compared to control subjects. Since the response to exogenous nitrates was similar in all groups, dysfunctional endothelium was implicated [22]. Hence, testing of brachial artery vasomotion could become a non-invasive and convenient approach to screen for and detect endothelial dysfunction in subjects at risk for CAD. There is indeed a good correlation between the presence of abnormal vasomotion in the brachial artery and in the coronary arteries [23].

In peripheral arteries, resistance vessel function is typically examined by measuring the blood flow responses using either venous strain gauge plethysmography or estimations of flow by transcutaneous Doppler ultrasonography. In healthy volunteers, infusion of the inhibitor of NO synthesis, L-NMMA into the brachial artery produces a 50% reduction in basal blood flow [24]. This suggests that a continuous release of NO contributes to the low resting vascular resistance in some tissues. The role of NO in the normal metabolic regulation of flow is also being examined: In healthy volunteers, brachial artery infusion of L-NMMA significantly decreases the peak hyperemic flow response to ischemia as well as the amount of repaid oxygen debt within 5 minutes of reperfusion [25]. These data provide initial evidence of NO's importance in metabolic regulation.

Since the endothelium is so uniquely positioned at the interface of the vessel wall and circulation, it is not surprising to see it affected by systemic disease processes. For example, patients with hypertension have decreased blood flow responses to infusions of ACh in the brachial artery. While normal control subjects demonstrate increased blood flow in response to ACh and a blunted response with the addition of L-NMMA, hypertensive patients showed no significant difference in response to ACh, with or without L-NMMA. These results provide evidence of a specific deficit in the endo-

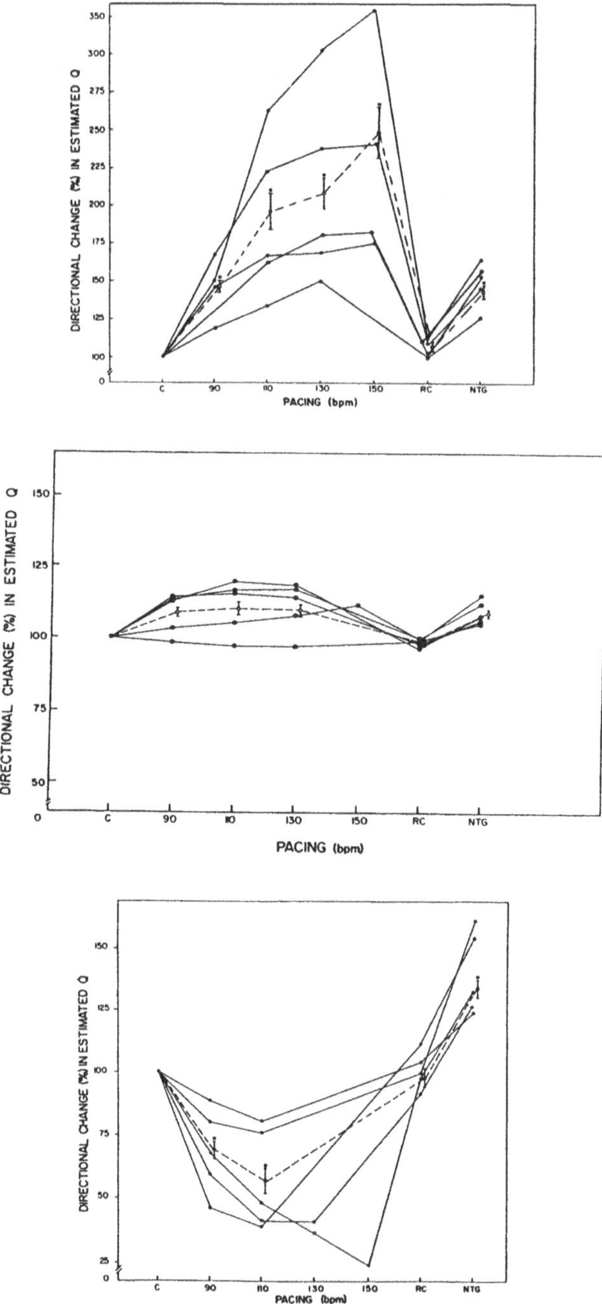

Figure 2.3. Plot of directional changes in coronary blood flow in response to rapid atrial pacing in normal arteries (Figure A), irregular arteries (Figure B) and arteries with severe angiographic narrowings (Figure C). Q, coronary blood flow; C, control; RC, repeat control; NTG, 50 μg intracoronary nitroglycerin; bpm, beats per minute. $^*P < 0.05$ for comparison to control. Solid lines are individual patient responses, whereas dashed line is mean response. Reproduced with permission. Circulation 81; p. 856–7,1990. American Heart Association.

thelium-derived nitric oxide system in the hypertensive population, which may play a role in the increased vascular resistance of these patients [26].

Endothelium: Future target for therapy?

It is now well accepted that endothelial dysfunction is an early marker of CAD and that it can be associated with a host of cardiovascular diseases. Understandably, there has been enormous interest in the reversal of this dysfunction. Three strategies are currently under investigation in humans. The first and most obvious is the treatment and reversal of risk factors, such as hypercholesterolemia. Reversal of dietary hypercholesterolemia in non-human primates restores endothelium-dependent relaxation of iliac arteries to normal [27]. A recent study examined whether treatment of hypercholesterolemic patients with angiographically normal coronary arteries can improve responses to acetylcholine. Twenty-five men with total cholesterol level of 6.2 mmol/L were treated with diet and cholestyramine for 6 months. Mean total cholesterol decreased from 7.1 to 5.1 mmol/L, LDL from 5.7 to 3.7 mmol/L with no change in HDL. Catheterization and vasomotion studies were performed at the beginning and termination of the study. Epicardial response to ACh infusion improved from a mean of 21.7% constriction to 6.2% dilation at follow-up [28]. Although interesting, these results were obtained in patient without CAD and could not be compared to a control group. Similar findings were reported in a interim analysis of an ongoing randomized, controlled study, involving patients with CAD. Results were available for the first 35 patients enrolled. Coronary vasomotor responses to ACh were significantly improved after a year of lipid lowering therapy as opposed to the unchanged responses in the control group treated with diet alone. Furthermore, the degree of improvement in vasomotion to ACh appeared to be related to the change in serum cholesterol [29]. Other risk factor modifications may also be beneficial. For example, in post-menopausal women, acute intravenous administration of conjugated estrogens improves coronary vasomotor response to ACh [30].

The second strategy used to improve endothelium-dependent dilation consists of specifically augment NO, either by supplying more substrate for its synthesis or by stabilizing the NO available. Intra-vascular administration of L-arginine, the substrate for NO synthesis, has been reported to restore ACh blood flow response in coronary arteries of hypercholesterolemic patients and to improve vasomotion of epicardial arteries [31]. Alternatively, NO inactivation by free oxygen radicals has also been investigated as a possible target of therapy: Infusion of recombinant human Cu-Zn superoxide dismutase (SOD) has been shown to significantly reduce the ACh induced vasoconstriction in epicardial arteries of patients with coronary atherosclerosis [32].

Thirdly, nitric oxide can be administrated by inhalation. However because of its lability, NO is inactivated in the pulmonary circulation. It has been used effectively to treat persistent pulmonary hypertension of the newborn [33], after mitral valve replacement [34] and in patients with the adult respiratory distress syndrome [35]. As a pulmonary vasodilator, nitric oxide has many advantages over the classical intravenous vasodilators. It is at least as effective in reducing pulmonary vascular resistance without provoking systemic hypotension which limits the use of the later. In addition, the theoretical risk of methemoglobin formation and toxicity has not been a problem in patients.

Many therapeutic interventions aimed at restoration of endothelial function need to be explored. At the present time however, the role of these interventions is promising but limited. More studies are required to define indications, efficacy and the effect on morbidity and mortality.

Conclusion

In the past 10 years, our understanding of vascular diseases has broadened to include not only the structural pathology that narrows the lumen but also to consider the coagulation, growth inhibition and vasomotor functions which are central to atherosclerosis and other diseases affecting the arterial wall. This has led to very potent advances in the treatment of stenoses (revascularization) and of acute thrombosis (thrombolysis). However, this new understanding of endothelial function in atherosclerosis will likely lead to strategies that can reverse endothelial cell dysfunctions in coronary lesions before catastrophic events occur, with improved patient outcome to follow.

References

1. Ambrose JA, Tannenbaum MA, Alexopoulos D *et al.* Angiographic progression of coronary artery disease and the development of myocardial infarction. J Am Coll Cardiol 1988; 12: 56–62.
2. Brown G, Albers JJ, Fisher LD *et al.* Regression of coronary artery disease as a result of intensive lipid-lowering therapy in men with high levels of apolipoprotein B. N Engl J Med 1990; 323: 1289–98.
3. Furchgott RF, Zawadzki JV. The obligatory role of endothelial cells in the relaxation of arterial smooth muscle by acetylcholine. Nature 1980; 288: 373–6.
4. Maseri A. Myocardial ischemia in man: current concepts, changing views and future investigation. Can J Cardiol 1986; Suppl. A: 225A–259A.
5. Meredith IT, Yeung AC, Weidinger FF *et al.* Role of impaired endothelium-dependent vasodilation in ischemic manifestations of coronary artery disease. Circulation 1993; 87: V–56–V–66.
6. Furchgott RF, Vanhoutte PM. Endothelium-derived relaxing and contracting factors. FASEB J 1989; 3: 2007–18.
7. Pohl U, Holtz J, Busse R, Bassenge E. Crucial role of endothelium in the vasodilator response to increased flow *in vivo*. Hypertension 1986; 8: 37–44.

8. Palmer RM, Ashton DS, Moncada S. Vascular endothelial cells synthesize nitric oxyde from L-arginine. Nature 1988; 333: 664–6.
9. Collins P, Lewis MJ, Henderson AH. Endothelium-derived factor relaxes vascular smooth muscle by cyclic GMP-mediated effects on calcium movements. In Vanhoutte PM (ed): Relaxing and contracting factors: biological and clinical research. Clifton, NJ: The Humana Press 1988: 267–83.
10. Harrison DG, Bates JN. The nitrovasodilators. New ideas about old drugs. Circulation 1993; 87: 1461–7.
11. Ludmer PL, Selwyn AP, Shook TL *et al.* Paradoxical vasoconstriction induced by acetylcholine in atherosclerotic coronary arteries. N Engl J Med 1986; 315: 1046–51.
12. Hodgson JM, Marshall JJ. Direct vasoconstriction and endothelium-dependant vasodilation. Mechanisms of acetylcholine effects on coronary blood flow and arterial diameter in patients with nonstenotic coronary arteries. Circulation 1989; 79: 1043–51.
13. Collins P, Burman J, Chung HI, Fox K. Hemoglobin inhibits endothelium-dependent relaxation to acetylcholine in human coronary arteries *in vivo*. Circulation 1993; 87: 80–5.
14. Lefroy DC, Crake T, Uren NG, Davies GJ, Maseri A. Effect of inhibition of nitric oxide synthesis on epicardial coronary artery caliber and coronary blood flow in humans. Circulation 1993; 88: 43–54.
15. Ross R. The pathogenesis of atherosclerosis: a perspective for the 1990s. Nature 1993; 362: 801–9.
16. Vita JA, Treasure CB, Nabel EG *et al.* Coronary vasomotor response to acetylcholine relates to risk factors for coronary artery disease. Circulation 1990; 81: 491–7.
17. Hodgson JM, Ravi N, Sheehan HM, Reddy KG. Endothelial dysfunction in coronary arteries precedes ultrasonic or angiographic evidence of atherosclerosis in patients with risk factors [abstract]. J Am Coll Cardiol 1992; 19 (Suppl A): 323A.
18. Sellke FW, Armstrong ML, Harrison DG. Endothelium-dependent vascular relaxation is abnormal in the coronary microcirculation of atherosclerotic primates. Circulation 1990; 81: 1586–93.
19. Zeiher AM, Drexler H, Saurbier B, Just H. Endothelium-mediated coronary blood flow modulation in humans. Effects of age, atherosclerosis, hypercholesterolemia and hypertension. J Clin Invest 1993; 92: 652–62.
20. Zeiher AM, Drexler H, Wollschläger H, Just H. Endothelial dysfunction of the coronary microvasculature is associated with impaired coronary blood flow regulation in patients with early atherosclerosis. Circulation 1991; 84: 1984–92.
21. Nabel EG, Selwyn AP, Ganz P. Paradoxical narrowing of atherosclerotic coronary arteries induced by increases in heart rate. Circulation 1990; 81: 850–9.
22. Celermajer DS, Sorensen KE, Gooch VM *et al.* Non-invasive detection of endothelial dysfunction in children and adults at risk of atherosclerosis. Lancet 1992; 340: 1111–5.
23. Uehata A, Gerhard MD, Meredith IT *et al.* Close relationship of endothelial dysfunction in coronary and brachial artery [abstract]. Circulation 1993; 88 (Suppl I): I–618.
24. Vallance P, Collier J, Moncada S. Effects of endothelium-derived nitric oxide on peripheral arteriolar tone in man. Lancet 1989; 997–1000.
25. Meredith IT, Hoffmann KE, Anderson TJ, Roddy MA, Ganz P, Creager MA. Post ischemic vasodilation in the human forearm is dependent on endothelium-derived relaxing factor [abstract]. Clin Res 1993; 41: 504 A.
26. Panza JA, Casino PR, Kilcoyne CM, Quyyumi AA. Role of endothelium-derived nitric oxide in the abnormal endothelium-dependent vascular relaxation of patients with essential hypertension. Circulation 1993; 87: 1468–74.
27. Harrison DG, Armstrong ML, Freiman PC, Heistad DD. Restoration of endothelium-dependent relaxation by dietary treatment of atherosclerosis. J Clin Invest 1987; 80: 1808–11.
28. Leung WH, Lau CP, Wong CK. Beneficial effect of cholesterol-lowering therapy on coronary endothelium-dependent relaxation in hypercholesterolemic patients. Lancet 1993; 341: 1496–500.

29. Anderson TJ, Meredith IT, Yeung AC, Lieberman EH, Selwyn AP, Ganz P. Cholesterol lowering therapy improves endothelial function in patients with coronary atherosclerosis [abstract]. Circulation 1993; 88 (Suppl I): I-368.
30. Lieberman EH, Gerhard M, Yeung AC *et al.* Estrogen improves coronary vasomotor responses to acetylcholine in post menopausal women [abstract]. Circulation 1993; 88 (Suppl I): I-79.
31. Dubois-Rande JL, Zelinsky R, Chabrier PE, Castaigne A, Geschwind H, Adnot S. L-arginine improves endothelium-dependent relaxation of conductance and resistance coronary arteries in coronary artery disease. J Cardiovasc Pharmacol 1992; 20 (Suppl 12): S211–3.
32. Meredith IT, Anderson TJ, Yeung AC *et al.* Superoxide dismutase restores endothelial vasodilator function in human coronary arteries *in vivo* [abstract]. Circulation 1993; 88 (Suppl I): I–467.
33. Kinsella JP, Neish SR, Shaffer E, Abman SH. Low-dose inhalation nitric oxide in persistent pulmonary hypertension of the newborn. Lancet 1992; 340: 819–20.
34. Girard C, Lehot JJ, Pannetier JC, Filley S, Ffrench P, Estanove S. Inhaled nitric oxide after mitral valve replacement in patients with chronic pulmonary artery hypertension. Anesthesiology 1992; 77: 880–3.
35. Rossaint R, Falke KJ, Lopez F, Slama K, Pison U, Zapol WM. Inhaled nitric oxide for the adult respiratory distress syndrome. N Engl J Med 1993; 328: 399–405.

PART TWO

QCA: Digital and cine coronary arteriography

3. Why and how should QCA systems be validated?

JOHAN H.C. REIBER, GERHARD KONING, CRAIG D. VON LAND & PIETER M.J. VAN DER ZWET

Summary

It has been clearly demonstrated that significant differences exist in the design and implementation of various QCA systems, as well as in the calculations of the derived clinical parameters. Therefore, extensive standardized validation studies must be carried out to demonstrate the strengths and weaknesses, as well as the clinical validity of QCA analytical software packages. In general, the following sequence of studies needs to be performed: 1) assessment of the accuracy and precision of the underlying edge detection technique with phantom, *in vivo* and postmortem models; 2) assessment of the reproducibility of the QCA procedure; and 3) assessment of the short-, medium- and long-term variabilities. Application of QCA in clinical research studies requires Quality Assurance in image acquisition (catheterization laboratory calibration) and image analysis (core laboratory calibration).

Introduction

Quantitative Coronary Arteriography (QCA) systems for either off-line or on-line purposes have been around for some time now. An extensive overview of the different approaches as of 1991 was published in [1]. This overview clearly demonstrated that significant differences exist in the design and implementation of these QCA systems. Very briefly, these differences included: 1) the calibration procedures; 2) the definition of the pathline of the coronary segment to be analyzed; 3) the edge detection algorithm used; 4) correction for the limited resolution of the X-ray system; 5) pincushion distortion correction; 6) calculation of the diameter function by different approaches (certainly not a trivial task!); 7) assessment of derived parameters with differences among others in user-defined and automatically determined reference diameters; and finally, 8) the validation procedures for which hardly any standardization existed.

As an example, the assessment of the arterial diameter function from the detected contours depends among others on the sampling distance and the direction of the scanlines (Figure 3.1). In this figure, a hypothetical example of an obstructed vessel is given together with the scanlines which represent the local width of the vessel. If course sampling is used, small irregularities may be missed entirely (upper example). In addition, the diameter measure-

J.H.C. Reiber and P.W. Serruys (eds): Progress in quantitative coronary arteriography, 33–48.

Arterial Diameter Function

Large pixel distance between diameters

Small pixel distance between diameters

Small pixel distance, reference centerline method

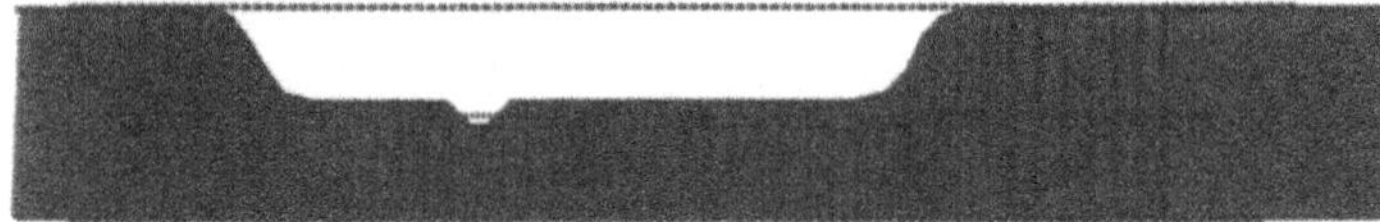

Figure 3.1. The calculation of the arterial diameter function is not a trivial task and depends among others on the sampling distance and the direction of the scanlines. The ideal situation is depicted in the lower example. For further details see text.

ments are taken perpendicular to the calculated centerline, which will result in overestimations at the entrance and exit of the obstructive region. With a small sampling distance, the small irregularity is recognized, but the overestimations are still present (middle example). Ideally, the sampling distance should be small (on the order of 0.1 mm) and the sampling direction perpendicular to the unknown centerline of the original, nonobstructed vessel segment as demonstrated in the lower example of Figure 3.1.

Whichever QCA analytical software package is being used, it will always produce numbers describing the morphology of the coronary segment analyzed. However, to demonstrate the strengths and weaknesses, as well as the clinical validity of such analytical packages, extensive standardized validation studies must be carried out. In a very first attempt to find out to which degree different QCA systems produce comparable results, a cinefilm of a plexiglass phantom with 11 tubular vessels was analyzed on four different QCA systems. The results in terms of the signed differences between the mean measured diameters and the true diameters for the 11 individual tubes are shown in Figure 3.2. This figure clearly demonstrates that indeed significant differences exist between these four systems, particularly for sizes below 1 mm (Systems E and H); all these systems have been used in clinical research

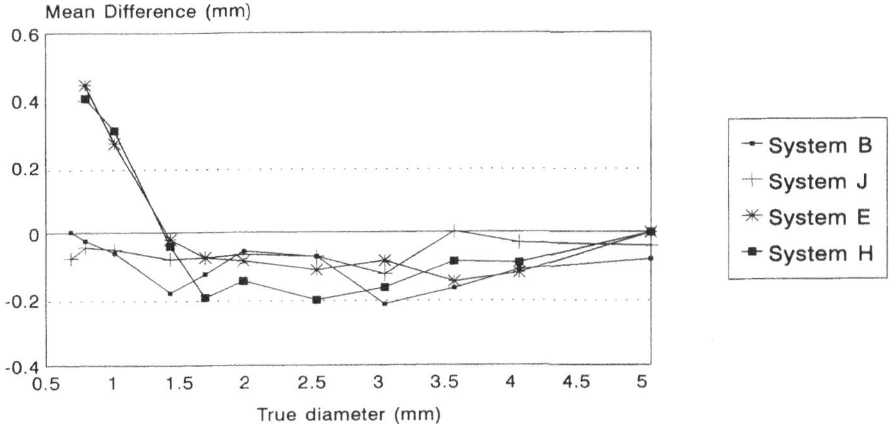

7" 70kV

Figure 3.2. Mean differences between measured and true diameters of a plexiglass phantom acquired on a homogeneous scatter medium (off patient) for four different QCA systems. The differences in mm are plotted along the ordinate and the true sizes of the 11 tubes along the abscissa. Systems E and H show large overestimations for the sizes below one mm.

trials. Further information on these intersystem and interlaboratory variabilities is presented by Glenn Beauman in Chapter 6 of this book [2].

On the basis of our experience with the development and validation of QCA analytical software packages, we feel that the following sequence of studies needs to be carried out for a thorough validation of a QCA package: 1) assessment of the accuracy and precision of the underlying edge detection technique; 2) assessment of the reproducibility of the QCA-procedure; and 3) assessment of the short-, medium-, and long-term variabilities. Furthermore, if one wants to exchange or compare data from different laboratories with the same or different QCA systems, or just wants to check the quality of the output of a particular institute, it is of great interest to study the interinstitute or -laboratory variability. This is, of course, of particular relevance in the large clinical research trials.

The details of the validation studies proposed will be described more extensively in the following sections and illustrated with material obtained with the QCA package on the CMS-system[1] and with the ACA-package on the DCI-system.[2] Finally, it should be mentioned that for laboratories involved in longitudinal coronary arteriographic studies a strictly controlled Quality Assurance (QA) program is of eminent importance; an example of such QA program will be given.

1. MEDIS Medical Imaging Systems, Nuenen, the Netherlands.
2. Philips Medical Systems, Best, the Netherlands.

Assessment of the accuracy and precision of the underlying edge detection technique

Before a QCA package can be applied in clinical research studies the limitations of the basic edge detection algorithm must be known. In other words, some of the following questions need to be addressed: are there any systematic errors in the measurements, and are these vessel size dependent; what is the variability in the measurements; etc. It is our belief that these questions can best be answered by using well-defined models of coronary vessels. For that reason we have developed the following sequence of tests in order of increasing complexity, which are suitable both for digital as well as cinefilm systems.

A. Evaluation studies using a plexiglass phantom on a homogeneous scatter medium (off patient)

For these purposes we have used a plexiglass phantom with 11 straight circular 'vessel' tubes ranging in size from 0.687 to 5.062 mm, which can be filled with various concentrations of the contrast medium and acquired at different kV-levels and image intensifier modes. This phantom was designed by R.L. Kirkeeide, Ph.D. from Houston, USA. As a scatter medium we have used a 10 cm stack of plexiglass or a similar water basin. A straight 'vessel' segment must be analyzed over a sufficient length, e.g. 2 cm. The derived diameter function provides a set of independent measurement values, from which a mean value and a standard deviation can be calculated. An example of an analysis of one of the smallest tubes with the CMS system is illustrated in Figure 3.3. In this example a mean diameter of 1.01 mm was found with a standard deviation in the measurements of 0.08 mm; the true tube size was 1.011 mm. If the contour detection results in an under- or overestimation of this mean diameter, this will be evident in the systematic error or accuracy for this segment defined as the average measured diameter minus the known true diameter.

It has been well accepted that the results from validation studies be described in terms of the mean signed differences (accuracy) and the standard deviation (precision) of these signed differences (measurement 1 – measurement 2; not absolute differences) between the actual and measured values or between the values from repeated measurements [1,3]. The precision *per segment* is defined by the standard deviation of the signed differences between each measured diameter in the diameter function of the segment and the measured average diameter of the segment; this standard deviation is a measure for the irregularity of the detected contours. In other words, this precision measure represents an uncertainty range for a diameter value measured at a discrete position, such as at the minimal lumen diameter (MLD).

To obtain an overall quality measure for the phantom, acquired under a certain imaging condition, the mean difference values can be averaged over

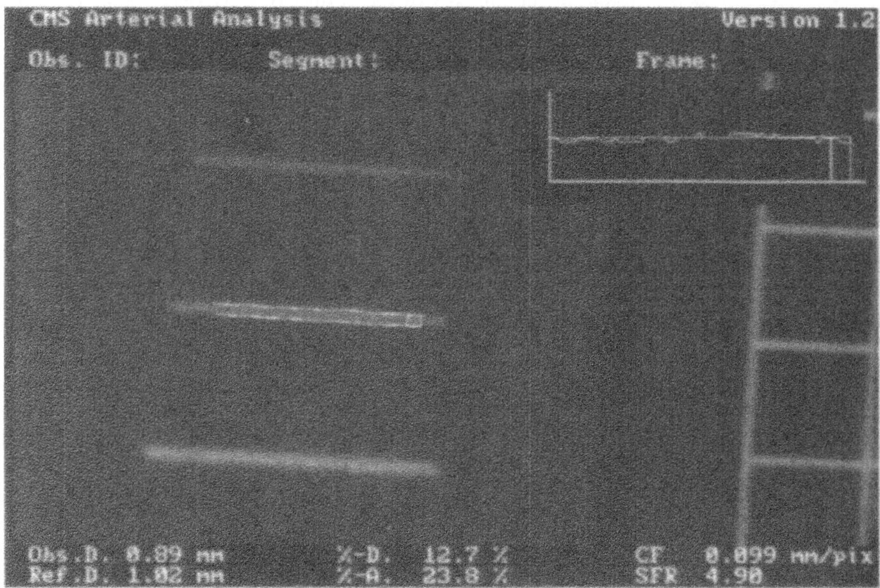

Figure 3.3. Results of automated contour detection and quantitative analysis of a vessel tube (true size 1.011 mm) in the plexiglass phantom with the CMS system. This resulted in an average diameter of 1.01 mm and a standard deviation of 0.08 mm. This standard deviation value is a measure for the irregularity of the detected contours.

all segments providing an overall accuracy value, and the pooled standard deviation provides an overall precision value [4]. It is important to realize that the overall precision should not be based on the standard deviations of the signed differences between the mean diameter value of a segment and its true value; this would result in too optimistic values! This can be illustrated with the example of Table 3.1. Here the signed differences between the average measured dimensions and the true diameters for the 11 vessel tubes are given, as well as the standard deviations of the differences. By carrying out the calculations as proposed above, this results in an overall systematic underestimation of only 0.015 mm and an overall precision of 0.096 mm. However, if we would have calculated the overall precision on the basis of only the signed differences of the mean measured and true diameters, a value of only 0.074 mm would have been found. This is clearly a much too optimistic interpretation of the results, due to the fact that the irregularities in the detected contours were not taken into account.

For an edge detection technique to be acceptable, the overall accuracy value should be close to zero, which means that no significant over- or underestimations, or systematic errors may occur; the overall precision in absolute vessel sizes should be on the order of 0.10–0.13 mm.

Table 3.1. Hypothetical example of the analysis of the results of a plexiglass phantom with 11 'vessel' tubes. For further details, see text.

True D (mm)	Measured D (mm)	M-T (mm)	s.d. (mm)
0.687	0.774	0.087	0.111
0.794	0.854	0.060	0.135
1.011	1.023	0.012	0.101
1.431	1.336	−0.095	0.107
1.696	1.685	−0.011	0.107
1.986	2.073	0.087	0.076
2.533	2.518	−0.015	0.098
3.046	3.016	−0.030	0.080
3.568	3.465	−0.103	0.085
4.062	3.933	−0.129	0.067
5.062	5.031	−0.031	0.067

Overall accuracy = $\Sigma_i[(M_i - T_i)/N] = -0.015$ mm. Overall precision = pooled s.d. = 0.096 mm. *Incorrect*: Overall precision = s.d. $\{M_i - T_i\} = 0.074$ mm. Abbreviations: M_i = mean measured diameter of segment i (i = 1,11), T_i = true diameter of segment i, N = total number of segments (here N = 11), s.d. = standard deviation.

However, this global analysis is not sufficient to demonstrate the success of a particular edge detection technique. The averaging process may hide local inaccuracies; for example, overestimations for the small vessel sizes may cancel out underestimations for the larger sizes. Therefore, it is of utmost importance to show the results for the individual vessel segments as well. An excellent way to do this, is by means of the difference plots as have been suggested by Bland and Altman [5]. Such a plot allows a rapid and easy interpretation of the efficacy of the edge detection technique for all the individual vessel sizes; 'local' inaccuracies will be readily apparent. As an example, the difference plot for the DCI system is shown in Figure 3.4. In this example for the phantom acquired at 7" image intensifier mode and at 90kV, an average systematic error of −0.028 mm was found and a pooled standard deviation of the measurements of 0.124 mm.

Precision numbers decrease when the degree of contour smoothing is increased. At first glance this would seem to be a positive characteristic of the contour detection algorithm. It is clear though, that by increasing the degree of contour smoothing the performance of the algorithm to accurately measure the minimal lumen diameter of an obstruction, particularly those of short severe obstructions, will deteriorate. The actually desired degree of contour smoothing is rather critical: too little smoothing results in very irregular contours, too heavy smoothing results in missing of abrupt changes in the vessel sizes at obstructions. It is therefore important that the algorithms are also tested on 'vessel' tube phantoms that contain obstructions. Preferably, these obstructions should taper to one single minimal diameter. If, on the contrary, phantoms are used that contain obstructions of constant diameter over a certain length, the minimum of all obstruction diameters is chosen, leading to a systematic underestimation of the MLD. Due to the

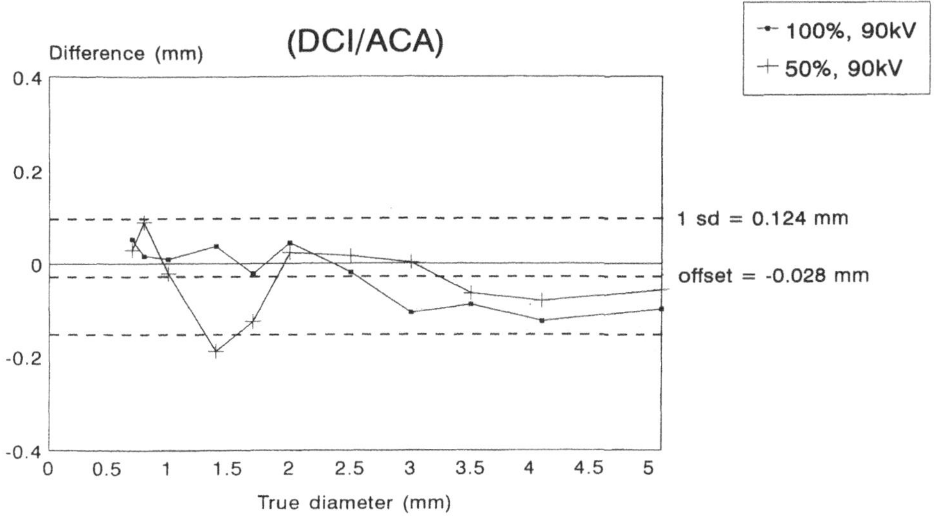

Figure 3.4. Difference plot for the DCI system according to the technique proposed by Bland and Altman. The true vessel sizes of the phantom are plotted along the horizontal axis and the signed difference between the average measured dimension and its corresponding true value along the vertical axis. A positive difference corresponds to an overestimation, a negative difference to an underestimation. In this example for the phantom acquired at 7" image intensifier mode and at 90kV, an average systematic error of −0.028 mm was found and a pooled standard deviation (dotted lines) of the measurements of 0.124 mm.

noise in the image, there will always be diameter values calculated below the actual vessel size as can be clearly appreciated from Figure 3.3. At this point in time, such a phantom is being designed in our laboratory.

B. Evaluation study of the plexiglass phantom on a nonhomogeneous background (on patient)

Under the previously described test setup, the phantom was positioned on a homogeneous scatter medium, being a stack of plexiglass. To allow for a clinically more realistic evaluation, as a next step this plexiglass phantom should be positioned on the chest of a patient over the heart and acquired during a routine catheterization procedure. The same analyses as described above can be carried out. This may result in an increase in the standard deviation values, due to the inhomogeneous background, usually lower signal-to-noise ratio, etc. However, the systematic errors should not be affected significantly. Figure 3.5 shows an example of a small vessel tube (true size 0.794 mm) with the inhomogeneous background analyzed with the Philips/DCI system. In this case a mean diameter of 0.818 mm was obtained with a standard deviation of 0.125 mm.

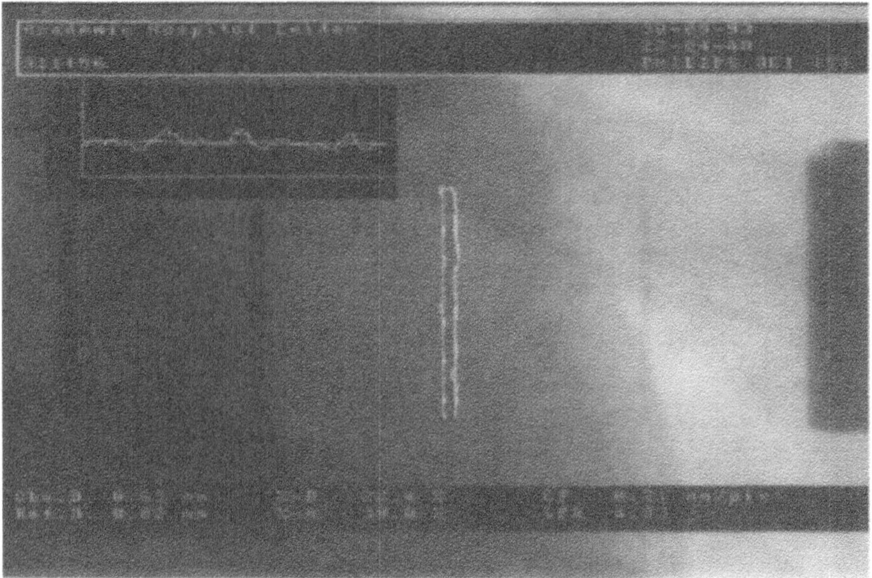

Figure 3.5. Results of the quantitative analysis of a small vessel tube (true size 0.794 mm) with the phantom superimposed onto a patient's chest. The irregularity of the contour as expressed in terms of the standard deviation value was found to be 0.125 mm. The mean measured diameter was 0.818 mm.

C. In vivo *animal study*

The next step is an *in vivo* animal study with hollow plastic cylinders of various luminal sizes inserted in the coronary arteries [6, 7]. Again the same analysis procedures as described earlier should be followed. Recently, *in vivo* animal studies have been carried out at the Leiden University Hospital. An example of a cinefilm image of a dog artery with a plexiglass cylinder having a luminal diameter of 0.70 mm is shown in Figure 3.6 with the results of the QCA/CMS-package superimposed. The mean diameter over the obstructive region was found to be 0.65 mm; due to X-ray noise influences the minimal lumen diameter was 0.53 mm. From a total of 21 measurements with various plugs a systematic error of −0.09 mm and a pooled standard deviation of 0.08 mm was found for the CMS system, and a systematic error of −0.01 mm and a pooled standard deviation of 0.14 mm for the DCI system.

D. Postmortem validation study

The final test to be carried out is a postmortem validation study [8]. For the Philips DCI/ACA package data from digital coronary arteriograms and

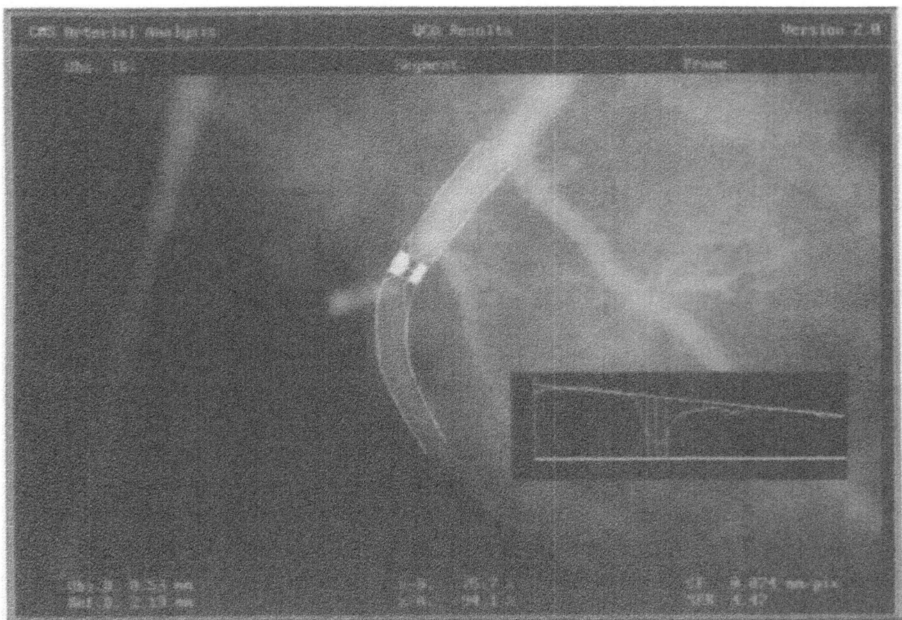

Figure 3.6. Example of a digital image of a dog artery with a plexiglass hollow cylinder positioned into the artery; the true luminal diameter of the plug was 0.70 mm. The mean measured diameter over the obstructive region was found to be 0.65 mm.

postmortem casts of 6 mongrel dogs were used. Vessel diameters were measured from the digital arteriograms at a total of 118 selected locations. Thin slices were cut from the casts at these same measurement locations, and the areas of the cross sections were obtained by manual tracing of the outline of each slice in an approximately 40x magnified image. From these cross-sectional areas, cast diameters were derived using the formula for circular cross sections. Cast diameters ranged in size from 0.69 to 3.30 mm. The systematic error between the measurements was found to be 0.058 mm ($p = 0.015$) and the standard deviation of the signed differences 0.255 mm ($r = 0.91$). The largest error sources were believed to be the slight differences in the selection of identical positions in the X-ray images and on the casts, and the 'out-of-plane' magnification for a number of vessel locations.

E. Densitometry

If densitometric validation studies are carried out, the hypothesis that the results are independent of the angiographic views in which these studies were acquired, must be tested. This may be done using a simple phantom with straight vessel tubes as proposed above for the diameter measurements. The results will then be indicative of the minimal variability in the densitometric analyses under optimal conditions. More complex phantoms should be tested in subsequent studies. However, so far densitometry has not resulted in reliable results, particularly from cinefilm [1]. It may be useful to revisit the densitometric approaches for the digital systems in which the entire transfer function of the X-ray system is better controlled and more stable than with the use of cinefilm.

Assessment of the reproducibility of the QCA procedure

Once the accuracy and precision of the edge detection technique have been established and found to be acceptable, the next issue is the assessment of the inter- and intraobserver variabilities on a set of routinely acquired coronary arteriograms. Frames to be analyzed will, in general, be selected by one of two users; the images selected for calibration do not need to be the same as the images in which the coronary segments are analyzed. For the inter-observer study, the selected frames are analyzed by the two observers independently from each other. For the intra-observer study, the same set of images are analyzed several weeks later by one of the two observers without using knowledge from the first analysis session [9]. From the inter- and intraobserver data, the mean signed differences (accuracy) and the standard deviation of these differences (precision) are calculated. Again the differences should not be statistically significantly different from zero, and the standard deviation values as small as possible. Precision values in absolute dimensions on the order of 0.10–0.14 mm are nowadays common. Examples of such analyses can be found in Ref. 9, as well as in the chapter by Reiber *et al.* in this book [10].

Assessment of the short-, medium- and long-term variabilities

The inter- and intraobserver variability measurements proposed above are obtained from selected frames of coronary arteriograms. Additional sources of variability are included with repeated acquisition of coronary arteriograms followed by quantitative analysis of these images [9]. Such studies will more closely resemble the situations in which these packages will be applied in clinical research studies. For these purposes we can define three kinds of studies, the socalled short-, medium- and long-term variability studies [9]. The short-term variability is defined by the variability in measured arterial dimensions from repeated acquisition and quantitative analysis of coronary arteriograms taken 5 minutes apart with unchanged geometry of the X-ray system. The medium-term variability is defined similarly with the first arteriogram taken at the beginning of the catheterization procedure and the second arteriogram taken at the end. Between these repeated arteriograms,

Table 3.2. Short- and medium-term variabilities of the DCI-ACA package as assessed from routine coronary arteriograms.

Parameter	Mean-value	Short-term (N = 41)		Medium-term (N = 40)		unit
		accur.	prec.	accur.	prec.	
Calibrat. factor	0.217	−0.002	0.007	0.003	0.012	mm/pixel
Obstruction diam.	1.69	0.00	0.19	0.03	0.18	mm
Reference diam.	3.18	−0.02	0.22	−0.02	0.34	mm
Percent diam. sten.	46.47	−0.57	5.61	−0.47	5.28	%

the X-ray system settings will be changed various times for the acquisition of other angiographic views (and e.g. of the left ventriculograms). This means that the X-ray system needs to be returned to the initial arteriographic view for the repeat study. Finally, the long-term variability is defined with the first and the second arteriograms taken at two separate catheterization sessions. The time period between the two sessions should not exceed 6 months to exclude the effects from progressive coronary artery disease.

It will be clear that standardized acquisition protocols need to be followed to minimize the contributions from the various error sources [9]. Standardization items include, among others, the use of a coronary vasodilator (e.g. 5 mg of isosorbide dinitrate sublingual, administered immediately prior to each of the arteriograms), preferably a nonionic contrast agent, maximal and reproducible breath holding by the patient, careful read-out and resetting of the rotation and angulation angles of the gantry, etc. From our experience, the short-, medium- and long-term variabilities in the absolute dimensions in absolute vessel dimensions will be on the order of 0.20 mm or higher. The outcome of the short- and medium-term variability study with the Philips DCI/ACA analytical package is presented in Table 3.2. From all the additional error sources that are introduced with the repeated acquisition procedures as compared to the simple reproducibility studies on the same images, we concluded that the increased variabilities in the absolute dimensions are most likely due to the variations in the calibration factor assessed on the basis of the contrast catheter [9].

Assessment of intersystem and interlaboratory variabilities

With the widespread use of QCA on different workstations and in different laboratories, the question comes up how well the results from these QCA-laboratories correlate. This is of particular relevance for Core-laboratories which at a certain point in time may wish to combine QCA data from similar trials for meta-analysis purposes, or otherwise want to compare data, e.g. from recanalization procedures carried out in different countries. Most likely systematic differences exist in the absolute dimensions between the two laboratories; hopefully, the two laboratories show the same trends between baseline and follow-up studies, although such claim must be proven first.

If two core-laboratories use the same equipment, differences will exist in the image quality of the coronary arteriograms, in the way the angiograms are analyzed in terms of the frame selection and the definition of the coronary segments, in the dedication and experience of the technicians in the actual analysis of the images, etc. In addition, the question must be raised whether the individual analyses are overread by a QCA specialist as part of the quality assurance program of the core-laboratory. Otherwise, two laboratories may use different QCA equipment, but otherwise have the same level of sophistication in the coronary arteriographic acquisition and analysis procedures. The worst situation is present of course, if two laboratories use different QCA-equipment, if they must process coronary arteriograms of different image quality, if they follow different approaches in the analysis procedures, etc. So far very little has been done to assess these intersystem and interlaboratory variabilities. Beauman *et al.* recently demonstrated from a comparison of plexiglass phantom studies among seven angiographic core laboratories (ACL's) that average differences from the true phantom diameters ranged widely among these laboratories (0.05–0.20 mm). In addition, automated analysis failure was recorded for 26% of attempts to analyze diameters <1.0 mm, which were largerly overestimated by the ACL's (0.10 ± 0.09 mm). For further information, the reader is referred to Chapter 6 of this book.

Training courses

It is well known that standardized analysis of coronary arteriograms is an extremely important factor in minimizing existing variabilities. For example, in cases of very diseased vessels the calculation of the automated reference diameter with the CMS/QCA and DCI/ACA packages is dependent upon the length of the segment analyzed. We believe that the users can get most out of these packages if the basic underlying principles are well understood. In practice, user manuals are not read, misplaced in the QCA-laboratory, etc. In an attempt to transfer the information about the basic principles of QCA, and about standardized acquisition and analysis procedures, in a more efficient manner, we have set up Quantitative Coronary and Left Ventricular Cine and Digital Angiography (QCLA) training courses at the University Hospital of Leiden. During these courses a great deal of attention is given to hands-on training on the equipment under the supervision of faculty members. This has shown to be very effective in transferring our QCLA

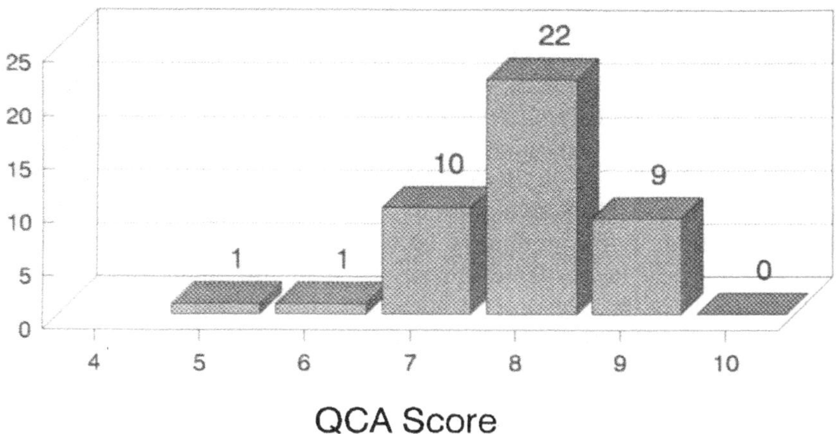

Figure 3.7. Results from QCLA-Course of January 1993. In this histogram the number of grades are plotted along the vertical axis, and the grades along the horizontal axis. Nine out of the total of 43 outcomes (i.e. 21%) was graded a 9, and 22 + 9 = 31 (72%) of the results were graded 8 or higher, i.e. the results fell within a range of 2 standard deviations of the Faculty results.

experience to the (potential) users. The following example illustrates the effectiveness of this kind of training.

As part of the hands-on training the course participants are asked to analyze preselected digital and cine images. These same frames had been analyzed previously by the faculty members so that each QCA-parameter (e.g. minimum lumen diameter MLD) can be characterized by a mean value and a standard deviation on the basis of the faculty outcomes. These ranges are then used to grade the outcomes of the participants. If the result as obtained by a course participant falls within the range defined by the mean value +/- one s.d., a grade of 9 is given. For results outside of this 1 s.d. range, but within a range of two s.d. a grade of 8 is given, etc. The results from one of our last QCLA-Courses is presented in Figure 3.7. This figure shows that after such a short training nine out of the total of 43 measurements (i.e. 21%) were graded a 9, and 72% an 8 or higher, i.e. 72% of the results fell within a range of 2 standard deviations of the Faculty results.

Quality assurance (QA) in longitudinal coronary arteriographic studies

This chapter is mainly devoted to the questions why and how QCA systems should be validated. One of the main applications of QCA systems is in longitudinal coronary arteriographic studies in which the vessel dimensions and particularly the degree of obstructions must be compared in great detail from baseline and follow-up arteriographic studies. The time between baseline and follow-up studies will in general be on the order of two to three years. The quality of these quantitative analyses naturally do not only depend upon the quality of the QCA systems, but even to a greater degree upon the quality of the underlying arteriographic image data. Images with little image contrast will result in a lower reliability in the detected contours; images can be so poor in quality that they cannot be analyzed at all. Significant changes in the film development process may have an effect on the contour detection. If the geometry of the X-ray system changes over time the vessels will not be projected anymore from the same directions which may particularly be problesome in stenosed vessels, etc. Many more causes for differences in the image analyses results could be summed up. It will be clear that these effects are particularly troublesome when these occur slowly over time such that they may go unnoticed, or may be detected after the study has been completed.

It has been clear that proper 'calibration' of the participating catheterization laboratories carried out on a regular basis (e.g. once every 3–4 months) will improve the consistency and reliability of the image data. Only if these conditions are met can corresponding segments from multiple views can be compared with precision. To determine the quality of the X-ray imaging chain and the possible changes therein over a study period, appropriate Quality Assurance (QA)[3] or calibration programs have been developed for catheterization laboratories [11]. Items which are measured include, among others:

1. accuracy and precision of the rotation and angulation read-out devices on the X-ray gantry;
2. accuracy and precision of tower height and table read-out devices;
3. resolution of the X-ray system based on a modulation transfer function (MTF) analysis and on the basis of line-pair phantoms with the MEDIS X-ray phantom;
4. determination of the large detail detectability (LDD) of the X-ray system using the MEDIS X-ray phantom;
5. signal-to-noise ratio in the phantom images;
6. spatial distribution and degree of pincushion distortion;
7. the quality of the cinefilm development process.

The derived data from these measurements are stored in a QA-database, allowing trend analysis from follow-up calibration procedures which are carried out at regular time intervals. As soon as it becomes evident that one of the parameters will fall outside of the normal ranges, preventive maintenance procedures can be initiated. In addition to these regular calibration procedures, the quality of cardiac catheterization laboratories can be measured using the same techniques prior to inclusion in a clinical trial (Quality Acceptance Program). In this way the principal investigator of such a trial and the

3. MEDIS Medical Imaging Systems, Nuenen, the Netherlands.

Table 3.3. Example of the grading of a catheterization laboratory as part of the regular Quality Assurance Program.

Signal to noise ratio	7
Contrast	7
Detail	7
Geometric distortion	8
Reproducibility geometry X-ray system	7
Stability film development	8
Overall impression	7.3

Table 3.4. Guidelines for accuracy and precision of a state-of-the-art QCA system.

	Accuracy (mm)	Precision (mm)
Plexiglass phantom		
off patient	<0.10	0.10–0.13
on patient	<0.10	0.10–0.13
In vivo study		0.10–0.20
Postmortem study		0.20–0.30
Inter/intra-observer variabilites		0.10–0.15
Short-term variabilities		0.15–0.25
Medium-term variabilities		0.20–0.30
Long-term variabilities		0.20–0.30

sponsor obtain objective criteria to choose those centers which are most suitable for participation in the trial.

Table 3.3 provides an example of the grading of a catheterization laboratory as part of the regular Quality Assurance Program.

Concluding remarks

From the above it will be clear that assessing the strengths and weaknesses and the validity of a new QCA analytical software package is not a trivial task. Proper validation studies ranging from phantom to repeated coronary arteriographic studies must be carried out. Proper statistical techniques, which are simple to interpret, must be used. For a QCA technique to be acceptable, the following guidelines for accuracy and precision values of absolute vessel dimensions can be established, whereby the accuracy values for the plexiglass phantom apply to each of the individual measurements (Table 3.4).

In addition to all these variability measurements, a great deal of attention must also be given to the user interface, to the amount of manual corrections that need to be carried out to the detected contours in routinely acquired arteriograms and the simplicity with which these corrections can be applied, to the success score in tracking complex lesions, etc. Quality Assurance in image acquisition (Cath. Lab. Calibration) and image analysis (Core Lab. Calibration) is a requirement for QCA clinical research studies.

Acknowledgement

The authors wish to thank mrs. B. Smit-van der Deure for her secretarial assistance in the preparation of this manuscript.

References

1. Reiber JHC. An overview of coronary quantitation techniques as of 1989. In Reiber JHC, Serruys PW (eds): Quantitative coronary arteriography. Dordrecht: Kluwer Academic Publishers 1991: 55–132.
2. Beauman GJ, Reiber JHC, Koning G, van Houdt R, Vogel RA. Comparison of QCA Core Laboratory Analyses: Inter-laboratory variability determined from common analyses of an arterial phantom. This volume.
3. Herrington DM, Walford GA, Pearson TA. Issues of validation in quantitative coronary angiography. In Reiber JHC, Serruys PW (eds): New developments in quantitative coronary arteriography. Dordrecht: Kluwer Academic Publishers 1988: 153–66.
4. Reiber JHC, van der Zwet PMJ, von Land CD *et al.* Quantitative coronary arteriography: equipment and technical requirements. In Reiber JHC, Serruys PW (eds): Advances in quantitative coronary arteriography. Dordrecht: Kluwer Academic Publishers 1993: 75–111.
5. Bland JM, Altman DG. Statistical methods for assessing agreement between two methods of clinical measurement. Lancet 1986; 1: 307–10.
6. Haase J, Di Mario C, Slager CJ *et al. In vivo* validation of on-line and off-line geometric coronary measurements using insertion of stenosis phantoms in porcine coronary arteries. Cathet Cardiovasc Diagn 1992; 27: 16–27.
7. Mancini GBJ. Morphologic and physiologic validation of quantitative coronary arteriography ulilizing digital methods. In Reiber JHC, Serruys PW (eds): New developments in quantitative coronary arteriography. Dordrecht: Kluwer Academic Publishers 1988: 125–41.
8. Van der Geest RJ, Morris KG, Cusma JT, Reiber JHC. Postmortem validation of the Automated Coronary Analysis (ACA) software package. Int J Card Imaging. In press.
9. Reiber JHC, van der Zwet PMJ, Koning G *et al.* Accuracy and precision of quantitative digital coronary arteriography: observer-, short-, and medium-term variabilities. Cathet Cardiovasc Diagn. 1993; 28: 187–98.
10. Reiber JHC, von Land CD, Koning G, van der Zwet PMJ, van Houdt RCM, Schalij MJ, Lespérance J. Comparison of accuracy and precision of quantitative coronary arterial analysis between cinefilm and digital systems. This volume.
11. Van der Zwet E, Reiber JHC. Quality control (calibration) of catheterization laboratories involved in longitudinal coronary angiographic studies. In Abstract book 5th International Symposium on Coronary Arteriography. Rotterdam: 1993: 196.

4. Percutaneous implantation of coronary stenosis phantoms in an anesthetized swine model to validate current quantitative angiography analysis systems

JÜRGEN HAASE, DAVID KEANE, CARLO DI MARIO, JAVIER ESCANED, YUKIO OZAKI, CORNELIS J. SLAGER, ROB VAN BREMEN, WILLEM J. VAN DER GIESSEN & PATRICK W. SERRUYS

Introduction

Computerized quantitative coronary angiography (QCA) has basically altered our approach to the assessment of interventional techniques and strategies aimed at the prevention of restenosis and progression of coronary artery disease [1, 2]. With an increasing number of QCA systems being developed, and a growing number of core laboratories for the analysis of multicenter angiographic studies, it has become crucial that the performance of QCA systems, upon which much of our scientific understanding has become integrally dependent, is evaluated in an objective and uniform manner [3].

QCA systems with a low level of precision may fail to detect small but significant differences in study populations while QCA systems with poor accuracy may provide misleading results of absolute measurements of obstruction diameter. The results of studies based on unreliable QCA systems may not be directly comparable to those of reliable systems. To render the results of angiographic trials meaningful and universally applicable, it is important that QCA systems be validated in a systematic and standardized fashion. Without a standardized approach to validation it becomes difficult to assess to what degree individual angiographic studies are reliable, and how much weight should be attributed to absolute values of minimal luminal diameter derived from individual QCA systems and the significance of their failure to detect relative changes in obstruction diameter. Furthermore, it is only by detailed validation studies, that systematic errors in QCA systems can be identified and thereby provide guidance for the refinement of algorithms in QCA software.

The present investigation was performed to determine accuracy, reliability and reproducibility offered by one digital and three cinefilm-based QCA systems currently in use and undergoing continuous refinement. Stenosis phantoms of known diameter mimicking the narrowings of human coronary arteries were used as a reference both in an *in vitro* plexiglass model as well as after serial inserion in the coronary arteries of pigs [4–6]. The QCA

J.H.C. Reiber and P.W. Serruys (eds): Progress in quantitative coronary arteriography, 49–65.

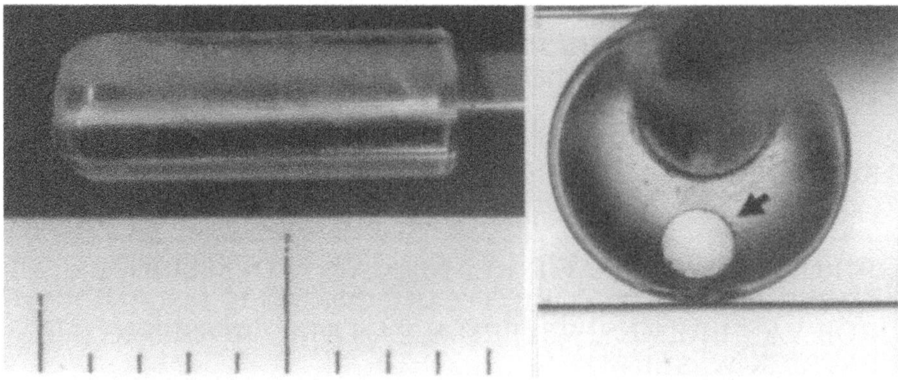

Figure 4.1. Catheter mounted cylindrical plexiglass stenosis phantom (length 8.4 mm, diameter 3.0 mm) in two projections. On the short axis view (right) the entrance of the 0.7 mm stenosis channel is indicated by an arrow.

systems were assessed by their measurement of the absolute value of 'minimal luminal diameter' or 'obstruction diameter' within the artificial stenoses which has previously been shown to be more reliable than relative measures of coronary artery dimensions based on the definition of a reference contour [7–9]. To assess the influence of different calibration techniques on the outcome of geometric measurements *in vivo*, calibration at the isocenter was compared with catheter calibration as conventionally used in clinical practice.

Methods

Stenosis phantoms

The stenosis phantoms used in the *in vitro* as well as *in vivo* model consisted of radiolucent acrylate or polyimide cylinders with precision-drilled eccentric circular lumens of 0.5, 0.7, 1.0, 1.4 and 1.9 mm in diameter (Figure 4.1). The outer diameters of the cylinders were 3.0 or 3.5 mm, and the length was 8.4 mm. Acrylate was used to produce the phantoms with small stenosis diameters (0.5, 0.7 mm), whereas the less fragile polyimide was better suited to the drilling of large stenosis diameters (1.0, 1.4, 1.9 mm). Optical calibration of the stenosis channels using 40–fold magnification gave a tolerance of 0.003 mm. Parallel to the stenosis lumen a second hole of 1.3 mm in diameter was drilled in the cylinders to attach them to the tip of 4 F Fogarty catheters (Vermed, Neuilly en Thelle, France). The central lumens of these catheters contained a removable metal wire, which was used for intracoronary insertion of the phantoms as well as for their positioning in the radiographic isocenter (Figure 4.2).

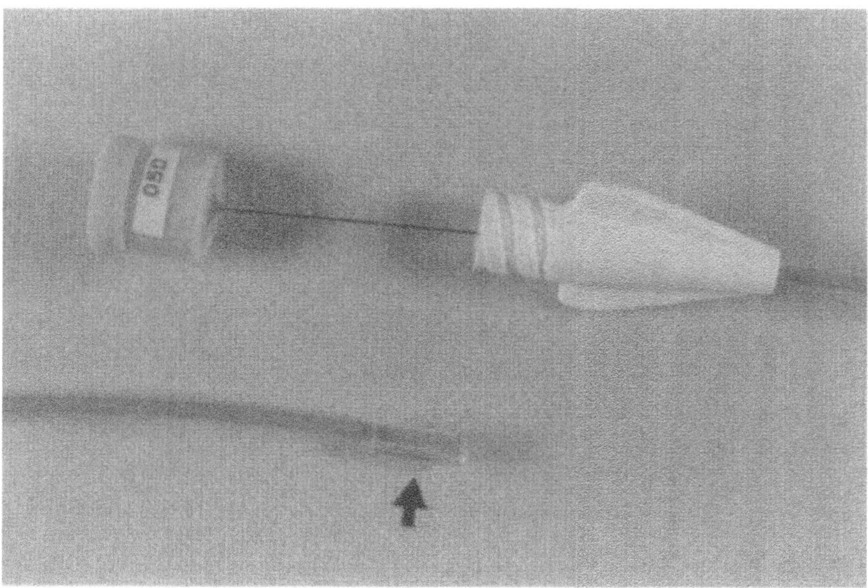

Figure 4.2. Phantom catheter with removable metal wire. At the tip of the catheter the 0.7 mm phantom is mounted (arrow).

In vitro *experiments*

The stenosis phantoms were serially inserted in the center of cylindrical acrylate models (diameter 25 mm, length 120 mm) with a concentric channel of 3.0 mm in diameter. The plexiglass channel including the artificial stenosis was then filled with contrast medium (iopamidol 370, Bracco, Milano, Italy; 370 mg iodine/ml) at a concentration of 100%. Digital as well as cinefilm acquisition was performed with an additional thickness of plexiglass blocks (12.5 cm anterior and 5 cm posterior to the models) to approximate the density of water. The addition of plexiglass blocks results in a more appropriate kV-level (75 kV) and in a scatter medium which more closely approximates the x-ray scatter in the humen thorax during fluoroscopy. Each phantom filled with contrast medium was recorded digitally as well as on cinefilm.

In vivo *experiments*

The experimental approach employing the catheter mounted stenosis phantoms in normal coronary arteries of anesthetized pigs has already been described in recent studies from our group [4–6]. Two different calibration methods were applied to geometric measurements. Calibration at the isocenter was carried out by radiographic acquisition of a drill-bit (diameter 3

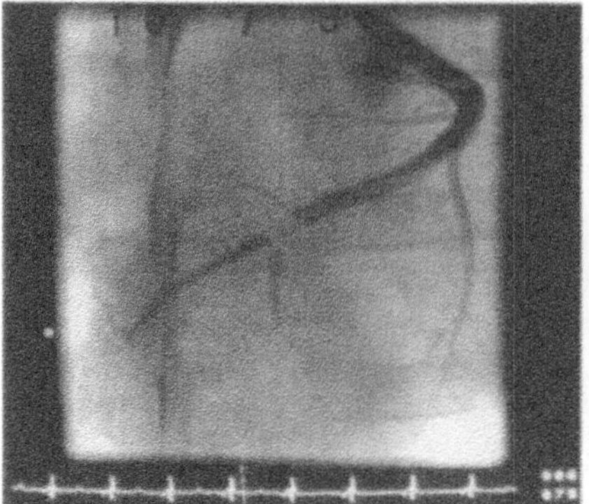
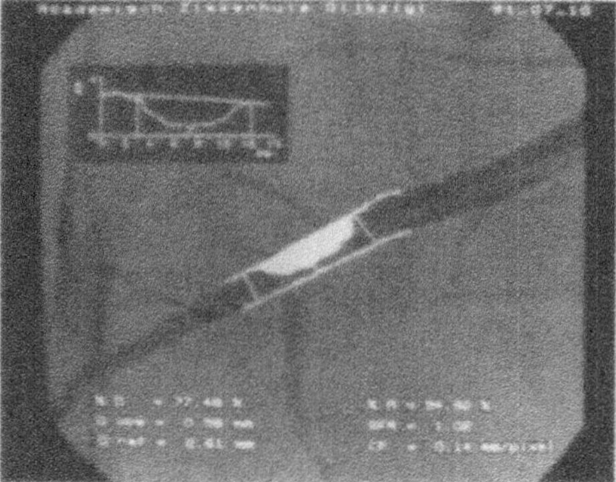

Figure 4.3. Angiographic visualization of the artificial coronary obstruction produced by an 0.7 mm stenosis phantom in the left anterior descending artery (left) with subsequent digital measurement of obstruction diameter (right).

mm) within the isocenter of the X-ray system before angiography. Catheter calibration was performed by acquisition of the unfilled tip of the contrast catheter as conventionally recommended for clinical routine [10]. The diameter of the non-tapering part of this catheter was assessed with a precision micrometer (no. 293–501, Mitutoyo, Tokyo, Japan; accuracy 0.001 mm), resulting in the respective calibration factor (mm/pixel). Using these two calibration procedures, two series of results were obtained allowing an estimation of the potential geometric error introduced by non-isocentric calibration.

Image acquisition and processing

The 5''-field mode of the image intensifier (focal spot 0.8 mm) was selected and the radiographic system settings were kept constant (kV, mA, X-ray pulse width) in each projection. All phantoms were imaged isocentrically in two projections and acquired digitally by the Philips Digital Cardiac Imaging system (DCI) as well as on 35–mm cinefilm using identical frame rates of 25 images/s. The DCI system employs a matrix size of 512 × 512 pixels. The horizontal pixel size was 200 μm and the density resolution was 8 bits (256 density levels). The images were stored on a 474 MB Winchester disk. From each digital angiogram which fulfilled the requirements of image quality for automated quantitation (no superimposition of surrounding structures, no major vessel branching at the site of the phantom position), a homogenously filled enddiastolic coronary image was selected and quantitative analysis of the stenosis phantom was performed on-line (Figure 4.3) with the Automated Coronary Analysis (ACA) analytical software package [11].

The corresponding 35–mm cineframes (CFE Type 2711, Kodak, Paris,

France) were used for off-line analysis with the previous and the recent version of the Cardiovascular Angiography Analysis System (CAAS I and CAAS II) [12, 13] as well as with the Cardiovascular Measurement System (CMS) [14].

Edge detection analysis

Ten *in vitro* and 19 *in vivo* frames were suitable for quantitative analysis of the artificial stenoses. A sufficiently long segment of the contrast filled lumen including the stenosis phantom was selected on all images; care was taken to define the same segment length on corresponding digital and cinefilm images.

Optical magnification of a region of interest is performed on the cinefilm-based QCA systems before digitization of the images into a 512 × 512 pixel matrix. On the DCI system as well as on the CMS the user is requested to define only a start and an end point of the vessel segment, and a centerline through the vessel is subsequently defined automatically. On the CAAS I and CAAS II the user defines a number of centerline points within the arterial segment which are subsequently connected by straight lines, serving as a first approximation of the vessel centerline. On all four QCA systems the basic automated edge detection techniques are similar; they are based on the first and second derivative functions applied to the brightness profiles along scanlines perpendicular to a model using minimal cost criteria [11, 12].

With CAAS, the edge detection algorithm is carried out in two iterations. First, the model is the initially defined centerline and second, the model is a recomputed centerline, determined automatically as the midline of the contour positions which were detected in the first iteration. With DCI and CMS, the edge detection algorithm is also carried out in two iterations and two spatial resolutions. In the first iteration the scan model is the initially detected centerline and edge detection takes place at the 512 × 512 matrix resolution. Here, the detected contours in the first iteration function as scan models. In the second iteration, a ROI centered around the defined arterial segment is digitally magnified by a factor of two with bilinear interpolation. Furthermore, on CAAS II, DCI and CMS, the edge detection algorithm is modified to correct for the limited resolution of the entire x-ray imaging chain. Thereby, the focal spot size related overestimation of vessel diameters smaller than 1.2 mm diameter is corrected for.

'Minimal luminal diameter' and 'obstruction diameter'

To objectively compare geometric measurements by all four QCA systems, no user interaction on the process of autometd contour detection was performed, and the absolute measure of 'minimal luminal diameter' or 'obstruction diameter' respectively, was used as a parameter of validation. In this

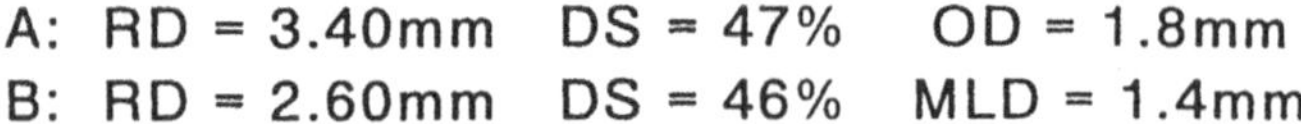

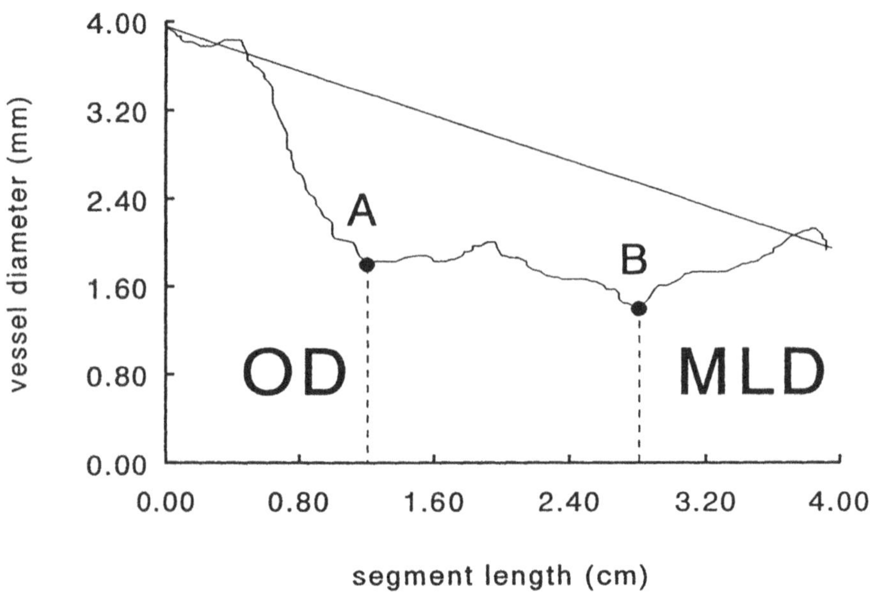

Figure 4.4. Definition of 'obstruction diameter' on DCI and CMS: schematic display of the diameter function curve of a coronary artery obstruction. The minimum of the diameter function curve is located at position B. Due to the tapering of the vessel, B is not necessarily identical with the site of maximum percent diameter stenosis represented by position A, where the obstruction diameter is defined (OD = obstruction diameter, MLD = minimal luminal diameter, RD = reference diameter, DS = percent diameter stenosis).

context, it has to be taken into account, that the geometric definitions of 'minimal luminal diameter' as used in CAAS I, and 'obstruction diameter' by DCI, CMS and CAAS II are not identical. On CAAS I, the classical parameter of 'minimal luminal diameter' is taken as the shortest distance between the two vessel contours, whereas on DCI and CMS, the so-called 'obstruction diameter' refers to the diameter measured at the site of maximum percent diameter stenosis, thereby taking into account the tapering of the vessel (Figure 4.4). On the CAAS II, a new definition of 'obstruction diameter' is introduced in order to avoid artificial minima of the diameter function curve produced by noise of the acquisition system. Here, 'obstruction diameter' is determined as the value measured at the 'geometric center' of the obstruction, which is defined as the middle between the two closest diameter values that excced the minimal luminal diameter of the stenosis by 5% (Figure 4.5).

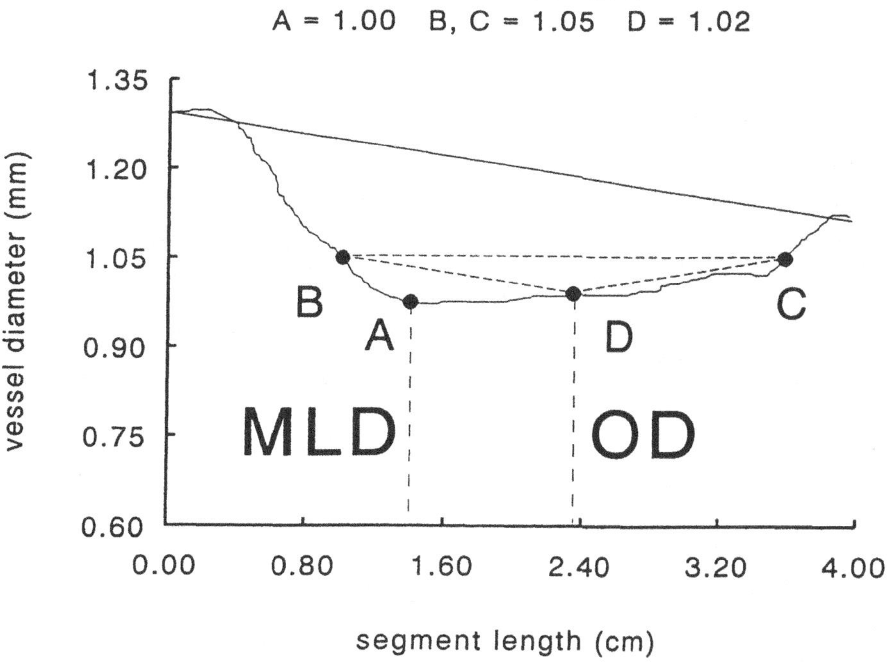

Figure 4.5. Definition of 'obstruction diameter' on CAAS II: schematic display of the so-called 'geometric center' of the obstruction, defined as the middle (D) between the two closest diameter values which exceed the minimal luminal diameter (A) of the stenosis by 5% (B, C). At position D, the 'obstruction diameter' (OD) is calculated (OD = obstruction diameter, MLD = minimal luminal diameter).

Statistical analysis

Using both calibration methods (calibration at the isocenter, catheter calibration), the individual data for minimal luminal diameter or obstruction diameter obtained by the respective system were compared with true phantom diameters by a t-test for paired values. The mean of the signed differences between measured diameters and individual reference values was considered an index of accuracy and the standard deviation of the differences an index of precision. The measured values were plotted against the true phantom diameters and linear regression analyses were applied. Precision values from both calibration techniques were compared using Pitman's test [15].

The standard deviation of the mean value from 15 or 30 geometric measurements on the same angiographic phantom was considered a measure of reproducibility. From two systems, these values were calculated separately

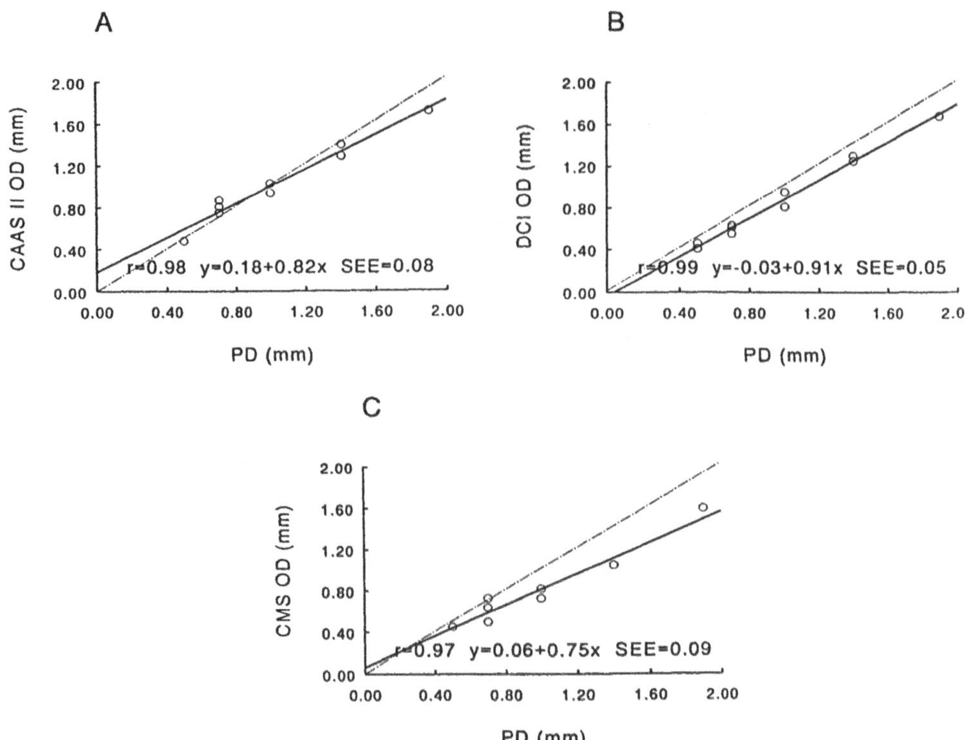

Figure 4.6. In vitro validation of geometric coronary measurements using 100% contrast medium: the individual obstruction diameter values (OD) obtained by CAAS II (A), DCI(B), and CMS(C) are plotted against the knowm diameters of the stenosis phantoms (PD). The graphs include the lines of identity as well as the individual results from the linear regression analyses.

for all five stenosis phantoms. The mean reproducibility was defined as the mean value from those five reproducibility values.

Results

A. In vitro *validation of obstruction diameter assessments*

With the new version of the CAAS, the *in vitro* assessment of obstruction diameters yielded an accuracy of 0.00 mm and a precision of ±0.11 mm. As illustrated by Figure 4.6A, there was a high correlation between obstruction diameter values and true phantom diameters (r = 0.98, y = 0.18 + 0.82x, SEE = 0.08) with a slight tendency to underestimate large phantom sizes.

Using the DCI, we obtained an accuracy of 0.11 mm and a precision of ±0.06 mm with an excellent correlation between measured values of obstruction diameter and referece diameters ($r = 0.99$, $= 0.03 + 0.91$, $SEE = 0.05$), as depicted in Figure 4.6B.

The corresponding cinefilm-based measurements on the CMS, gave an accuracy of 0.18 mm and a precision of ±0.14 mm with relatively good correlation ($r = 0.97$, $y = 0.06 + 0.75x$, $SEE = 0.09$), as illustrated by Figure 4.6C. The difference in variability from DCI and CMS measurements was statistically significant ($p < 0.05$).

B. In vivo *validation of obstruction diameter assessments*

Assessment of Minimal Luminal Diameter on CAAS I

The results of *in vivo* validation using CAAS I are illustrated by Figure 4.7A. Calibrated at the radiographic isocenter, the assessment of minimal luminal diameter gave an accuracy of −0.07 mm and a precision of ±0.21 mm with a non-significant trend towards overestimation of small phantom diameters ($r = 0.91$, $y = 0.30 + 0.79x$, $SEE = 0.19$). Using catheter calibration (Figure 4.7B), the corresponding measurements yielded an accuracy of 0.09 mm with a precision of ±0.23 mm and tended to underestimate large phantom sizes ($r = 0.89$, $y = 0.19 + 0.74x$, $SEE = 0.19$).

Assessment of obstruction diameter on CAAS II

As demonstrated by Figure 4.7, the overestimation of small phantom diameters is less pronounced with CAAS II. Using this version with calibration at the isocenter (Figure 4.7C), the assessment of obstruction diameters gave an accuracy of −0.01 mm and a precision of ±0.18 mm with high correlation between measured values and true phantom diameters ($r = 0.94$, $y = 0.22 + 0.82x$, $SEE = 0.15$). With catheter calibration (Figure 4.7D), an accuracy of 0.14 mm and a precision of ±0.17 mm was obtained. In this series, the measurement points of the smallest phantom diameters lay rather close to the line of idendity, while large diameters were significantly underestimated ($p < 0.05$) producing a relatively low slope of the regression line ($r = 0.96$, $y = 0.14 + 0.76x$, $SEE = 0.12$).

Assessment of obstruction diameter on DCI

Using calibration at the isocenter, the assessment of obstruction diameters by the digital system (Figure 4.8A) gave an accuracy of 0.08 mm and a precision of ±0.15 mm with high correlation between measured values and true phantom sizes ($r = 0.96$, $y = 0.08 + 0.86x$, $SEE = 0.14$). Catheter calibration (Figure 4.8B) yielded an accuracy of 0.18 mm and a precision of ± 0.21 mm ($r = 0.92$, $y = 0.09 + 0.76x$, $SEE = 0.17$). The tendency towards underestimation of phantom diameters with calibration at the isocenter ($p < 0.05$) was more pronounced when catheter calibration was applied ($p < 0.01$).

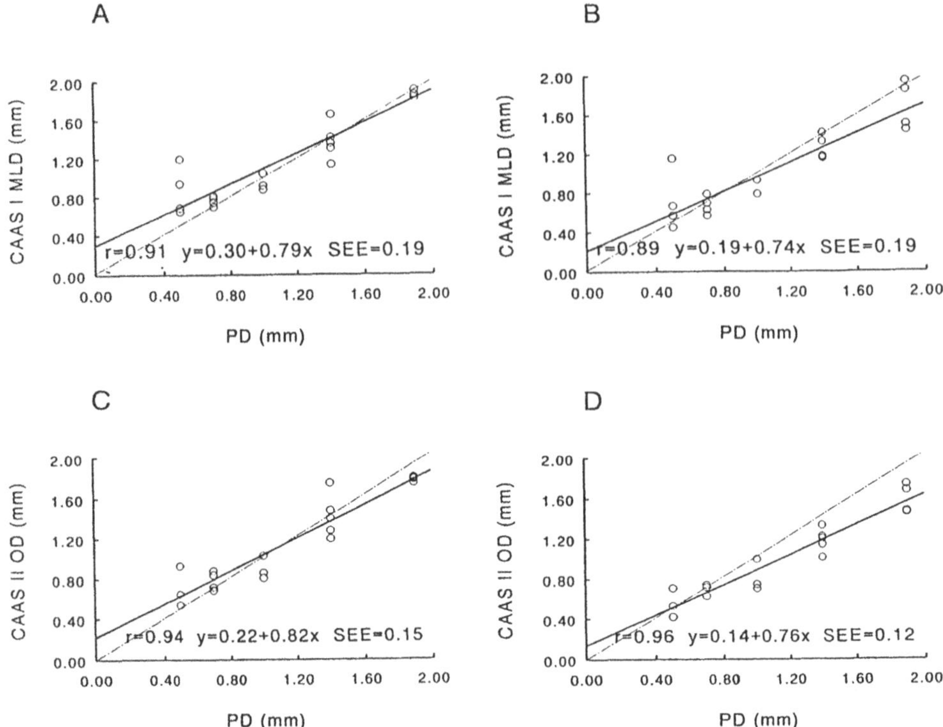

Figure 4.7. In vivo validation of geometric coronary measurements by CAAS I and CAAS II: the plot of measured minimal luminal diameter values (MLD) or obstruction diameter values (OD) against known phantom diameters (PD) obtained by CAAS I with calibration at the isocenter are displayed in graph A, the corresponding plot with catheter calibration is displayed in graph B. Graphs C and D show the results from CAAS II using calibration at the isocenter and catheter calibration, respectively.

Assessment of obstruction diameter on CMS

The corresponding cinefilm-based measurements on the CMS are displayed in Figure 4.8C and D. Calibrated at the radiographic isocenter (Figure 4.8C), the assessment of obstruction diameters yielded an accuracy of 0.18 mm and a precision of ±0.23 mm ($r = 0.89$, $y = 0.02 + 0.83x$, SEE = 0.22). The underestimation of large phantom sizes was statistically significant ($p < 0.01$). Compared with DCI, the CMS measurements showed a higher degree of variability ($p < 0.05$). Using catheter calibration (Figure 4.8D), we found an accuracy of 0.26 mm and a precision of ±0.24 mm ($r = 0.89$, $y = 0.06 + 0.72x$, SEE = 0.19) with an even more pronounced tendency to underestimate true phantom diameters ($p < 0.001$).

The resluts from the *in vitro* and *in vivo* validation using CAAS I, CAAS II, DCI and CMS, are summarized in Tables 4.1 and 4.2, respectively.

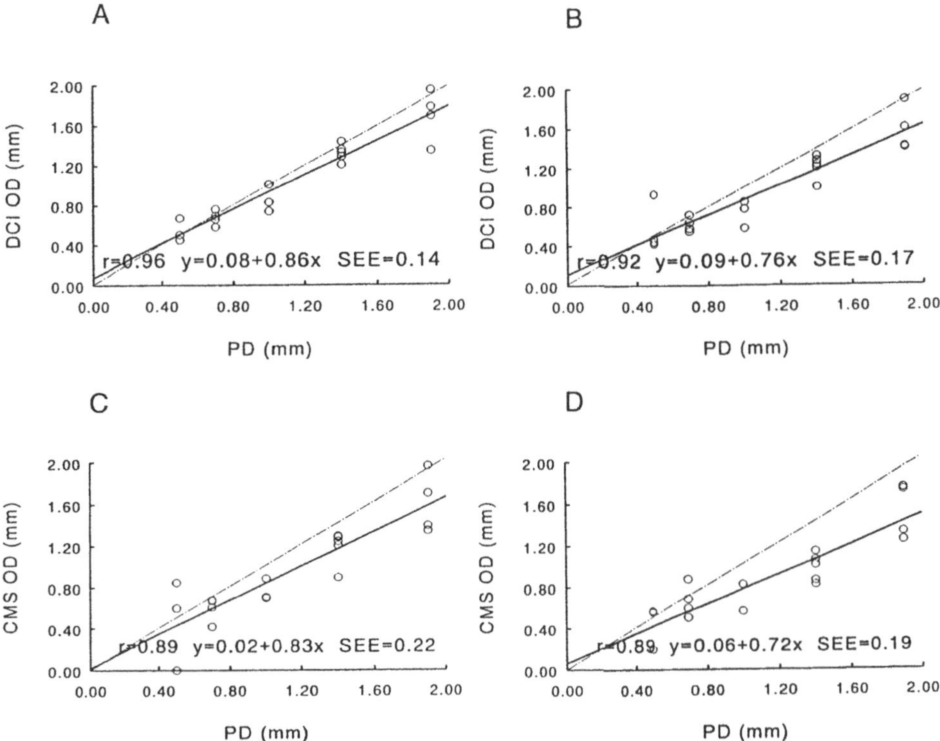

Figure 4.8. In vivo validation of geometric coronary measurements by DCI and CMS: the plot of measured obstruction diameter values (OD) against known phantom diameters (OD) obtained by DCI with calibration at the isocenter are displayed in graph A, the corresponding plot with catheter calibration is displayed in graph B. Graphs C and D show the results from CMS using calibration at the isocenter and catheter calibration, respectively.

Table 4.1. In vitro validation of quantitive coronory analysis systems.

System	Accuracy	Precision	Difference	Correlation	Linear regression Analysis	Standard error of estimate
CAAS II	0.001	0.11	N.S.	r = 0.98	y = 0.18 + 0.82x	SEE = 0.08
DCI	0.11	0.06	N.S.	r = 0.99	y = -0.03 + 0.91x	SEE = 0.05
CMS	0.18	0.14	$p < 0.01$	r = 0.97	y = 0.06 + 0.75x	SEE = 0.09

Reproducibility of geometric coronary measurements

The results from 30 repeated obstruction diameter assessments of each stenosis phantom on the recent version of the CAAS and from 15 repeated measurements with the CMS are depicted in Figure 4.9. Using CAAS II (Figure 4.9A), the variability of measurements was ±0.07 mm with the 1.4 mm phantom, ±0.09 mm with the 0.5 mm, 0.7 mm, and 1.0 mm phan-

Table4.2. In vivo validation of quantitive coronory analysis systems.

System	Calibration	Accuracy	Precision	Difference	Correlation	Lin. regression Analysis	SEE
CAAS I	Isocenter	−0.07	0.21	N.S.	r = O.91	y = 0.30 + 0.79x	0.19
	Catheter	0.09	0.23	N.S.	r = 0.89	y = 0.19 + 0.74x	0.19
CAAS II	Isocenter	−0.01	0.18	N.S.	r = 0.94	y = 0.22 + 0.82x	0.15
	Catheter	0.14	0.17	p > 0.05	r = 0.96	y = 0.14 + 0.76x	0.12
DCI	Isocenter	0.08	0.15	p < 0.05	r = 0.96	y = 0.08 + 0.86x	0.14
	Catheter	0.18	0.21	p < 0.001	r = 0.92	y = 0.09 + 0.76x	0.17
CMS	Isocenter	0.18	0.23	p < 0.01	r = 0.89	y = 0.02 + 0.83x	0.22
	Catheter	0.26	0.24	p < 0.001	r = 0.89	y = 0.06 + 0.72x	0.19

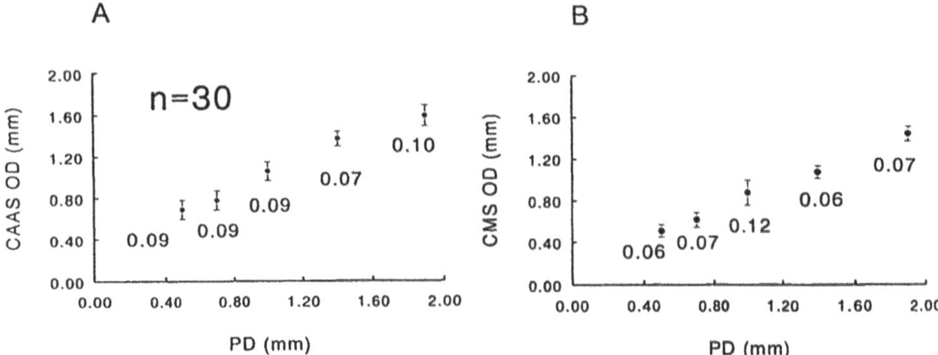

Figure 4.9. Reproducibility of the CAAS II (A) and the CMS system (B): mean values from 30 measurements of obstruction diemeter obtained by the CAAS II and from 15 measurements obtained by the CMS on one representative frame of each size of the stenosis phantoms (0.5, 0.7, 1.0, 1.4, 1.9 mm) are plotted with the respective standard deviation as a measure of reproducibility against the true phasntom diameters.

toms, and ±0.10 mm with the 1.9 mm stenosis phantom, resulting in a mean reproducibility of ±0.09 mm. From CMS (Figure 4.9B), the variability of measurements was ±0.06 mm with the 0.5 and 1.4 mm phantom, ±0.07 mm with the 1.9 mm phantom, and ±0.12 mm with the 1.0 mm phantom, resulting in a mean reproducibility of ±0.08 mm.

Discussion

Continuous improvement of software packages and their adaption to different imaging systems implies potential changes of accuracy, precision and reliability of autometad geometric coronary measurements [6]. To maintain quality control, each new version of a quantitative coronary analysis system should undergo *in vitro* and *in vivo* validation in a way that allows the user to objectively compare the respective systems [16]. *In vitro* test series can easily be standardized, however, their results are not always representative for the outcome of computerized measurements on angiographic images from human coronary artery dimensions, since beam scattering from surrounding tissue and the potential influence of motion blurr are unpredictable. On the other hand, an identical scaling of measured diameters for *in vitro* and *in vivo* validation is desirable if the impact of these factors on the reliability of automated measurements should be investigated.

To solve this problem, a unique experimental approach has been applied using identical stenosis phantoms for *in vitro* testing as well as for serial insertion in porcine coronary arteries with subsequent quantitative analysis of the respective angiographic images [4–6]. This experimental approach served for the comparative validation of the previous and the recent version of the Cardiovascular Angiography Analysis System (CAAS I and CAAS II), the Automated Coronary Analysis Package of the Digital Cardiac Imaging system (DCI) as well as for the Cardiovascular Measurement System (CMS).

In the primary description of the CAAS system (CAAS I), an accuracy of −0.03 mm and a precision of ±0.09 mm is reported from *in vitro* assessment of minimal luminal diameter using plexiglass phantoms [17]. The focal spot size related tendency to overestimate small luminal diameters [18] was not yet corrected in this first version. CAAS II, however, offering special algorithms to correct for this overestimation, gave an accuracy of 0.00 mm and a precision of ±0.11 mm in our series. The improvement of measurement reliability is confirmed by the results from our *in vivo* validation [5]. While CAAS I gave an accuracy of −0.07 mm and a precision of ±0.21 mm with calibration at the isocenter ($r = 0.91$, $y = 0.30 + 0.79x$, $SEE = 0.19$), corresponding measurements with CAAS II yielded an accuracy of −0.01 mm and a precision of ±0.18 mm ($r = 0.94$, $y = 0.22 + 0.82x$, $SEE = 0.15$). As illustrated by Figure 4.6B and D, catheter calibration, on the other hand, reveals a tendency towards underestimation of large diameters with both versions, although less pronounced with CAAS II. The high level of reproducibility throughout the range of all phantom sizes, as demonstrated with the recent version, is comparable to current digital as well as cinefilm-based quantitative coronary analysis systems [19].

The same experimental approach was used to compare the cinefilm-based CMS with the DCI system. This comparison was of particular interest, because the edge detection software of the CMS has primarily been developed for the Automated Coronary Analysis package of the Philips Digital Cardiac Imaging system and was tuned later on for the application to cinefilm. The measurement of obstruction diameter using the *in vitro* trial revealed a change of accuracy values from 0.11 to 0.18 mm when the edge detection algorithm designed for digital images is applied to conventional cineframes. This loss of accuracy is combined with a significant underestimation of true phantom diameters ($p < 0.01$) which is particularly evident with large phantom diameters as illustrated by a decrease of the slope of the regression line from 0.91 to 0.75 in Figure 4.6B and 6C, respectively. Furthermore, we observed an increase of variability from ±0.06 mm to ±0.14 mm ($p < 0.05$).

The result of this *in vitro* comparison is confirmed by the outcome of our animal experiments in which we serially implanted the same stenosis phantoms into porcine coronary arteries.

Calibrated at the radiographic isocenter (corresponding to the *in vitro* trial), we found a change in accuracy values from obstruction diameter measurements from 0.08 mm to 0.18 mm and an increase of variability from ±0.15 mm to ±0.23 mm ($p < 0.05$) when the algorithm was applied to cinefilm images. The underestimation of true phantom diameter values which has already been present with digital measurements ($p < 0.05$) was more pronounced when the edge detection algorithm was applied to the corresponding cineframes ($p < 0.01$). When the imaging systems were calibrated on the angiographic catheter, we found a change of accuracy values from 0.18 mm (digital measurements) to 0.26 mm (cinefilm-based measurements), while the variability increased from ±0.21 mm to ±0.24 mm. It appears from Figure 4.8B and D that these differences are explained by a higher degree of scatter as well as by a more pronounced underestimation of large phantom diameters.

The variable shape of human coronary artery stenoses [20] has prompted the use of non-circular stenosis phantoms for the validation of quantitative coronary angiographic analysis systems. This approach seems to be particularly relevant for the measurement of minimal luminal cross sectional area by densitometry [21]. Cylindrical phantoms which have been used for our experiments however, fulfill the requirements for the application of two-dimensional geometric measurements and therefore are eminently satisfactory as a surrogate of coronary obstructions.

In order to be able to compare *in vivo* results with those obtained from *in vitro* assessments, we performed geometric measurements using two calibration methods: calibration at the radiographic isocenter which is used for *in vitro* settings, and catheter calibration which represents the calibration technique conventionally used in clinical practice [17].

The use of angiographic catheters for the calibration of quantitative coronary analysis systems may influence the outcome of luminal diameter measurements, because varying catheter composition may result in varying X-ray attenuation [22] and therefore in differences in the automated detection of the contour points. In our *in vivo* study, only one type of catheter was used for calibration and thus the influence of different materials on the process of calibration was excluded. Another geometric error is introduced if the planes of calibration and measurement are not identical [23]. This error can be circumvented by out of plane correction as proposed by Wollschläger [24], or by calibration at the isocenter of the X-ray system.

The results of the present study show that, in general, the values of both digital and cinefilm measurements using catheter calibration are smaller than those using calibration at the isocenter. Theoretically, a greater distance between image intensifier and catheter tip than between image intensifier and isocenter would result in out-of-plane magnification producing smaller calibration factors. A similar effect might have been produced by pincushion distortion for which DCI and CMS are not correcting. Both factors could explain smaller values of measurement when catheter calibration was applied.

In spite of the above mentioned disadvantages, the adaption of the edge detection algorithm from digital to cinefilm-based analysis did not affect the high reproducibility of automated geometric coronary measurements. The reproducibility of obstruction diameter measurements with the CMS system ranged from ±0.06 mm to ±0.12 mm which corresponds to the reproducibility of the digital system [19, 25] and is comparable to the values obtained from the new version of the CAAS (Figure 4.8).

In principle, the use of 'minimal luminal diameter' or 'obstruction diameter' for validation of quantitative coronary angiography systems may be criticized. The size of the stenosis channel theoretically could be underestimated if the measurements of the automatic edge detection algorithm are influenced either by the presence of cellular debris collected in the phantom lumen during insertion, or by the development of micro-thrombosis, or by the presence of noise from the acquisition system. These occurrences may also explain the underestimation of the true lumen by different techniques [26]. In our experimental study, the minimal luminal diameter or obstruction diameter has been selected for the comparative validation of various quantitative coronary analysis systems because it represents a non-arbitrary measurement obtained by fully automated analysis of the entire coronary segment.

In conclusion, the present comparative investigation has demonstrated that geometric coronary measurements can be applied with a high degree of reliability. Superior *in vivo* results are obtained when systems are calibrated using a well defined structure at the rediographic isocenter. Conventional catheter calibration, in general, results in a slightly lower level of accuracy and precision. Furthermore, the transformation of an edge detection algorithm from a digital to a cinefilm-based system can lead to an impairment of measurement accuracy which is independent from calibration techniques. Tuning of an algorithm for the application to another imaging system should be guided by the results of simultaneous *in vitro* and *in vivo* validation studies in order to maintain a high level of measurement reliability.

References

1. Serruys PW, Luijten HE, Beatt KJ. Incidence of restenosis after successful coronary angioplasty: a time-related phenomenon. A quantitative angiographic study in 342 consecutive patients at 1, 2, 3 and 4 months. Circulation 1988; 77: 361–71.
2. De Feyter PJ, Serruys PW, Davies MJ, Richardson P, Lubson J, Oliver MF. Quantitative coronary angiography to measure progression and regression of coronary atherosclerosis. Value, limitations, and implications for clinical trials. Circulation 1991; 84: 412–23.

3. Reiber JHC, Serruys PW. Quantitative coronary angiography. In Marcus ML, Schelbert HR, Skorton DJ, Wolf GL (eds): Cardiac imaging – a companion to Braunwald's heart disease, 1st ed. Philadelphia: W.B. Saunders Company 1991: 211–80.
4. Haase J, Di Mario C, Slager CJ *et al. In vivo* validation of on-line and off-line geometric coronary measurements using insertion of stenosis phantoms in porcine coronary arteries. Cathet Cardiovasc Diagn 1992; 27: 16–27.
5. Haase J, Escaned J, van Swijndregt EM *et al.* Experimental validation of geometric and densitometric coronary measurements on the new generation cardiovascular angiography analysis system (CAAS II). Cathet Cardiovasc Diagn 1993; 30: 104–14.
6. Haase J, van der Linden MMJM, Di Mario C, van der Giessen WJ, Foley DP, Serruys PW. Can the same edge detection algorithm be applied to on-line and off-line analysis systems? Validation of a new cinefilm-based geometric coronary measurement software. Am Heart J 1993; 126: 312–21.
7. Beatt KJ, Serruys PW, Hugenholtz PG. Restenosis after coronary angioplasty: new standards for clinical studies. J Am Coll Cardiol 1990; 15: 491–8.
8. Beatt KJ, Luijten HE, de Feyter PJ, van den Brand M, Reiber JHC, Serruys PW. Change in diameter of coronary artery segments adjacent to stenosis after percutaneous transluminal coronary angioplasty: failure of percent diameter stenosis measurement to reflect morphologic changes induced by balloon dilatation. J Am Coll Cardiol 1988; 12: 315–23.
9. Haase J, Nugteren SK, van Swijndregt EM *et al.* Digital geometric measurements in comparison to cinefilm analysis of coronary artery dimensions. Cathet Cardiovasc Diagn 1993; 28: 283–90.
10. Reiber JHC, Kooijman CJ, den Boer A, Serruys PW. Assessment of dimensions and image quality of coronary contrast catheters from cineangiograms. Cathet Cardiovasc Diagn 1985; 11: 521–31.
11. van der Zwet PMJ, von Land CD, Loois G, Gerbrands JJ, Reiber JHC. An on-line system for the quantitative analysis of coronary arterial segments. Comp Cardiol 1990; 157–60.
12. Reiber JHC, Kooijman CJ, Slager CJ *et al.* Coronary artery dimensions from cineangiogram – methodology and validation of a computer-assisted analysis procedure. Comp Cardiol 1984; 131–41.
13. Gronenshild E, Janssen J. A compact system for quantitative cardiovascular angiography analysis. In Lun KC *et al.* (eds): Medinfo 1992. Elsevier Science Publishers 1992, 795–800.
14. Reiber JHC. Personal communication 1992.
15. Snedecor GW, Cochran WG. Statistical Methods, 6th ed. Ames: The Iowa State University Press 1967, 196.
16. Keane D, Haase J, van Swijndregt EM *et al.* Comparative validation of quantitative coronary angiography systems: results and implications from a multicenter study using a standardized approach. Submitted.
17. Reiber JHC, Kooijman CJ, Slager CJ *et al.* Coronary artery dimensions from cineangiogram – methodology and validation of a computer-assisted analysis procedure. Trans Med Imaging 1984; MI-3: 131–41.
18. Beier J, Oswald H, Fleck E. Edge detection for coronary angiograms – error correction and impact of derivatives. Comp Cardiol 1992; 513–6.
19. Reiber JHC, van der Zwet PMJ, Koning G *et al.* Quantitative coronary measurements from cine and digital arteriograms; methodology and validation results [abstract]. 4th International Symposium on Coronary Arteriography, Rotterdam, June 23–25, 1991: Abstract book: 36.
20. Thomas AC, Davies MJ, Dilly S, Dilly N, Franc F. Potential errors in the estimation of coronary arterial stenosis from clinical arteriography with reference to the shape of the coronary arterial lumen. Br Heart J 1986; 55: 129–39.
21. Nichols AB, Gabrieli CFO, Fenoglio JJ Jr, Esser PD. Quantification of relative arterial stenosis by cinevideodensitometric analysis of coronary arteriograms. Circulation 1984; 512–22.
22. Fortin DF, Spero LA, Cusma JT, Santoro L, Burgess R, Bashore TM. Pitfalls in the

determination of absolute dimensions using angiographic catheters as calibration devices in quantitative angiography. Am J Cardiol 1991; 68: 1176–82.

23. Gould KL. Quantitative coronary arteriography. In Gould KL (ed): Coronary artery stenosis, 1st ed. New York: Elsevier Science Publishing 1991: 93–107.
24. Wollschläger H, Zeiher AM, Lee P, Solzbach U, Bonzel T, Just H. Optimal biplane imaging of coronary segments with computed triple orthogonal projections. In Reiber JHC, Serruys PW (eds): New developments in quantitative coronary arteriography, 1st ed. Dordrecht: Kluwer Academic Publishers, 1983: 13–21.
25. Koning G, Zwet PMJ van der, Padmos I *et al.* Short- and medium-term variability of the DCI/ACA package [abstract]. 4th International Symposium on Coronary Arteriography, Rotterdam. Abstract book: 168.
26. Mancini GBJ, Simon SB, McGillem MJ, LeFree MT, Friedman HZ, Vogel RA. Automated quantitative coronary arteriography: Morphologic and physiologic validation *in vivo* of a repid digital angiographic method. Circulation 1987; 75: 452–460.

5. Comparison of accuracy and precision of quantitative coronary arterial analysis between cinefilm and digital systems

JOHAN H.C. REIBER, CRAIG D. VON LAND,
GERHARD KONING, PIETER M.J. VAN DER ZWET,
RONALD C.M. VAN HOUDT, MARTIN J. SCHALIJ &
JACQUES LESPÉRANCE

Summary

In this chapter we have compared the accuracy and precision of two state-of-the-art analytical software packages for quantitative coronary arteriography (QCA) developed in our laboratory. The two packages are the QCA package (Versions 1.11 and 1.2) on the film-based Cardiovascular Measurement System (CMS), and the ACA package (Version 1.0) on the Philips Digital Cardiac Imaging System (DCI). In these studies the accuracy is defined as the systematic error described in terms of the mean signed difference between actual and measured values of phantoms or catheters, or between the values from repeated measurements; ideally the systematic errors should be as small as possible. The precision or random error is described in terms of the standard deviation of these signed differences; ideally these random errors should be as small as possible as well. In this chapter four comparative studies have been described.

First, to assess the accuracy and precision of the intrinsic edge detection algorithms, images of a plexiglass phantom with eleven tubular 'vessels' (sizes 0.68–5.06 mm) were acquired under a variety of imaging conditions and analyzed using both systems. The phantoms were placed on a homogeneous background (scatter medium) as well as on a nonhomogeneous background (patient anatomy). This last approach simulates clinical conditions best and resulted in an overall accuracy of −0.05 mm and −0.03 mm, and an overall precision of 0.10 mm and 0.11 mm for the QCA/CMS and the ACA/DCI, respectively.

Second, to ensure the accuracy of absolute measurements on the two systems, a study was also performed to assess the suitability of Cordis and Mallinckrodt, 6F and 7F contrast catheters for calibration purposes. Again, a variety of imaging conditions were used, including filling with saline, 50% contrast and 100% contrast agent with the catheters on a scatter medium (*in vitro* study). In addition, an *in vivo* study was carried out for the Cordis catheters. It was concluded that all these catheters satisfied the basic requirements for QCA, with significantly smaller coefficients of variations in the *in vivo* study for the cinefilm analyses.

J.H.C. Reiber and P.W. Serruys (eds): Progress in quantitative coronary arteriography, 67–85.

Third, an *in vivo* animal study with plexiglass plugs (0.5–1.57 mm) inserted into the coronary arteries was carried out as the ultimate test for a QCA package. Preliminary results indicated precision values of 0.08 mm and 0.10 mm for the QCA/CMS and ACA/DCI, respectively.

Fourth, a direct comparison of cinefilm and digital coronary angiographic data was performed. For identical frames random errors in minimum lumen and reference diameters were found to be 0.16 mm and in percentage diameter stenosis 5.69%. Corresponding systematic errors were −0.06 mm, 0.03 mm and 2,55%, respectively; correlation coefficients ranged from 0.84 to 0.96.

From these data it may be concluded that QCA can be performed with state-of-the-art analytical software packages from cinefilm (CMS) as well as from digital (DCI) with comparable accuracy and precision, even for small vessel sizes below 1.2 mm. Our data indicate that cinefilm allows a slightly better precision (by 10–15%).

Introduction

In the past questions have been raised whether digital angiography with matrix sizes of 512^2 pixels would give comparable accuracy and precision in the assessment of quantitative arterial dimensions as 35 mm cinefilm, which serves as the gold standard in quantitative coronary arteriography (QCA). Because of the intrinsic high resolution of the cinefilm and the fact that optical zooming can be applied for the selection of regions of interest (ROI's), expectations were that cinefilm would do significantly better. On the other hand, it should not be forgotten that the accuracy and precision of QCA results depend upon a large number of factors, among others the intrinsic image quality, the characteristics of the cinefilm-to-video converter [1] for film-based systems, and last, but not least, the quality and robustness of the analytical software packages.

In attempts to come up with appropriate answers to this question, several investigators have compared cinefilm and digital quantitative coronary arteriography. An extensive overview of most of these comparative studies on digital and cinefilm approaches was given in [2]. From these data it could be concluded that analysis of digital and film-based coronary angiograms as carried out with the systems used in these studies was essentially equivalent. However, since these studies were performed the quality of the X-ray imaging chains has continued to improve, as well as the quality of the analytical software packages.

In this chapter we will, therefore, present comparative results using two state-of-the-art analytical software packages developed in our laboratory, the QCA package on the cinefilm-based Cardiovascular Measurement System

CMS[1] [3, 4] and the Automated Coronary Analysis (ACA) package implemented on the Philips DCI[2] [5–7]. For this comparison we have carried out three kinds of validation studies using: 1) a plexiglass phantom acquired on a homogeneous background (scatter medium) and on a nonhomogeneous background (patient anatomy) to assess the accuracy and precision of the intrinsic edge detection algorithms; 2) coronary contrast catheters (Mallinckrodt and Cordis) to check the applicability of these catheters for calibration purposes; and 3) an *in vivo* animal study with plexiglass plugs of known sizes inserted into the coronary arteries, which is the ultimate test for a QCA package. In addition, the results from a direct comparison of cinefilm and digital coronary angiographic data carried out at the Montréal Heart Institute will be presented. Before describing the protocols and results of these studies, the basic principles of the two packages mentioned above will be explained.

Basic Principles of QCA Analytical Software Packages

The CMS workstation is based on a powerful 80486/33 MHz processor, a CAP-35E telecine converter featuring a zoom lens (optical magnification up to 6–fold) and CCD camera, and a frame grabber for digitizing the optically magnified analog video images from the telecine converter at a size of 512 × 512 × 8 bits (PAL) or 512 × 480 × 8 bits (NTSC). By panning the optical system any region-of-interest (ROI) of the 35 mm cinefilm can be projected onto the CCD-chip at the selected optical magnification. In practice, the magnification is chosen at approximately 2.3 fold, resulting in a recommended pixel size in the range of 0.08–0.1 mm/pixel; the edge detection software has been optimized for this range of pixel sizes.

The DCI is a digital cardiac imaging system that allows the real-time digitization and storage of angio-cardiographic images at a matrix size of 512 × 512 × 8 bits (PAL) or 512 × 480 × 8 bits (NTSC). The plumbicon video tube connected to the output screen of the image intensifier is read out in progressive scan mode. Maximum acquisition speed is 60/50 (USA/Europe) frames/s monoplane or 2 × 30/25 f/s biplane. The DCI-S is based on 80286 technology, the newer DCI-SX on 80486 technology.

For a quantitative coronary analysis package to be applicable in a routine clinical environment, a number of requirements must be met:

1. minimal user-interaction in the selection and processing of a coronary segment to be analyzed;
2. minimal editing of the automatically determined results. The user should seldom feel the need to edit the intermediary results, such as the detected contours of the arterial segments;

1. MEDIS Medical Imaging Systems, Nuenen, the Netherlands.
2. Philips Medical Systems, Best, the Netherlands.

3. a short processing time in the order of 15 seconds;
4. high accuracy and precision in the assessment of the morphological data. This to be demonstrated by extensive phantom and routinely acquired clinical studies.

A great deal of effort has been put into minimizing the amount of required user-interaction, into developing a robust edge detection algorithm, and the presentation of all the clinically relevant parameters, while keeping the processing time below 15 seconds. We feel that the current versions of the ACA/DCI (V1.0 on the DCI-SX) and the QCA/CMS-packages (Versions 1.11 and 1.2) satisfy these requirements for images of acceptable quality, with acceptable at this point based on a subjective interpretation. Naturally, the success score will decrease when there is little contrast in the image, when there are severe overlappings, with noisy images, etc. On the other hand, the edge detection algorithm that we have developed (Minimum Cost Algorithm (MCA)) has been shown to be more robust than any other algorithm in images with low signal-to-noise ratio [8]. Although the basic principles of the implemented edge detection algorithms are similar in design for the two image modalities, each of these has been optimized for the individual modality. Cinefilm and digital recordings have their own imaging characteristics, requiring individual algorithmic tunings.

Both the QCA/CMS and ACA/DCI packages are very similar in design and user-interface. We are convinced that simply defining the start and end point of the coronary segment to be analyzed is the best procedure for segment selection. In the next step, an arterial path through the segment of interest is computed automatically [6, 9]. The contour detection procedure is carried out in two iterations: the first one relative to the detected pathline, and the second one relative to the individual left and right vessel contours detected in the first iteration. To correct for the limited resolution of the entire X-ray system, the Minimum Cost contour detection technique is modified in the second iteration based on an analysis of the point spread function of the imaging chain, which is of particular importance for the accurate measurement of small vessels. Calibration of the image data is performed on a nontapering part of the contrast catheter following a similar edge detection procedure as for the arterial segment; however, in this case, additional information is used in the edge detection process, knowing that this part of the catheter is characterized by parallel boundaries.

From the left- and right-hand contours of the arterial segment a diameter function is determined, on the basis of which the following parameters are automatically calculated: the site of maximal percent diameter stenosis, the obstruction diameter, the corresponding automatically determined reference diameter and the extent of the obstruction. Additionally derived parameters include obstruction symmetry, area of the atherosclerotic plaque and functional information in terms of the radiographic Stenotic Flow Reserve (SFR-) value and transstenotic pressure gradients. The CMS provides in addition (sub)segment related data, such as the mean and standard deviation of diameter measurements, and projected vessel areas in the proximal, obstructed and distal segments.

Study Protocols

Plexiglass Phantom Study

To determine the accuracy and precision of the edge detection algorithms on the two systems, a plexiglass phantom with eleven tubular 'vessel' sizes, ranging from 0.687 mm to 5.062 mm, filled with different contrast agent concentrations (100% and 50%), acquired at different kV-levels (70 and 90 kV) using a small X-ray focus, and at the 5″ and 7″ image intensifier modes, was analyzed. For the first part of this study, this phantom was placed on a 10 cm block of plexiglass functioning as scatter medium; this is the socalled off-patient situation with a homogeneous background. For calibration purposes, the phantom was replaced by a cm-grid allowing a highly reliable calibration factor. Since the cm-grid was positioned at the same level as the phantom relative to the image intensifier, errors due to out-of-plane magnification were eliminated.

To obtain a more clinically relevant situation with a nonhomogeneous background, the plexiglass phantom filled with 100% contrast was also positioned on the chest of a patient and over the heart, and acquired at the 5″ and 7″ image intensifier modes; again for calibration purposes a cm-grid was positioned on the chest next to the phantom. This situation was denoted 'on-patient'.

Calibration on Catheters

In the quantitative assessment of coronary arterial dimensions from cine and digital coronary arteriographic images, the coronary contrast catheters are almost exclusively used as the calibration device. For a catheter to be acceptable for QCA studies, it must satisfy certain criteria; the criteria that we have set will be described further on in this section. Over the last several years there have been strong requests from the clinicians to use smaller size (i.e. 6F and even 5F) catheters.

Our test procedure required that the last 7 cm of the catheters were taped to a block of plexiglass with dimensions $10 \times 10 \times 10$cm. The height of the X-ray table was adjusted such that the catheters were acquired in the angiographic isocenter. For this comparative study three different fillings of the catheters were used:

- only saline (socalled empty catheters);
- 175 mgI/cc (50% concentration);

- 350 mgI/cc (100% concentration; socalled full catheters).

Each situation was filmed at three different kilovoltages of the X-ray tube (approximately 60 kV, 75 kV and 90 kV) and at two image intensifier modes (5″ and 7″). For calibration purposes, a cm-grid was filmed on top of the plexiglass block after removal of the catheters.

The following catheters were used in this study:

A. *Mallinckrodt*[3]

- 6F Judkins right nylon catheter with a Softouch^R tip with improved image quality specifications.
- 7F ST Multipurpose B2 nylon catheter with a Softouch^R tip.

B. *CORDIS*[4]

- 6F Super Torque^{TM} Judkins left femoral catheter (polyurethane catheter).
- 7F High Flow^{TM} Judkins left femoral catheter (polyamide carrier).

Each catheter segment was analyzed with the arterial analysis edge detection software in order to obtain the necessary statistical data; in other words, the calibration module of the edge detection program including the a priori assumption about the catheter shape was not used for these purposes. Calibration was performed exclusively on the cm-grid using a manual digital caliper [10], available on the CMS and DCI systems.

For each analyzed catheter segment the mean diameter and standard deviation of the angiographically measured sizes were computed from the derived diameter function; the standard deviation is a measure for the irregularity of the detected boundaries. Catheters with a poor radiopaqueness will lead to very irregular contours associated with a large standard deviation. To describe the overall results for a particular catheter as assessed under certain or all imaging conditions, the overall mean diameter and pooled standard deviation from the individual standard deviation values were calculated.

In addition to the *in vitro* study described above, an *in vivo* catheter study was carried out for the two types of Cordis catheters. For each type, five angiographic runs were collected from several diagnostic patient studies. In these studies precaution was taken to visualize the catheter parallel to the image intensifier to prevent foreshortening. Also, care was taken to prevent overlap of the catheter with strongly inhomogeneous structures which could influence the detection of the borders of the catheter. Images of the catheters were acquired filled with saline, as well as with 100% contrast medium concentration. All angiographic runs were acquired at a frame speed of 25 f/s using the small X-ray focus and the 7″ image intensifier mode.

3. Mallinckrodt Medical GmbH, Hennef, Germany.
4. Cordis Europe NV, Roden, the Netherlands.

Requirements for catheters acceptable for QCA

To be acceptable for quantitative coronary arteriographic calibration procedures, we require that a catheter meets the following criteria: in *in vitro* studies the absolute average difference in the angiographically measured mean diameters of the catheter with respect to the true value should be smaller than 5% under each of the individual circumstances and smaller than 3.5% as averaged over all said conditions (which are: saline filling and 100% contrast medium filling, 5″ and 7″ image intensifier sizes, and 60, 75 and 90 kV-levels). Under these circumstances, the pooled standard deviation of the angiographically measured size of the catheter should be on the order of 0.1 mm or smaller.

In *in vivo* studies two times the pooled standard deviation of the derived calibration factors should be smaller than 5% of the average calibration factor; in other words, two times the coefficient of variation should be less than 5%. In practice, this means that in 95% of the cases the error in the calibration factor would be limited to 5%.

In vivo *plexiglass plugs*

The ultimate test for a QCA system is the analysis of clinical images of obstructions with known dimensions. For this purpose small plexiglass plugs were fabricated in our mechanical workshop. The following outer diameters were made available: 2.5, 3.0 mm and 3.5 mm, and inner diameters 0.5, 0.69, 0.70, 1.32, 1.33 and 1.57 mm; the length of each plug was approximately 7.5 mm. The actual inner diameters were measured with a microscope with a precision of 0.001 mm (Courtesy Cordis Europe NV). The plugs were introduced with a catheter into the coronary arteries of dogs. Images were acquired on cinefilm as well as in digital format with the DCI-SX system.

From the dog studies, frames were selected which showed the plugs with least overlap with other structures such as catheters, and with optimal contrast filling. In each case a long coronary segment including the plug was analyzed. From the obstructive region, the mean diameter and the standard deviation of the diameter measurements were assessed; the mean diameter was compared with the known true diameter of the plug. Calibration was performed in the usual way on the 7F contrast catheter. The accuracy of this study was therefore defined by the average difference of the true values and the measured mean values; a positive difference corresponds with an overestimation, a negative difference with an underestimation. In addition, a regression analysis was carried out. The overall precision was defined by the pooled standard deviation of the standard deviation values of the individual obstruction measurements. In other words, the pooled standard deviation is a measure for the irregularities of the detected boundaries over the obstructive region.

Comparison of clinical cinefilm and digital angiographic studies

Dr. Jacques Lespérance from the Montréal Heart Institue compared the QCA results from 62 coronary stenoses (pre-PTCA) analyzed both with the QCA/CMS and ACA/DCI analytical software packages (pers. comm.). Initially, frames to be analyzed on both the DCI and CMS were selected in the catheterization laboratory on the DCI (Same frame). Later on, the CMS technician performed a second frame selection (Best frame) without knowledge of the first choice of frames on the DCI, replicating her usual approach for cinefilm frame selection. In some cases the frames by the two approaches were the same. In the second frame selection particular attention was paid to optimal contrast filling of the vessel, minimal overlap with other sidebranches, etc., similarly as is done in longitudinal QCA research studies. In the Best Frame selection, the CMS results from the Best Frame were compared with the DCI results from the Same Frame.

Results

Plexiglass phantom study

Figure 5.1 is an example of the analysis with the CMS of a phantom vessel positioned on the homogeneous scatter medium (off patient). The mean measured diameter was 1.01 mm, the standard deviation 0.06 mm and the true size of the vessel 1.011 mm. The overall results are presented in Table 5.1. It is evident that all accuracy values were smaller than or equal to 0.10 mm with the negative sign indicating an average underestimation. The overall accuracy or systematic error for the QCA/CMS was −0.09 mm and for the ACA/DCI − 0.03 mm, respectively. Under each of the four different situations the QCA/CMS precision or random error was slightly better than the ACA/DCI precision. The overall precision for the QCA/CMS was 0.08 mm and for the ACA/DCI 0.10 mm, respectively.

The individual results of the vessel tubes for the four radiographic settings are given in Figure 5.2A for the QCA/CMS and in Figure 5.2B for the ACA/DCI, respectively according to the presentation techniques proposed by Altman and Bland [11]. The true values of the vessel tubes are given along the horizontal axis and the differences between the true dimensions and measured mean diameters along the vertical axis with overestimations denoted by positive differences and underestimations by negative differences. From Figure 5.2A it can be concluded, that no systematic overestimations occur for the smallest sizes (<1.2 mm) and that all measurements fall within the range of 0 and −0.22 mm. This is consistent with the overall underestimation by −0.09 mm. The ACA/DCI data (Figure 5.2B) show a slightly different pattern, again with minimal overestimation for the smallest sizes (<1.2 mm) and all values ≤4 mm falling within the range of +0.10 and −0.13 mm.

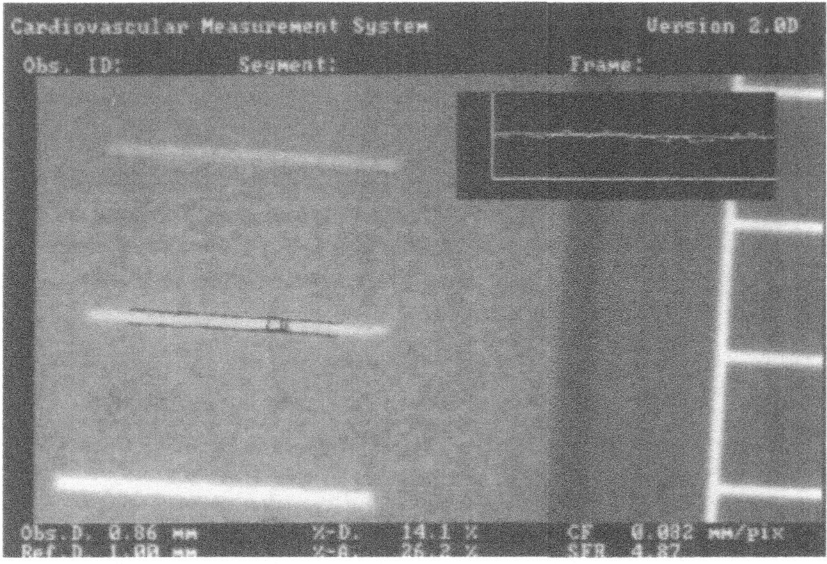

Figure 5.1. Example of the QCA/CMS analysis of a phantom vessel with the homogeneous scatter medium (off patient). The measured mean diameter was 1.01 mm, the standard deviation 0.06 mm and the true tube size 1.011 mm.

Table 5.1. Results of the plexiglass phantom study with the homogeneous background (off patient) for the QCA/CMS and ACA/DCI analyses.

Radiographic settings	QCA/CMS		ACA/DCI	
	Accur.	Prec.	Accur.	Prec.
5″, 72 kV	−0.08	0.06	−0.02	0.08
5″, 89 kV	−0.08	0.09	−0.04	0.12
7″, 70 kV	−0.10	0.07	−0.02	0.08
7″, 90 kV	−0.09	0.09	−0.03	0.12
Overall	−0.09	0.08	−0.03	0.10

Note: The radiographic settings refer to the image intensifier size (5 and 7 inch) and the load (kiloVoltage) of the X-ray generator.

The higher offset for the largest value (5.062 mm) cannot be explained at this point in time and needs further investigation.

For the situation with the phantom positioned on a patient chest (on patient; inhomogeneous background) the results are presented in Table 5.2, separately for the 5″ and 7″ images, as well as overall. Again, the overall accuracy values were excellent at −0.05 mm for the QCA/CMS and −0.03 mm for the ACA/DCI. Overall precision values were slightly, al-

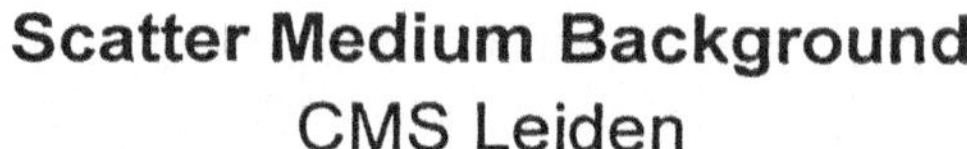

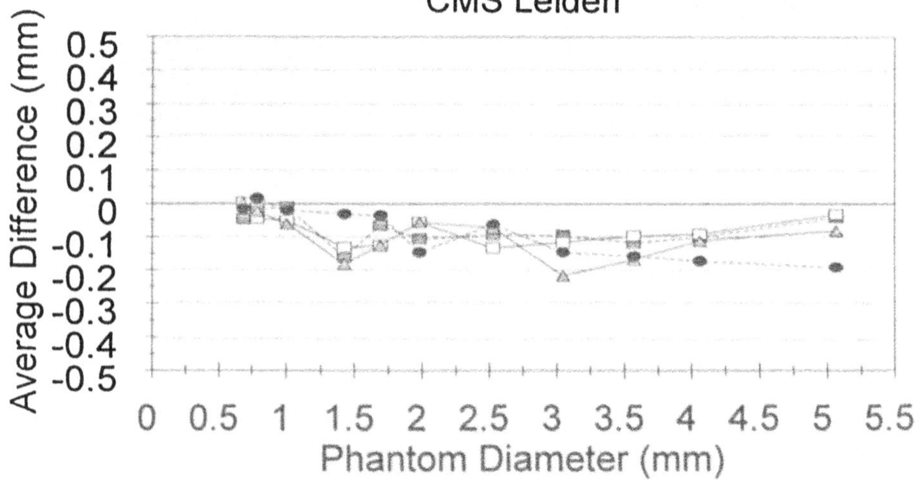

5" 70kV 5" 90kV 7" 70kV 7" 90kV

Scatter Medium Background

DCI Leiden

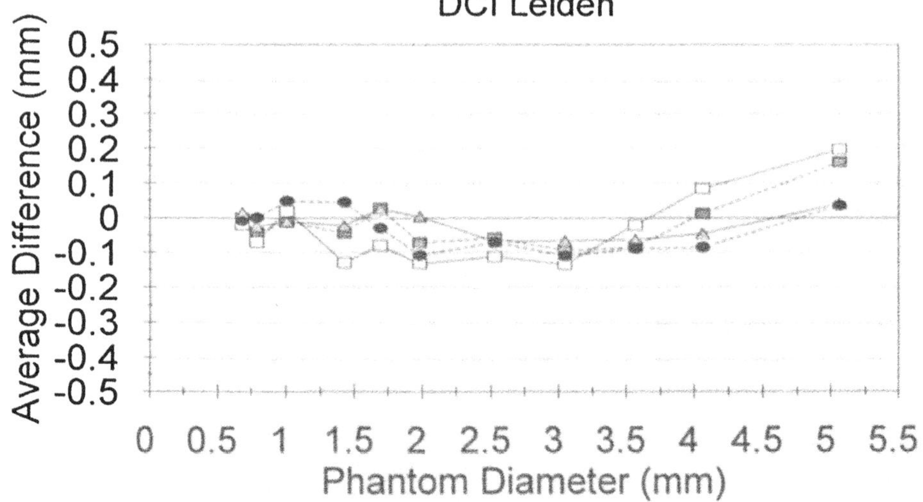

5" 70kV 5" 90kV 7" 70kV 7" 90kV

Table 5.2. Results of the plexiglass phantom study with the patient anatomy as background (on patient) for the QCA/CMS and ACA/DCI analyses.

Radiographic settings	QCA/CMS		ACA/DCI	
	Accur.	Prec.	Accur.	Prec.
5"	−0.08	0.10	−0.07	0.11
7"	−0.03	0.10	0.01	0.11
Overall	−0.05	0.10	−0.03	0.11

Note: The radiographic settings refer to the image intensifier size (5 and 7 inch).

though not significantly, higher than in the off-patient situation, now at 0.10 mm for the QCA/CMS and 0.11 mm for the ACA/DCI, respectively. Again, the individual results are presented in Figure 5.3A for the QCA/CMS and Figure 5.3B for the ACA/DCI, respectively. Figure 5.3A shows that the measurements at the 7" II tend to give slightly larger vessel sizes than for the 5" II. The same phenomenon can be seen from Figure 5.3B for the ACA/DCI.

Calibration on catheters

The results for the 6F and 7F Mallinckrodt catheters for the QCA/CMS are given in Table 5.3A and for the ACA/DCI in Table 5.3B, respectively. From Table 5.3A (CMS) it is clear that both 6F and 7F Mallinckrodt catheters satisfy the basic requirements as stated earlier. In this case the accuracy values of each of the individual conditions remain below 2.8%, whereas the overall precision data are ≤0.10 mm. Also the digital analyses (Table 5.3B) satisfy these requirements with the individual accuracy values remaining below 4.4% and the precision values better than 0.13 mm. When comparing Tables 5.3A and 5.3B, it becomes evident that the precision values for the 100% contrast measurements are slightly better for QCA/CMS than for ACA/DCI; the same is true for the 6F tip filled with saline. The other situations are very much comparable. On the other hand, the systematic errors are smaller for the ACA/DCI for the 50% contrast situation.

The results of the *in vitro* study for the 6F and 7F Cordis catheters for the QCA/CMS are given in Table 5.4A and for the ACA/DCI in Table 5.4B, respectively. From Table 5.4A (QCA/CMS) it is evident that all the individual absolute accuracy values remain below 3.5%, and the precision values below 0.09 mm. For the digital measurements the absolute systematic errors

Figure 5.2. Individual systematic errors in the measurement of the plexiglass vessel tubes under various imaging conditions with homogeneous background (off patient) for the CMS (top) and the DCI (bottom), respectively according to the techniques by Altman and Bland [11].

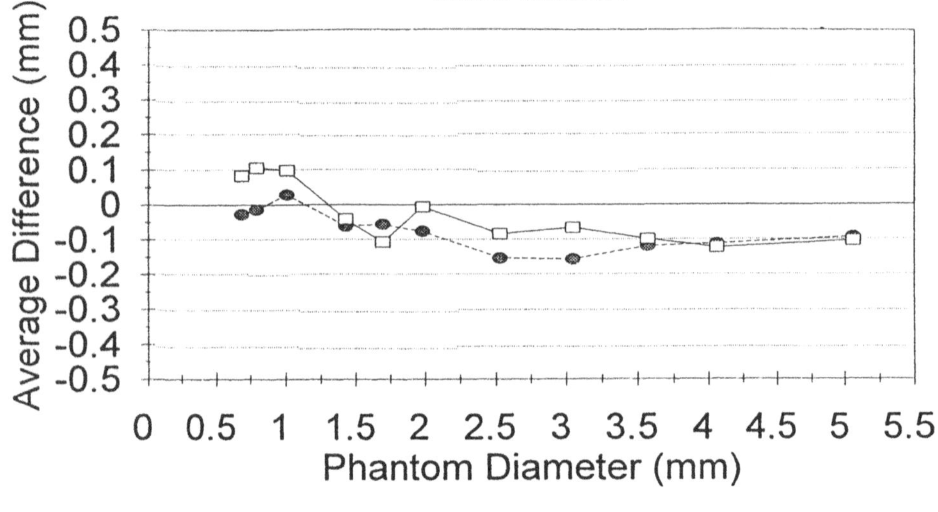

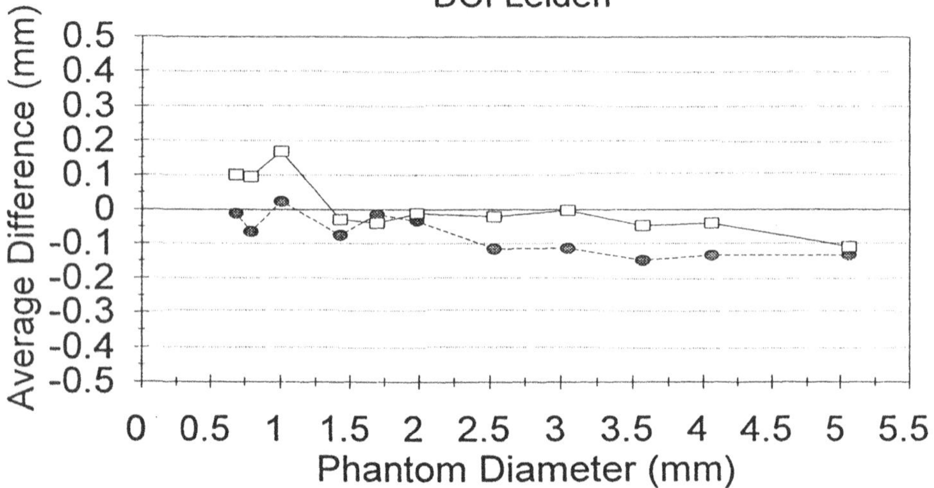

Figure 5.3. Individual systematic errors in the measurement of the plexiglass vessel tubes under various imaging conditions with inhomogeneous background (on patient) for the CMS (Figure A) and the DCI (Figure B), respectively according to the techniques by Altman and Bland [11].

Table 5.3A. Accuracy and precision values for the 6F and 7F Mallinckrodt Softouch® tip catheters under 100% and 50% contrast filling and with saline as measured with the CMS.

		Cinefilm QCA/CMS		
	True size (mm)	100% contrast	50% contrast	Saline
6F tip	1.98	1.94 ± 0.09 (−1.6%)	1.94 ± 0.09 (−1.6%)	1.97 ± 0.08 (−0.1%)
7F tip	2.26	2.28 ± 0.09 (1.1%)	2.32 ± 0.10 (2.6%)	2.32 ± 0.08 (2.8%)

Notes: QCA measurements averaged over three kV-levels (60, 75, 90 kV). True sizes were measured with an electronic caliper.

Table 5.3B. Accuracy and precision values for the 6F and 7F Mallinckrodt Softouch® tip catheters under 100% and 50% contrast filling and with saline as measured with the DCI.

		Digital ACA/DCI		
	True size (mm)	100% contrast	50% contrast	Saline
6F tip	1.98	1.89 ± 0.12 (−4.4%)	1.95 ± 0.08 (−1.1%)	1.96 ± 0.11 (−0.8%)
7F tip	2.26	2.24 ± 0.13 (−1.0%)	2.25 ± 0.10 (−0.3%)	2.31 ± 0.08 (2.3%)

Notes: QCA measurements averaged over three kV-levels (60, 75, 90 kV). True sizes were measured with an electronic caliper.

Table 5.4A. Accuracy and precision values for the 6F and 7F Cordis catheters under 100% and 50% contrast filling and with saline as measured with the CMS.

		Cinefilm QCA/CMS		
	True size (mm)	100% contrast	50% contrast	Saline
6F tip Super Torque	1.99	1.92 ± 0.07 (−3.5%)	1.98 ± 0.08 (−0.5%)	1.96 ± 0.08 (−1.5%)
7F tip High Flow	2.22	2.15 ± 0.08 (−3.2%)	2.18 ± 0.09 (−1.8%)	2.20 ± 0.07 (−0.9%)

Notes: QCA measurements averaged over three kV-levels (60, 75, 90 kV). True sizes were measured with an electronic caliper.

are smaller (<2.0%) and the random errors or precision values slightly higher (<0.12 mm) than for cinefilm. In this study we found consistently smaller random error values from the film measurements than from the digital measurements.

Table 5.4B. Accuracy and precision values for the 6F and 7F Cordis catheters under 100% and 50% contrast filling and with saline as measured with the DCI.

		Digital ACA/DCI		
	True size (mm)	100% contrast	50% contrast	Saline
6F tip Super Torque	1.99	2.00 ± 0.12 (0.5%)	1.95 ± 0.10 (−2.0%)	1.99 ± 0.11 (0%)
7F tip High Flow	2.22	2.22 ± 0.11 (0%)	2.21 ± 0.10 (−0.5%)	2.22 ± 0.12 (0%)

Notes: QCA measurements averaged over three kV-levels (60, 75, 90 kV). True sizes were measured with an electronic caliper.

Table 5.5A. *In vivo* study Cordis catheters. Variability in calibration factors (CF) assessed from routine coronary arteriograms expressed as (2 s.d./average CF) × 100%.

	Cinefilm QCA/CMS		
	Contrast	Saline	Overall
6F tip Super Torque	2.10	2.10	2.10
7F tip High Flow	1.44	1.25	1.86

Table 5.5B. *In vivo* study Cordis catheters. Variability in calibration factors (CF) assessed from routine coronary arteriograms expressed as (2 s.d./average CF) × 100%.

	Digital DCI/ACA		
	Contrast	Saline	Overall
6F tip Super Torque	3.88	3.48	3.98
7F tip High Flow	2.07	2.56	2.46

In vivo *study Cordis catheters*

The results of the *in vivo* study on the variability of the calibration factors expressed as (2.s.d./average CF) × 100% are given in Table 5.5A for the QCA/CMS measurements and in Table 5.5B for the ACA/DCI measurements, respectively. Earlier it was stated that catheters suitable for QCA should be associated with a variability as defined above of less than 5%. From Table 5.5A (QCA/CMS) it is apparent that the variability numbers are all far less than 5% and better for the saline than the 100% contrast filled catheters. For the ACA/DCI (Table 5.5B) the variabilities are slightly larger, but still amply below the 5%.

Table 5.6. Accuracy and precision values of the *in vivo* plug studies.

	QCA/CMS	ACA/DCI
N	21	17
Accuracy (mm)	−0.091	−0.024
Precision (mm) (pooled s.d.)	0.08	0.10
Regression line	y = 0.85x + 0.07	y = 1.05x − 0.08
Correlation coeff.	0.96	0.97

Table 5.7. Mean and standard deviations for differences between digital (ACA/DCI) and cinefilm (QCA/CMS) coronary measurements (N = 62); i.e. DCI minus CMS.

	Minimum diameter (mm)	%-D stenosis	Interpolated Ref. diameter (mm)
Same frame	−0.06 ± 0.16 DCI = 0.07 + 0.88CMS; r = 0.83	2.60 ± 5.73 DCI = 21.5 + 0.70CMS; r = 0.84	0.03 ± 0.16 DCI = 0.04 + 1.00CMS; r = 0.97
Best frame	−0.06 ± 0.18 DCI = 0.21 + 0.76CMS; r = 0.80	2.59 ± 5.98 DCI = 22.5 + 0.68CMS; r = 0.79	0.04 ± 0.17 DCI = 0.07 + 1.00CMS; r = 0.96

In vivo *plexiglass plugs*

On the CMS a total of 21 images were analyzed, and on the DCI 17 images. The accuracy, pooled standard deviation values, as well as the regression analyses are presented in Table 5.6. Accuracies and precisions are excellent and of the same order as the results from the 'vessel' phantom on a homogenous background (scatter medium) and on patient anatomy. Although the slopes of the regression lines for the two segments are different, the correlation coefficient are very similar at 0.96 and 0.97.

Comparison of clinical cinefilm and digital angiographic studies

In Table 5.7 the results are given for the cinefilm/digital comparative study on clinical data carried out at the Montréal Heart Institute. Results are given in mean signed differences (DCI-CMS) and the standard deviation of these differences, as well as in terms of the regression lines through the data points and the correlation coefficients.

From Table 5.7 it can be concluded that there is an excellent correlation between the two modalities with very small systematic errors (≤0.06 mm) and random errors (approximately 0.17 mm) for both the obstruction and reference diameters. Apparently, there is a slight underestimation (negative difference) of MLD and overestimation (positive difference) of percent diameter stenosis for on-line ACA/DCI versus off-line cinefilm QCA/CMS measurements. The smaller systematic differences in the reference diameters on the other hand, show slight overestimations for ACA/DCI versus QCA/CMS. Searching for the best frames apparently introduced a slight additional error for the interpolated reference diameter. The random errors are only slightly higher than the inter- and intra-observer variabilities that have been found for the two systems individually. The random error of percent diameter stenosis is almost equal to values found in these observer variability studies. Surprisingly is the excellent slope (= 1.00) of the regression lines for the interpolated reference diameter measurements.

Discussion

In this chapter we have described our experiences and results in the comparison of quantitative angiographic measurements from 35 mm cinefilm and digital images using two state-of-the-art analytical software packages (QCA/CMS and ACA/DCI) developed in our laboratory. Earlier studies carried out by other investigators on other systems had shown little differences in the outcomes.

The first study that we described was the ultimate test on the edge detection algorithms carried out with a plexiglass phantom on a homogeneous (scatter medium) and nonhomogeneous (patient anatomy) background. From the results presented in Tables 5.1 and 5.2 it could be concluded that both QCA/CMS and ACA/DCI show small systematic errors (QCA/CMS < -0.09 mm; ACA/DCI < -0.03 mm) and an excellent precision (QCA/CMS < 0.10 mm; ACA/DCI < 0.11 mm). It was apparent that for both systems, the random errors were slightly higher in the nonhomogeneous background situation as compared to the homogeneous background, as was to be expected. From Figure 5.2 it is also clear that the correction procedures that have been developed to correct for the limited resolution of the X-ray imaging chain and thereby correct for the otherwise occurring overestimations for sizes below 1.2 mm work well.

Calibration of the image data on the basis of the contrast catheters is one of the most important steps in the QCA procedures. The use of high quality, qualified, catheters is a must in QCA-studies. So far we have extensively studied Mallinckrodt and Cordis catheters and could conclude that these satisfy the basic requirements for QCA.

The variability in the calibration factors assessed from routine coronary arteriograms expressed as 2 times the coefficient of variation for Cordis 6F Super Torque and 7F High Flow Cordis catheters demonstrated that the random errors were all less than 5%, with those from cinefilm roughly 40–50% smaller that those from digital data.

Both the *in vitro* and *in vivo* studies show minimal differences between contrast-filled and contrast-empty catheters. In both the Mallinckrodt and

Cordis studies the radiographic sizes of the saline-filled catheters as measured with the QCA/CMS were slightly higher than those for the 100% contrast fillings. This is consistent with data from the CMS provided by J. Lespérance from the Montréal Heart Institute (Figure 5.4). In a total of 128 measurements on empty and full catheters (120 Schneider 8F, 2 Schneider 7F and 6 Medtronic 8F) the average empty calibration factor was 0.0916 ± 0.006 mm/pixel and the average full calibration factor 0.0908 ± 0.007 mm/pixel (mean difference: 0.0008 ± 0.004 mm/pixel); this represents a difference of only 0.87%! The same phenomenon could be seen in our digital analysis for the Mallinckrodt catheters, whereas no differences were found for the Cordis catheters with the ACA/DCI package. Based on these data we may conclude that there is no reason for calibration on empty catheters only.

Furthermore, our data demonstrate that it is indeed possible to use 6F catheters for QCA calibration purposes, if properly manufactured taking into account a sufficient degree of radiopaqueness [3]. However, it must be stressed that other or new catheters can only be accepted for QCA after an extensive testing with the associated QCA analytical software packages. Although not supported with objective data in this study, we have been convinced from our experiences that the current state of the analytical software do *not* allow 5F catheters to be used for calibration purposes; there are just too few pixels available for a reliable measurement.

Although currently limited information is available from our animal experimental *in vivo* plug study, the first results are very encouraging. The systematic errors are negligible and the precision values of the same order of magnitude as found from the plexiglass 'vessel' phantom studies. If this trend remains consistent as we gather more *in vivo* material, this would mean that properly carried out phantom studies could truly substitute the far more expensive and laborious animal experimental studies.

Finally, the direct comparison between cinefilm and digital data as carried out in Montréal demonstrated minimal differences in the obstruction diameters and in the interpolated reference diameters; the slope for the reference diameters was 1.00! The random errors or precision values in the comparisons of the same frames from these two different image carriers (Table 5.7), were only slightly higher than the known inter-observer variabilities of the individual systems. This statistical analysis was based on pre-PTCA data with the severities of the obstructions ranging from about 40% to 80%. Although this is a limited range of values, further evaluations at the Montréal Heart Institute for the post-PTCA data with severities ranging from 5% to 60% confirmed these excellent results and actually resulted in even higher correlation coefficients ($r \geq 0.91$) and better slopes (0.97–1.03) for the three variables. The systematic and random errors in the QCA parameters in this post-PTCA analysis were almost identical to the ones presented in Table 5.7.

In summary, QCA can be performed with state-of-the-art analytical software packages from cinefilm (CMS) as well as from digital (DCI) with comparable accuracy and precision, even for small vessel sizes below 1.2 mm.

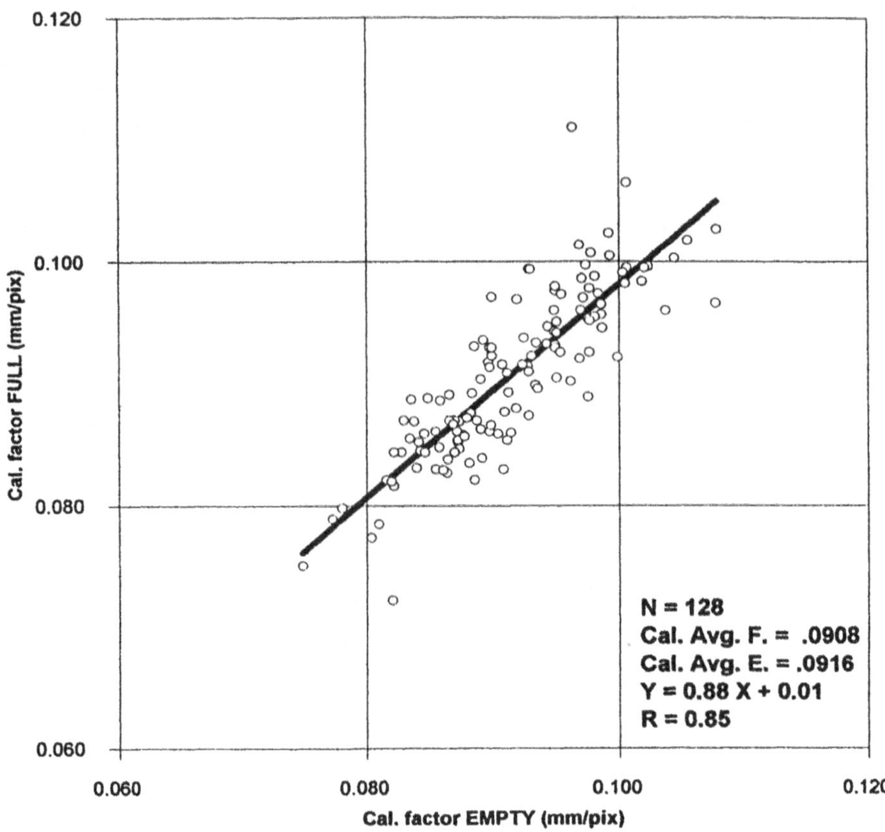

Figure 5.4. Comparison of calibration factors assessed from 128 measurements on empty and full catheters.

All our validation studies indicate that cinefilm allows a slightly better precision (by 10–15%). This is, among others, due to the differences in pixel sizes between the two approaches, being at the average 0.09 mm/pixel for CMS and 0.23 mm/pixel for DCI.

Acknowledgements

The authors wish to thank Mrs. B. Smit-van der Deure for her secretarial assistance. H. Buys of the mechanical workshop, Department of Cardiology, University Hospital Leiden fabricated the plexiglass plugs. The precise measurements of these plugs was carried out at Cordis Europe NV in Rhoden, the Netherlands under the supervision of Jan Weber, M.Sc.

References

1. Reiber JHC. An overview of coronary quantitation techniques as of 1989. In Reiber JHC, Serruys PW (eds): Quantitative coronary arteriography. Dordrecht: Kluwer Academic Publishers 1991: 55–132.
2. Mancini GBJ. Digital coronary angiography: advantages and limitations. In Reiber JHC, Serruys PW (eds): Quantitative coronary arteriography. Dordrecht: Kluwer Academic Publishers 1991: 23–42.
3. Koning G, Zwet PMJ van der, Land CD von, Reiber JHC. Angiographic assessment of dimensions of 6F and 7F Mallinckrodt Softouch[R] coronary contrast catheters from digital and cine arteriograms. Int J Card Imaging 8, 1992: 153–61.
4. Reiber JHC, Zwet PMJ van der, Land CD von *et al.* Quantitative coronary arteriography: equipment and technical requirements. In Reiber JHC, Serruys PW (eds): Advances in quantitative coronary arteriography. Dordrecht: Kluwer Academic Publishers 1992: 75–111.
5. Reiber JHC, Zwet PMJ van der, Land CD von *et al.* On-line quantification of coronary arteriograms with the DCI system. Medicamundi 1989; 34: 89–98.
6. Zwet PMJ van der, Land CD von, Loois G, Gerbrands JJ, Reiber JHC. An on-line system for the quantitative analysis of coronary arterial segments. Comp Cardiol 1990; 157–60.
7. Reiber JHC, Zwet PMJ van der, Koning G *et al.* Accuracy and precision of quantitative digital coronary arteriography; observer-, as well as short- and medium-term variabilities. Cath Cardiovasc Diagn 1992; 28: 187–98.
8. Gerbrands JJ. Segmentation of noisy images. Thesis, Delft University of Technology, 1988.
9. Zwet PMJ van der, Pinto IMF, Serruys PW, Reiber JHC. A new approach for the automated definition of path lines in digitized coronary angiograms. Int J Card Imaging 5, 1990: 75–83.
10. Koning G, Reiber JHC, Land CD von, Loois G, Meurs B. van. Advantages and limitations of two software calipers in quantitative coronary arteriography. Int J Card Imag 7, 1991: 15–30.
11. Bland JM, Altman DG. Statistical methods for assessing agreement between two methods of clinical measurement. Lancet 2, 1986: 307–10.

6. Angiographic core laboratory analyses of arterial phantom images: Comparative evaluations of accuracy and precision

GLENN J. BEAUMAN, JOHAN H.C. REIBER, GERHARD KONING, RONALD C.M. VAN HOUDT & ROBERT A. VOGEL

Summary

Quantitative coronary arteriography (QCA) is commonly regarded as a reproducible and accurate method of assessing coronary anatomy. Centralized, quantitative core laboratory analysis of clinical study images has consequently become the standard for determining interval change in coronary anatomy. QCA systems and laboratory methods, however, are known to vary among core facilities and the effect of such differences on the variability of quantitative assessments among angiographic core laboratories (ACL) has not been studied. We evaluated QCA variability among seven active ACL, using four differing QCA systems by comparing analyses performed on a common set of phantom cinefilm images. Phantom analyses were performed in an automated, un-edited fashion on images of a plexiglass arterial phantom containing eleven precision drilled lumens (0.68–5.06 mm). Phantom images were acquired under varying radiographic conditions (5″ and 7″ image intensifier magnifications at 70 and 90 kV with uniform (scatter medium) and non-uniform (patient anatomy) backgrounds). Over the range of phantom diameters, analysis differences from actual luminal dimensions ranged widely (+0.42 to −0.45 mm) among ACL.

Smallest systematic errors and most comparable results were found in the middle diameter range between 1.2 and 2.8 mm. In the smallest lumen range (<1.2 mm) some systems severely overestimated the true sizes or were unable to analyze these images in an automated fashion. The greatest variability among ACL was found in the measurement of diameters of scatter medium background images >2.8 mm. Under these conditions, 36% of averaged measurement differences resulted in an absolute systematic error >0.2 mm; for patient anatomy images this was only 7%. From random error measurements it could be concluded that QCA systems provide smoother contours for larger diameters.

Interlaboratory variability among ACL was small when like QCA systems were employed. However, significant analyses differences were found between ACL using differing QCA systems. Our data demonstrate that there is a great need for establishing uniform performance standards for quantitative core laboratories.

J.H.C. Reiber and P.W. Serruys (eds): Progress in quantitative coronary arteriography, 87–104.

Introduction

Automated quantitative coronary arteriography (QCA) has become an important tool to the study of coronary artery disease. Automated analyses has been applied to clinical study images using computer systems which integrate various hardware and software components to illuminate, digitize, and analyze coronary anatomy from cinefilm [1]. Many systems now operate from a personal computer and, as a result of this user friendly format, centralized angiographic laboratories have proliferated. The edge detection algorithms of commercially available QCA systems are commonly validated for accuracy and reproducibility against plexiglass arterial phantoms and implantable stenoses of known dimension [2]. Edge detection algorithms and system components, however, vary among QCA systems and although the variability of visual assessment techniques have been widely reported, little is known of the variability among angiographic core laboratories (ACL) or QCA systems [3–9]. We have therefore compared ACL analyses of a common set of plexiglass phantom images to evaluate the variability among ACL and QCA systems.

Background

We have previously reported on the variability between ACL related to differences in core laboratory methods [10]. Those evaluations compared analyses of randomly selected clinical images performed by two ACL, using different QCA systems. We found that site specific methods of frame selection resulted in variability between laboratory analyses that was similar to the variability that intrinsically exists between frames in various points in the cardiac cycle and was considered to exert minimal influence on inter-laboratory variability. On the other hand, operator influences such as visual verification and corrections of automatically determined arterial profiles, as well as operator based parameter definitions were implicated as significant sources of inter-laboratory variability.

Although the focus of our investigation centered on operator based influences, there were also indications that intrinsic differences between QCA systems may be a significant source of inter-laboratory variability. Figure 6.1 shows a same frame analysis comparison between the two laboratories, where the parameters of minimal lumen diameter (MLD) and percent diameter stenosis (% DS) were determined in each laboratory using the same methodology. In that comparative analysis, MLD measurements were found to be significantly different (0.23 ± 0.37 mm, $p < 0.05$) between ACL and widely variable [10]. In fact, the range of diameters for which each system has been shown to be most accurate (1.0–2.0 mm) contained the widest variability for measurements of a single diameter (MLD). Based on these differences between laboratories, we further pursued an evaluation of inter-laboratory variability using a set of common phantom images to determine systematic and random differences between ACL and QCA systems.

Methods

The study was conducted using a common set of arterial phantom images, comparing analyses performed by seven active angiographic core laboratories, each using one of four commercially available, automated edge detection, QCA systems. Each of the seven quantitative coronary arteriography core laboratories performed independent and blinded evaluations of the phantom images. Table 6.1 lists the participating centers and the quantitative system plus the software version of the analytical package used by each. All QCA systems have been extensively validated and are described in detail elsewhere [1, 11–20].

A plexiglass arteriographic phantom, containing eleven precision drilled lumens of uniform dimension (R.L. Kirkeeide, Ph.D., Houston, Texas), was filled with 100% contrast medium (Renografin 76, Mallinckrodt Medical., St. Louis, Missouri) and imaged under varying radiographic parameters using a catheterization laboratory imaging system (Poly-Diagnost C, Optimus 2000, Philips Medical Systems, Best, the Netherlands). Images were acquired at 5″ and 7″ image intensifier magnifications, with 70 and 90 kV energy outputs over 10 cm of plexiglass scatter medium. Two additional cine acquisitions were made (5 and 7 inch image intensifier modes) with the phantom positioned over a patients's chest (variable kV). During each acquistion the X-ray table was panned so that each phantom lumen could be visualized at the center of the image field. Luminal diameters of the phantom ranged from 0.687 to 5.062 mm and were validated for accuracy (±0.001 mm) using a laser micrometer (Cordis Europa N.V., Roden, the Netherlands). Figure 6.2 is an example of the phantom positioned over a patient's chest.

Individual cine frames, considered optimal for analysis by a qualified observer, were identified in each acquisition sequence for each phantom lumen. Frames were considered optimal based on edge sharpness (focus) and orientation at the center of the imaging field.

The film was then forwarded to each participating laboratory with a protocol specifying the pre-selected frames and details that would assure uniform evaluation of the film. Laboratories were requested to position the specified frames on cine film projectors and digitize the images in a fashion consistent with their usual core laboratory practice. Each laboratory thereby analyzed the same set of individual phantom images (6 radiographic acquisitions; 4 with scatter media, 2 with patient anatomy; 11 lumens, 66 individual analyses). The central most portion of each lumen (a length of approximately two centimeters) was the targeted segment for each analysis. Results were reported as the average diameter ±standard deviation for the analysis segment, derived typically from between 150 and 200 diameter values per segment. A

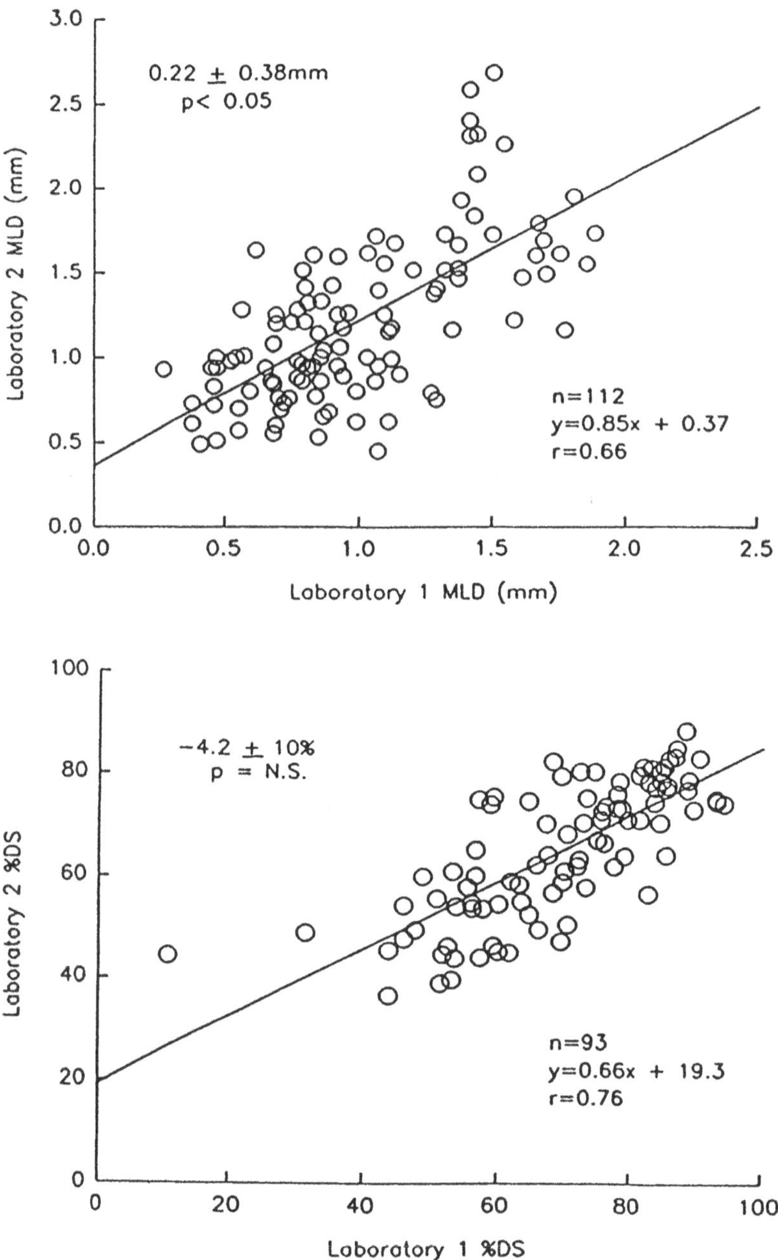

Figure 6.1. Inter-laboratory variability-same frame, same methods. These plots show inter-laboratory comparisons of minimal lumen diameter (MLD) and percent diameter stenosis analyses (% DS) when the same frame and the same parameter assessment techniques are used.

Table 6.1. Particpating QCA core laboratories and quantitative systems.

Core laboratory	Quantitative system	Software version
University of Maryland	ADAC Labs.	ARTREK V10
University Hospital Leiden	CMS-MEDIS	CMS V 1.0
Washington Hospital Center	IMAGECOMM	ARTREK V 1.32
Duke University Hospital	DUQUES	VMS Fortran V. 2
Montreal Heart Institute	CMS-MEDIS	CMS V 1.11
Rhode Island Hospital	ADAC Labs.	ARTREK V10
Thomas Jefferson University	IMAGECOMM	ARTREK V 1.32

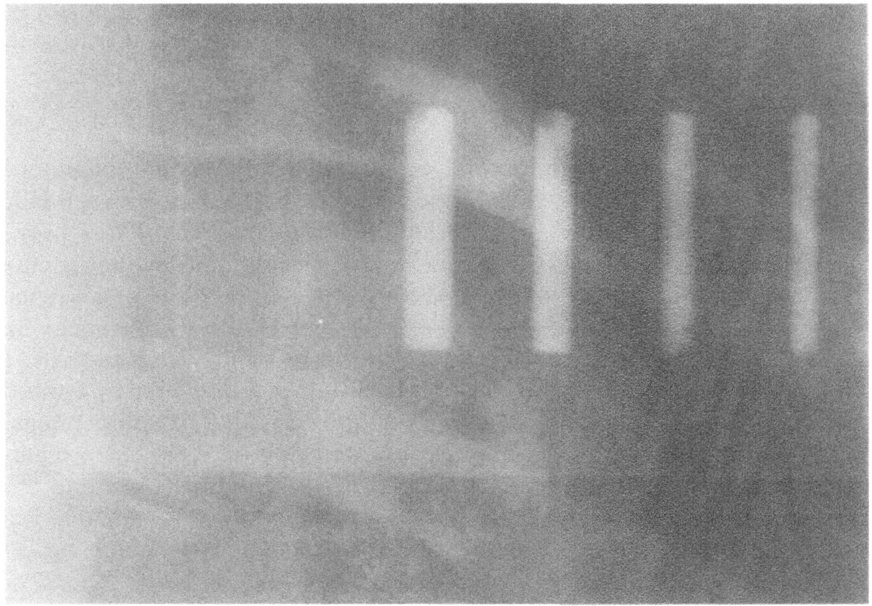

Figure 6.2. Plexiglass arterial phantom filmed over patient anatomy.

rectangular centimeter grid, filmed at corresponding radiographic parameters was provided for calibration purposes. Laboratories were requested to report only automated analysis results with *no manual edge point correction*. The data thereby, represents the results of each QCA system/laboratory's digitization and automated edge detection, essentially free of operator bias.

Statistical methods

Calculations of average signed difference between the mean measured and true lumen diameters were used to assess the overall systematic error or accuracy. Random error or precision for each lumen was defined by the standard deviation of the measured diameters. This standard deviation describes the irregularity of the detected contours. The pooled standard deviation was calculated to describe overall precision for specific ranges of phantom diameters.

The systematic error defined above is based on signed differences of mean measured diameters and true values. Positive and negative differences may cancel each other, resulting in a very small or zero systematic error for the entire phantom. To assess the degree of these differences, an average absolute difference measure has been introduced as well. The student T-test was used to evaluate statistical significance ($p < 0.05$). Linear regression correlation was used to describe the relationship between laboratories.

Accuracy and precision of ACL analyses

The difference of each mean luminal estimate from the actual diameter was determined for each of the 44 separate analyses performed by each laboratory. Figure 6.3A–D shows these results for the cine sequences acquired with the scatter media as background. The true phantom diameters are plotted along the horizontal axis and differences between the mean detected diameter and its true size, along the vertical axis. Positive differences correspond to overestimations and negative differences to underestimations. Few luminal measurements varied from the actual luminal diameter by more than ±0.2 mm when determined from images acquired with a 5″ image intensifier mode. Ten percent of all the analyses (77 data points; 7 ACL, 11 phantom lumens) performed on images acquired at 70 kV (Figure 6.3A) and 5% of all analyses at 90 kV (Figure 6.3B) images fell outside of a ±0.2 mm range. Luminal measurements determined from 7″ field images were less accurate. When measured from images acquired at 70 kV (Figure 6.3C), 27% of analyses were different from the actual diameter by more than ±0.2 mm and 22% of the analyses at 90 kV (Figure 6.3D) images fell outside this range.[1] It should be noted that the percentages of errant measurements (> ±0.2 mm) reported above were not equally distributed among the ACL and QCA systems.

An average difference for each phantom lumen was calculated from the differences determined from analyses of images of each radiographic variable. These data are shown in Figure 6.4A and B for images with uniform (scatter media) and non-uniform (patient anatomy) backgrounds, respectively. Averaged differences are again plotted along the vertical axis against the true luminal diameters along the horizontal axis. When averaged over

1. Although ±0.2 mm is a relatively broad measure of QCA system accuracy, based on comparative validation studies, this range may be a fair representation of 95% confidence limits (2 standard deviations) for all QCA systems used in this study.

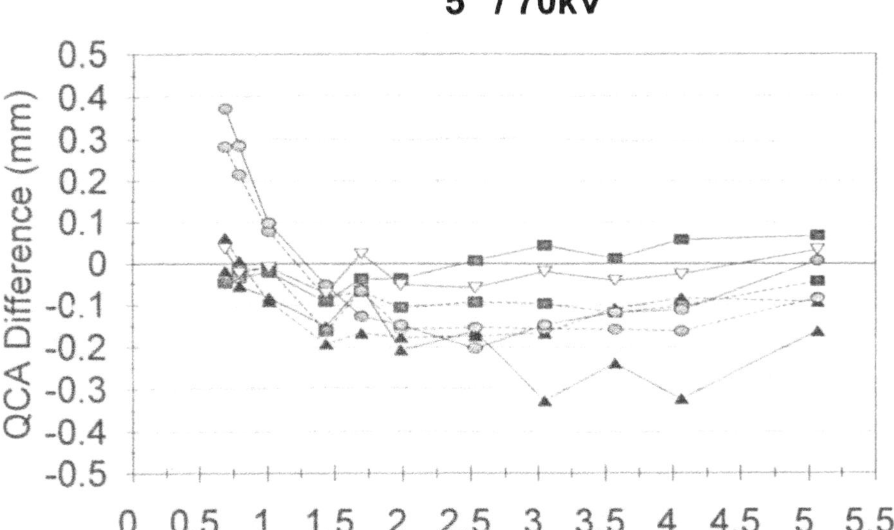
5" / 70kV
QCA Difference (mm)
0.5
0.4
0.3
0.2
0.1
0
-0.1
-0.2
-0.3
-0.4
-0.5
0 0.5 1 1.5 2 2.5 3 3.5 4 4.5 5 5.5
Phantom Diameter (mm)

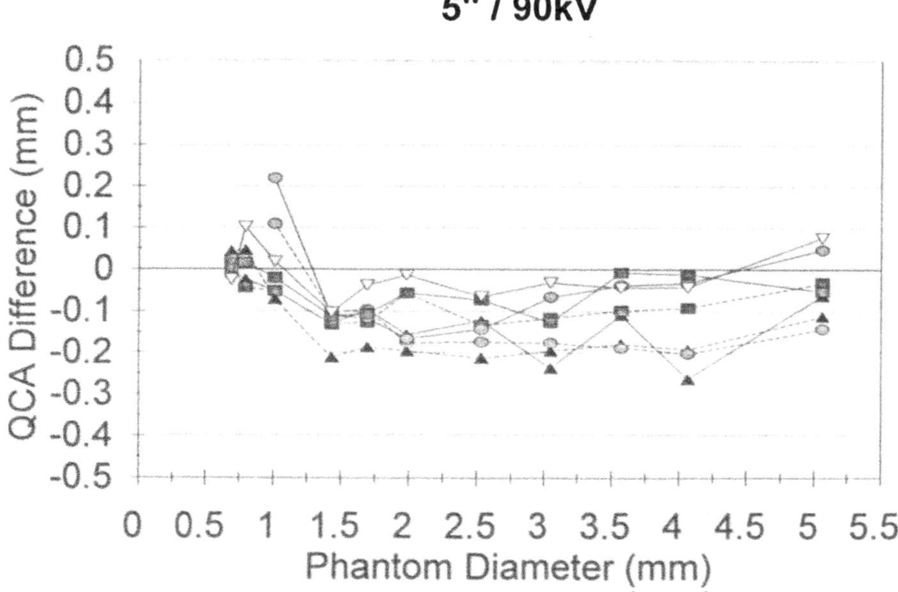
5" / 90kV
QCA Difference (mm)
0.5
0.4
0.3
0.2
0.1
0
-0.1
-0.2
-0.3
-0.4
-0.5
0 0.5 1 1.5 2 2.5 3 3.5 4 4.5 5 5.5
Phantom Diameter (mm)

Figure 6.3.A, B.

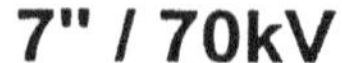

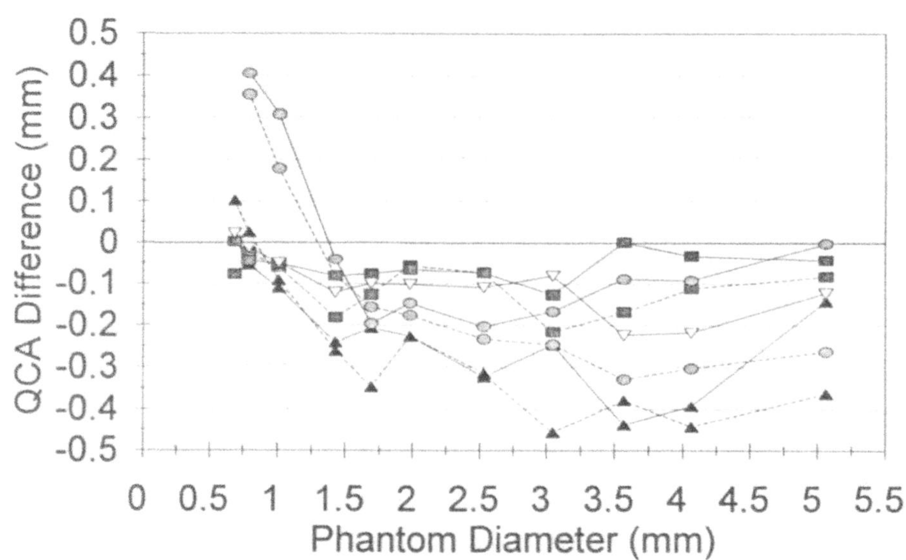

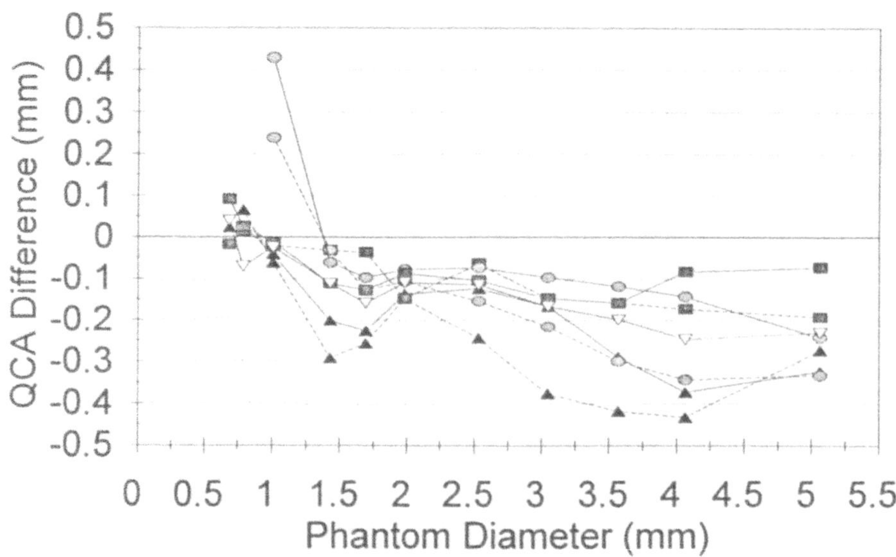

Figure 6.3. Analysis differences from actual phantom diameters for images with scatter medium as background for different image intensifier modes (5 and 7 inch) and kV levels (70 and 90 kV). Same QCA systems are represented by the same symbols, while ACL are differentiated by differing plot lines. The true values of the eleven vessel tubes are plotted along the horizontal axis and the individual differences between the mean diameter and its true size along the vertical axis. A positive difference corresponds to an overestimation, a negative difference to an underestimation.

the range of radiographic variables, phantom analyses among ACL were more comparable and followed similar patterns. Diameters ≤1.2 mm (3 lumens) were largely over-estimated by two ACL and diameters >1.2 mm were generally under-estimated. Diameters >1.2 mm and <2.8 mm (4 lumens) were most accurately analyzed by all ACL, with 93% (52 of 56) of averaged analysis differences falling within ±0.2 mm of the actual diameter. However, larger variability among ACL & QCA systems was noted for diameters outside of this range. Tables 6.2A and 6.2B categorize ACL accuracy for specific ranges of phantom diameters for phantom images with uniform (scatter medium) and non-uniform (patient anatomy) backgrounds, respectively. Phantom diameters were divided into 3 groups, sizes <1.2 mm (3 lumens), between 1.2 and 2.8 mm (4 lumens), and > than 2.8 mm (4 lumens). Within each group, luminal measurements were categorized into 3 ranges of accuracy: absolute systematic errors within 0.1 mm, between 0.1 and 0.2 mm, and greater than 0.2 mm. In addition, failed automated analyses were also tabulated. (To preserve anonymity, ACL are listed by letter, in random order. Their sequence bares no correlation to the order in which they appear in Table 6.1). Obviously, greater ACL accuracy is associated with smaller systematic errors, in other words, the higher the number in the left column for each of the three ranges, the better a system performs. Predictably, difficulties were encountered in the measurement of diameters <1.2 mm. This was especially apparent for images with non-uniform background (patient anatomy) where three ACL were unable to adequately analyze the two smallest phantom diameters in an automated fashion. Even when measured against a uniform background (scatter medium), 14% (3 of 21) of averaged differences were found to be errant of the true diameter by >0.2 mm. Surprisingly, the greatest variability among ACL was found in the measurement of diameters of scatter medium background images >2.8 mm. Under these conditions, 36% (10 of 28) of averaged measurement differences resulted in an absolute systematic error >0.2 mm in contrast to measurements on the patient anatomy images where for the same range of diameters only 7% (2 of 28) were errant by >0.2 mm.

Table 6.3 lists the average absolute differences between the mean measured diameters and the true values of the lumens and the earlier defined pooled standard deviations for the phantom diameter ranges described in Table 6.2A and 6.2B for the analyses performed on images with non-uniform (patient anatomy) background. Standard deviations were not available from two ACL. Overall the greatest absolute accuracy was obtained in the measurements of diameters falling in the middle range (>1.2 mm and <2.8 mm), while measurements of the larger diameters were found to be least accurate. Smaller pooled standard deviations for measurements of larger diameters was a consistent trend among ACL, suggesting QCA systems provide smoother contours (less variable measurements) for larger diameters. Measurements of the smallest diameters were the most variable, i.e. having the largest random errors.

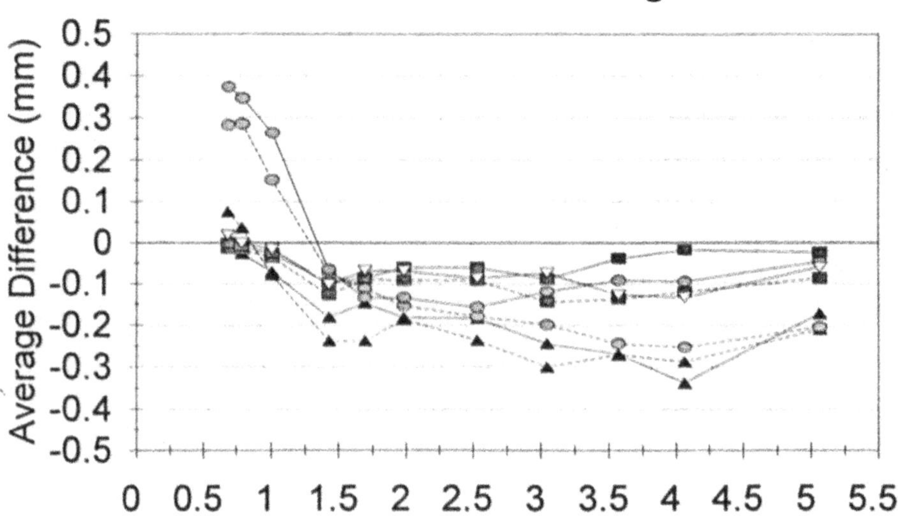

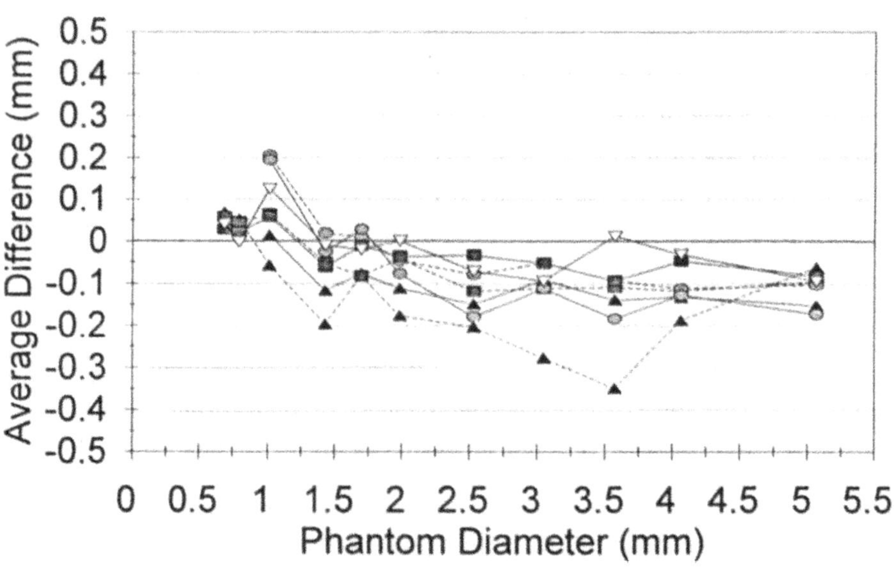

Figure 6.4. Laboratory/system average difference from true phantom diameters. Figure A shows the results with uniform background (scatter medium) and Figure B with nonuniform background (patient anatomy). Same symbols and connecting plotlines as in Figure 6.3. Again, the true values of the eleven vessel tubes are plotted along the horizontal axis and the individual differences between the mean diameter and its true size along the vertical axis. A positive difference corresponds to an overestimation, a negative difference to an underestimation.

Table 6.2A. Analysis accuracy for phantom images with uniform (scatter medium) backgrounds.

	Range of phantom diameters (mm)											
	<1.2 mm (N = 3)				>1.2 < 2.8 mm (N = 4)				>2.8 mm (N = 4)			
ACL	$\Delta < 0.1$	$0.1 < \Delta \leqslant 0.2$	$\Delta > 0.2$	ϕ	$\Delta < 0.1$	$0.1 < \Delta \leqslant 0.2$	$\Delta > 0.2$	ϕ	$\Delta < 0.1$	$<0.1 < \Delta \leqslant 0.2$	$\Delta > 0.2$	ϕ
A	3	–	–	–	3	1	–	–	1	3	–	–
B	3	–	–	–	–	4	–	–	–	1	3	–
C	–	1	1	1	1	3	–	–	–	1	3	–
D	3	–	–	–	3	1	–	–	2	2	–	–
E	3	–	–	–	4	–	–	–	4	–	–	–
F	3	–	–	–	–	1	3	–	–	–	4	–
G	–	–	2	1	1	3	–	–	3	1	–	–

Abbreviations: $\Delta < 0.1$ = averaged absolute analysis differences <0.1 mm, $0.1 < \Delta \leqslant 0.2$ = averaged absolute analysis differences between 0.1 and 0.2 mm, $\Delta > 2.0$ = averaged absolute analysis differences >0.2 mm, ϕ = failed automated analysis, ACL = Angiographic Core Laboratory.

Table 6.2B. Analysis accuracy for phantom images with non-uniform (patient anatomy) backgrounds.

	Range of phantom diameters (mm)											
	<1.2 mm (N = 3)				>1.2 < 2.8 mm (N = 4)				>2.8 mm (N = 4)			
ACL	$\Delta < 0.1$	$0.1 < \Delta \leqslant 0.2$	$\Delta > 0.2$	ϕ	$\Delta < 0.1$	$0.1 < \Delta \leqslant 0.2$	$\Delta > 0.2$	ϕ	$\Delta < 0.1$	$<0.1 < \Delta \leqslant 0.2$	$\Delta > 0.2$	ϕ
A	3	–	–	–	3	1	–	–	1	3	–	–
B	1	–	–	2	1	3	–	–	1	3	–	–
C	–	–	1	2	4	–	–	–	2	2	–	–
D	2	1	–	–	4	–	–	–	4	–	–	–
E	3	–	–	–	4	–	–	–	4	–	–	–
F	3	–	–	–	1	2	1	–	1	1	2	–
G	–	1	–	2	3	1	–	–	–	4	–	–

Abbreviations: $\Delta < 0.1$ = averaged absolute analysis differences <0.1 mm, $0.1 < \Delta \leqslant 0.2$ = averaged absolute analysis differences between 0.1 and 0.2 mm, $\Delta > 2.0$ = averaged absolute analysis differences >0.2 mm, ϕ = failed automated analysis, ACL = Angiographic Core Laboratory.

Table 6.3. Averaged absolute differences (mm) and pooled standard deviations (mm) for ACL analyses of phantom images with non-uniform (patient anatomy) background.

	Range of phantom diameters (mm)		
ACL	<1.2 mm (N = 3)	>1.2 < 2.8 mm (N = 4)	>2.8 mm (N = 4)
A	0.060 ± 0.14	0.073 ± 0.09	0.108 ± 0.07
B	0.055 ± ?	0.113 ± ?	0.128 ± ?
C	0.204 ± 0.18	0.048 ± 0.16	0.096 ± 0.15
D	0.059 ± 0.10	0.041 ± 0.07	0.062 ± 0.06
E	0.051 ± 0.12	0.036 ± 0.09	0.069 ± 0.07
F	0.058 ± 0.04	0.164 ± 0.07	0.218 ± 0.07
G	0.194 ± ?	0.089 ± ?	0.148 ± ?

ACL = Angiographic Core Laboratories.

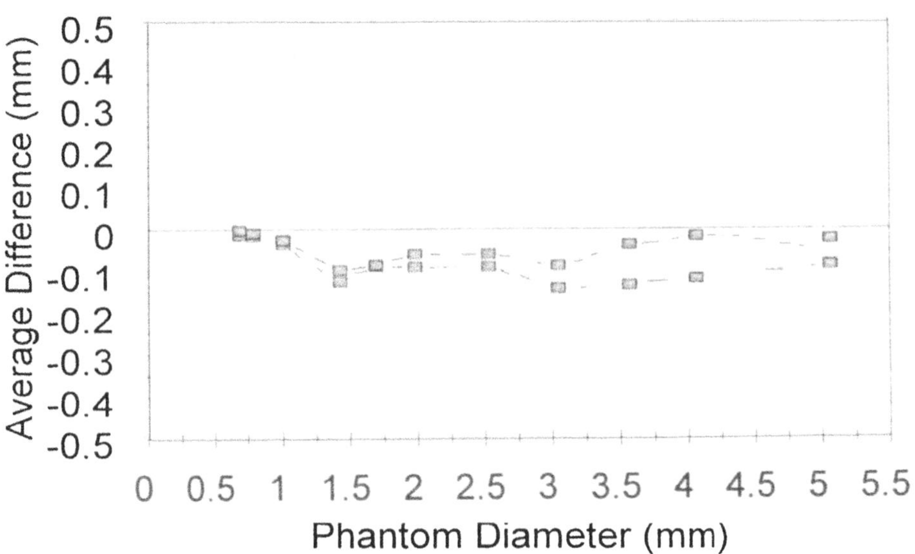

Figure 6.5A.

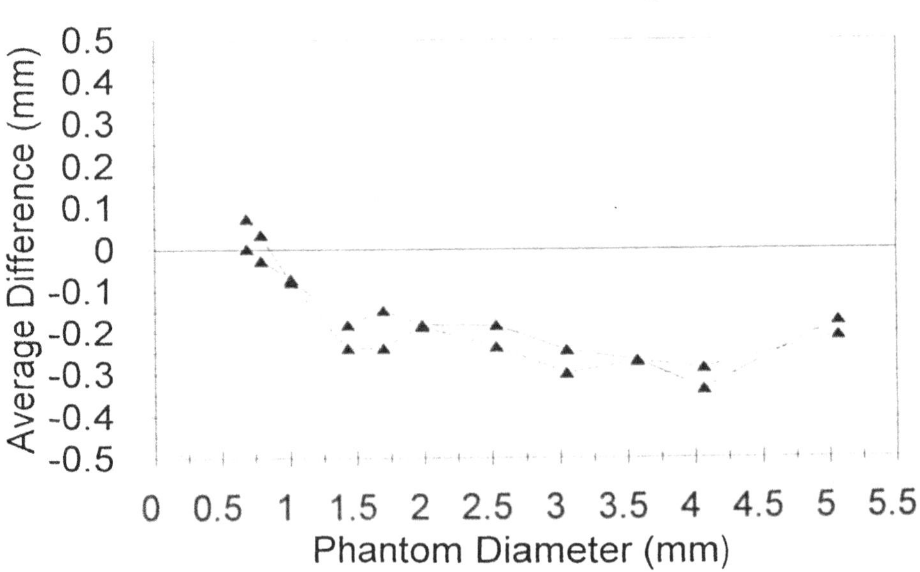

Figure 6.5B.

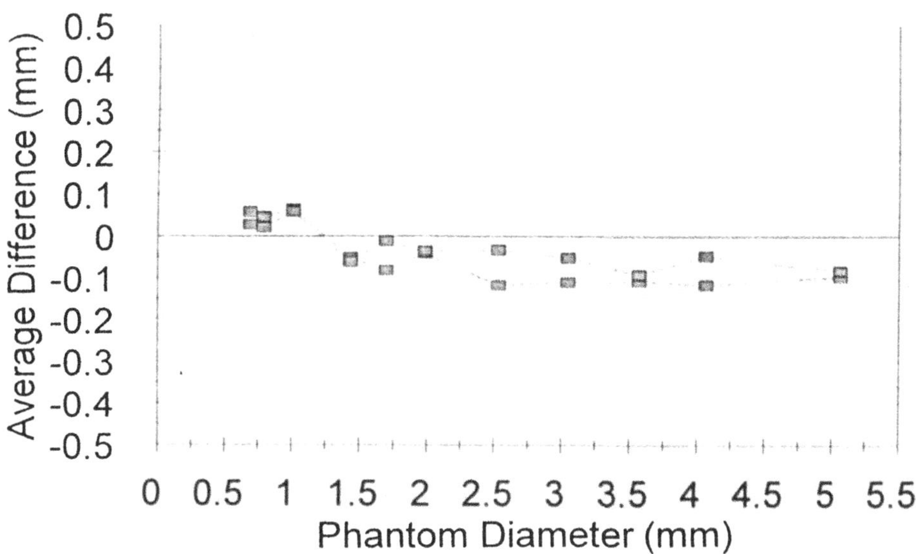

Figure 6.5A.

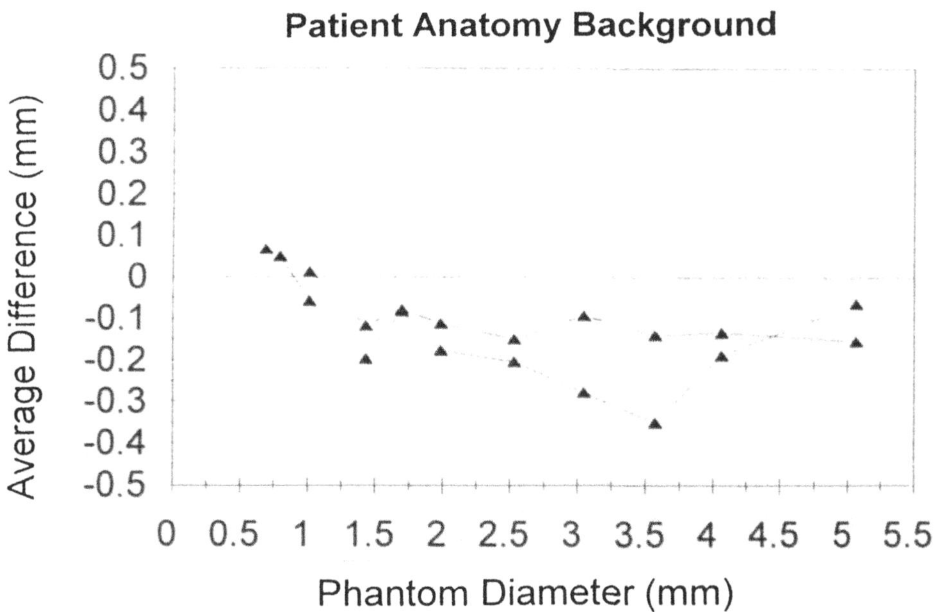

Figure 6.5B.

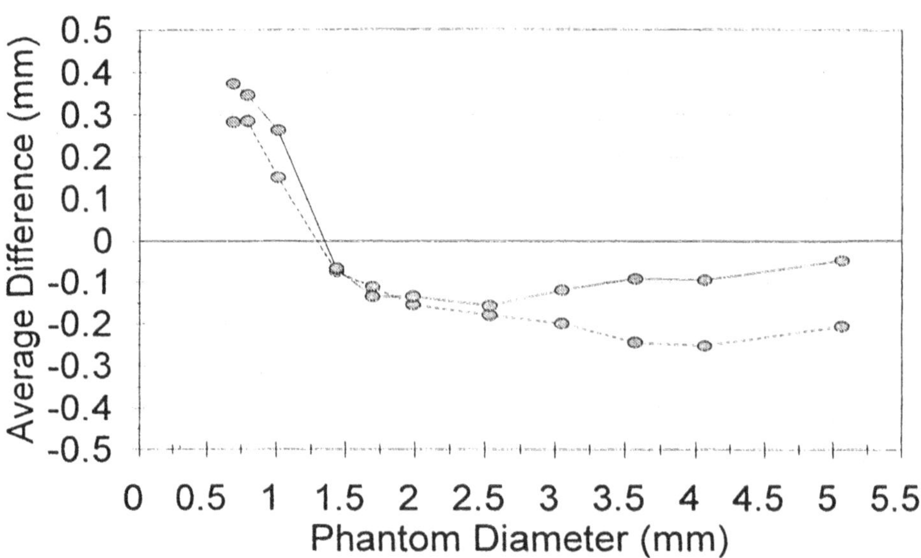

Figure 6.5C.

Figure 6.5A–F describe inter-laboratory analysis comparisons of ACL using the same QCA system. These data are the same as those given in Figures 6.4A and B, however, now separated clearly for the different QCA systems. The plots on the left correspond to analyses performed on images with uniform background (scatter medium) and those on the right with non-uniform background (patient anatomy). Analysis differences between ACL using the same system were found to be small and non-significant, however inter-system analysis comparisons showed significant differences ($p < 0.05$).

Discussion

The automated edge detection algorithms that were used in the study are similarly based on densitometric evaluations of profiles through a contrast filled lumen. Each algorithm determines lumen edge using hybrid first and second derivative calculations. Substantial differences in the approaches exist however. Sampling intervals, spatial continuity, weighted pixel value, and contour search techniques vary among the different systems [9]. In addition, image magnification and digitization, the initial step in the analysis process, was accomplished using varying image acquisition components (projectors, lenses, video camera and frame grabbers). Each of these factors has an effect on the intrinsic variability between laboratories and QCA systems.

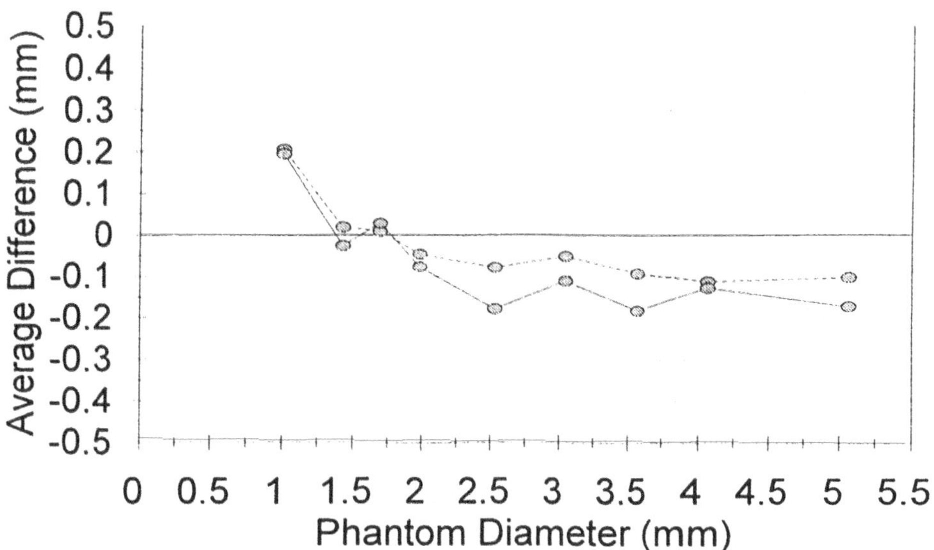

Figure 6.5C.

Figure 6.5. Average differences from actual phantom diameters combined in each plot for two systems of the same kind but installed in different ACL. The same symbols, plot lines and formats as in Figures 6.3 and 6.4. Plots on the left correspond to analyses performed on images with uniform background (scatter medium) and those on the right with non-uniform background (patient anatomy).

Analysis inaccuracy has been described for QCA analyses of diameters <1.2 mm, due to limited spatial resolution of X-ray systems. This was again demonstrated in this study by the number of failed automated analyses and analysis differences greater than 0.2 mm for lumens within this range (Tables 6.2A and 6.2B). Some QCA systems have incorporated point-spread function corrections to help address this limitation.

It should be noted that in this study luminal measurements were reported as mean diameter values. This approach has been shown to be less accurate, in this range, than identifying a single luminal diameter (MLD) which is a more common practice for defining the stenotic parameter [21]. This experiment however, was not designed to assess percent stenosis or stenotic diameter, but rather the systematic and random errors in the measurement of straight 'arteries' by automated edge detection techniques.

More concerning was the inaccuracy shown for the larger diameters (2.8–5.0 mm). In contrast to measurements in the smallest range, measurements of larger diameters were underestimated and ranged widely between ACL. The implications of these findings are substantial. As a result of overestimations of the smallest diameters combined with underestimations of the larger diameters, these data suggest that substantial inaccuracy could be present in the measurement of more severe clinical lesions. Comparison of quantitative and visual stenosis measurements suggests this is the case [21]. Interestingly, less underestimation of larger diameters was observed in the analysis of phantom images with variable background (patient anatomy) than with uniform background (scatter medium) for which no clear explanation exists at this time.

The smallest lumens provide the least amount of image contrast between object and background, thereby potentially resulting in irregular contours by any edge detection algorithm. In contrast the largest lumens provide the greatest background to object contrast ratio's and therefore less variable edge detection is to be expected. As coronary arteries have, in general, relatively smooth boundaries, most automated QCA systems incorporate some kind of edge smoothing or interpolation techniques to filter the unnaturally jagged edges described by hybrid first and second derivative calculations. This would seem to be a desirable characteristic of a contour detection algorithm. However, by increasing the degree of smoothing, system accuracy may be compromised for vessels with very irregular morphology. In the assessment of smooth and uniform diameters, as was the case in this study, we found that the random errors of the measurements decreased with the size of the vessel (Table 6.3). Table 6.3 further shows that some ACL provided measurements that were both accurate and precise over the whole range of phantom diameters, while others were either less accurate or precise over certain ranges.

Although analysis accuracy (averaged differences) was found to vary widely between ACL over the range of radiographic variables, analysis differences between systems were minimal in the analysis of images acquired at 5" magnification (Figure 6.3A and B). Under these conditions, ≥90% of all analyses, (performed over the entire range of phantom diameters) were found to be accurate within ±0.2 mm. These data suggest that images acquired at larger image intensifier magnifications are more optimally suited to automated quantitative analysis.

From the plots comparing analyses performed by the same QCA systems (Figure 6.5), we may conclude that site specific methods had minimal influence on the analysis differences between ACL when similar QCA systems were used. Moreover, these data clearly indicate that analysis results obtained from ACL using differing QCA systems should not be combined in meta analyses of clinical studies.

Study limitations

Operator dependant factors in the analysis process were minimized to more purely define system hardware and software differences. Frames were preselected and only automated analyses were reported. It was however, not possible to eliminate the operator dependant process of frame digitization. The digitization process involves subjective operator control of various acquisition components (light source, optical magnification, etc.) and may contribute significantly to the quality of the image ultimately subjected to the analysis process. This source of variability can be eliminated once it is possible to transfer digital files containing image data between various systems. Currently this is hampered by the non-standardized way image data are stored. This obstacle is one of the next to be undertaken in the continued comparative evaluation of quantitative systems/laboratories. However, until such time when this hurtle is overcome, these factors remain an undefined influence in the variability among ACL.

Calibration factors used for the phantom evaluations were obtained from linear measurements performed on a centimeter grid. Some of the quantitative systems we evaluated were developed using predominately catheter calibration methods. Centimeter grid methodology is an uncommon to calibration among core laboratory evaluations of clinical images. However, this approach provided a uniform method of system calibration, independent of digitization process, computer software, and variabilities associated with catheter based methods. An *in-vivo* phantom model may be necessary to provide a more realistic evaluation of inter-system variability related to clinical conditions.

Conclusion

Among ACL, phantom analyses were widely variable over a broad range of luminal diameters filmed under various radiographic conditions. Significant over- and underestimations were observed for the smallest and largest diameters, respectively. Interlaboratory variability among ACL was small when like QCA systems were employed. However, significant analyses differences were found between ACL using differing QCA systems. Our data demonstrate that there is a great need for establishing uniform performance standards for quantitative core laboratories.

Acknowledgement

This study was supported in part by grants from the National Heart Lung & Blood Institute, Bethesda, Maryland and the Veterans Administration, Washington D.C.

References

1. Reiber JHC, Zwet PMJ van der, Land CD von, Koning G, Meurs B van, Buis B, Voorthuisen AE van. Quantitative coronary arteriography: equipment and technical require-

ments. In Reiber JHC, Serruys PW (eds): Advances in quantitative coronary arteriography. Dordrecht: Kluwer Academic Publishers 1992: 75–111.

2. Reiber JHC, Koning G, von Land CD, van der Zwet PMJ. Why and how should QCA systems be validated. In Reiber JHC, Serruys PW (eds): Quantitative coronary arteriography. Dordrecht: Kluwer Academic Publishers. This volume.
3. Detre KM, Wright E, Murphy ML, Takaro T. Observer agreement in evaluating coronary angiograms. Circulation 1975; 52: 979–86.
4. Zir LM, Miller SW, Dinsmore RE, Gilbert JP, Harthorne JW. Interobserver variability in coronary arteriography. Circulation 1976; 53: 627–32.
5. DeRouen TA, Murphy JA, Owen W. Variability in the analysis of coronary arteriograms. Circulation 1977; 55: 324–8.
6. Sanmarco ME, Brooks SH, Blankenhorn DH. Reproducibility of a consensus panel in the interpretation of coronary arteriograms. Am Heart J 1978; 96: 430–7.
7. Fisher LD, Judkins MP, Lespérance J *et al.* Reproducibility of coronary arteriography reading in the Coronary Artery Surgery Study CASS). Cathet Cardiovasc Diagn 1982; 8: 565–75.
8. Meier B, Gruentzig AR, Goebel N, Pyle R, von Gosslar W, Schlumpf F. Assessment of stenoses in coronary angioplasty: inter- and intraobserver variability. Int J Cardiol 1983; 3: 159–69.
9. Reiber JHC. An overview of coronary quantitative techniques as of 1989. In Reiber JHC, Serruys PW (eds): Quantitative coronary arteriography. Dordrecht: Kluwer Academic Publishers 1991: 55–132.
10. Beauman GJ, Reiber JHC, Koning G, Vogel RA. Variability of QCA core laboratory assessments of coronary anatomy. In Reiber JHC, Serruys PW (eds): Advances in quantitative coronary arteriography. Dordrecht: Kluwer Academic Publishers 1992: 137–59.
11. Cusma JT, Spero LA, Morris KG, Tcheng JE,Bashore TM. Quantitative analysis of cardiac images: application in the clinical environment. Medica Mundi 1991; 36: 16–35.
12. Hermiller JB, Cusma JT, Spero LA, Fortin DF, Harding MB, Bashore TM. Quantitative and qualitative coronary angiographic analysis: review of methods, utility, and limitations. Cath Cardiovac Diagnosis 1992; 25: 110–31.
13. Skelton TN, Kisslo KB, Mikat EM, Bashore TM. Accuracy of digital angiography for quantitation of normal coronary luminal segments in excised, perfused hearts. Am J Cardiol 1987; 59: 1261–5.
14. Mancini GBJ, Simon SB, McGillem MJ, LeFree MT, Friedman HZ, Vogel RA. Automated quantitative coronary arteriography: morphologic and physiologic validation *in vivo* of a rapid digital angiographic method. Circulation 1987; 75: 452–60.
15. Klein LW, Agarwal JB, Rosenberg MC *et al.* Assessment of coronary artery stenoses by digital subtraction angiography: a patho-anatomic validation. Am Heart J 1987; 113: 1011–7.
16. LeFree MT, Simon SB, Mancini GBJ, Vogel RA. Digital radiographic assessment of coronary arterial diameter and videodensitometric cross sectional area. Proc SPIE 1986; 626: 334–41.
17. Lespérance J, Waters D. Measuring progression and regression of coronary atherosclerosis in clinical trials: problems and progress. Int J Card Imaging 1992; 8: 165–73.
18. Land CD von, Koning G, Zwet PMJ van der, Reiber JHC. Comparison of accuracy and precision of quantitative coronary arterial analysis between cinefilm and digital systems. In Reiber JHC, Serruys PW (eds): Quantitative coronary arteriography. Dordrecht: Kluwer Academic Publishers. This volume.
19. Koning G, Zwet PMJ van der, Land CD von, Reiber JHC. Angiographic assessment of dimensions of 6F and 7F Mallinckrodt Softouch® coronary contrast catheters from digital and cine arteriograms. Int J Card Imaging 1992; 8: 153–161.
20. Popma JJ, Eichhorn EJ, Dehmer GJ. *In vivo* assessment of a digital angiographic method to measure absolute coronary artery diameters. Am J Cardiol 1989; 64: 131–8.
21. Beauman GJ, Vogel RA. Accuracy of individual and panel visual interpretations of coronary arteriograms: Implications for clinical decisions. J Am J Coll Cardiol 1990; 16: 108–13.

7. Task force of the ESC on digital cardiovascular imaging

RÜDIGER SIMON

Summary

Digital cardiac imaging in the catheterization laboratory has become a new modality that has gained widespread acceptance in the cardiological community. Concerned about the lack of quality control and standardization in this field, the European Society of Cardiology has installed a Task Force to investigate the problems involved with digital imaging and provide recommendations for present use and future development in this field.

Multiple sessions of this Task Force together with expert cardiologists and industry representatives have resulted in a number of basic recommendations for digital cardiac imaging that has inbetween been approved by the Board of the ESC and will be published in the near future. Part of the result of these expert discussions is presented in this paper.

The last decade has seen a remarkable change in the methodology of cardiac angiography. Due to rapid progress in computer and imaging technology, the on-line digital acquisition, processing and storage of entire angiocardiographic investigations has become feasible. The new technology of digital imaging in the catheterization laboratory is rapidly gaining widespread application, since it provides significant advantages for diagnostic and especially for interventional procedures [1–3].

The advent of these new facilities, however, had also raised questions such as:

- How do we control the quality of this new imaging modality?
- What should be the standards for image acquisition, processing and archiving?
- How do we store the tremendous amount of image data encountered with each investigation?
- How do we exchange image data between different systems?

For a long time, the 35 mm cinefilm has been the uniformly accepted medium for image storage and image exchange in angiocardiography. The improved quality of digitally acquired and processed angiographic video images has now raised the pertinent and logical question, whether or not the cinefilm should and can be replaced by electronic image storage, thus doing away with its disadvantages. Instead of the film development procedure with its

J.H.C. Reiber and P.W. Serruys (eds): Progress in quantitative coronary arteriography, 105–110.

inherent pitfalls and the necessity for large archival space and the 'by hand' archiving procedure, electronic storage could be immediate, much more space-efficient and combined with automated computerized archiving procedures. So far, however, no standard medium has emerged that could be used easily for the widespread exchange of digital images between systems of different manufacturers, different laboratories and different institutions. Nonetheless, an accelerating movement to cineless catheterization laboratories can be observed in Europe as well as in the USA and in Japan. In many new installations, video cassette systems such as Umatic or super VHS tapes have been used as a replacement for the cinefilm. Instead of improved image quality, however, this results in a degradation of image quality as compared to cinefilm, especially when copies are made from these cassettes, due to the restricted bandwidth of currently available tape recorders. In addition, the longevity of magnetic tape registration may be questioned creating legal problems in a number of European countries where archiving is requested for at least 10 years.

The European Society of Cardiology has become concerned about this development. It therefore has installed a Task Force on Digital Imaging in Cardiology (DIGICARE) in 1992 to review the current situation together with expert cardiologists and representatives of the industrial companies involved in angiographic imaging (see Appendix).

During the reviewing process it has become evident, that the following major complexes are of primary importance:

1. The process of digital image acquisition and processing during the procedure
2. On-site archiving and review
3. Off-site review and data exchange
4. Quality control

Although all these complexes are clearly interrelated, they may be investigated separately.

Digital imaging during procedure and on-site-archiving and review

Different industrial companies have developed and presented systems for the accomplishment of these two tasks. It has become clear, that they can be achieved following different strategies. The Task Force has felt, that in this area, general recommendations should be formulated to set some basic marks for future development.

1. *Spatial resolution*

In order to allow for a quality of digitally processed images at least as good as film pictures, a discerneability of at least 2.5 line pairs per mm using a high contrast phantom at a 5 inch image intensifier input screen is the minimal acceptable scenario. This will render matrix sizes smaller than 512 by 512 pixel obsolete.

2. *Frame rate*
In adult cardiology a maximum acquisition rate of 25 frames per second in Europe or 30 frames per second (US-system) will be sufficient for the bulk of the investigations. For pediatric use, a higher acquisition rate (up to 50 or 60 frames per second) may be required.

3. *X-ray exposure*
State of the art digital systems should offer the advantage of X-ray dose reduction for fluoroscopy as well as high quality acquisition implementing reduced X-ray pulse rates in combination with digital gap filling.

4. *Storage requirements*
Storage has to be performed during acquisition in a way to allow for immediate playback after acquisition. This storage has to take place on a non-volatile medium for reasons of safety. Immediate playback must be possible in real time and without any detectable loss in image quality compared to acquisition. Storage capacity has to be sufficient to provide complete storage of entire diagnostic as well as interventional procedures. According to present experience, this will mean more than 3,000 images in complicated cases.

5. *Image processing*
Image processing has to be available on-site during retrieval (and desirable also during acquisition), and should include changes in enhancement filter setting, zooming and inverse presentation. Other options such as different modes of subtraction are desirable.

6. *Quantitative assessment*
Quantitative assessment should be possible for ventricular function and dimensions of coronary lesions in the catheterization laboratory.

7. *Viewing stations*
To enable the dynamic viewing of acquired digital angiograms without using the catheterization laboratory facilities, viewing stations have to be provided that operate either directly connected to the digital imaging equipment in the cath-lab or from storage media. The handling of these viewing stations has to be simple and the presentation of images has to be quick. The quality of images has to be without any detectable loss as compared to acquisition.

8. *On-site archiving*
The archiving of digitally acquired images has to match the following requirements: quick and easy accessibility, longevity and durability of storage media, and lower space requirements as compared to the traditional film archive.

Table 7. 1. Requirements media that could replace the cinefilm for storage and exchange.

1. Quality	Image quality at least as good as with cinefilm
2. Capacity	Should be sufficient to store all images of at least onepatient's investigation
3. Speed	Real time acquisition and retrieval (25 frames/s or faster)
4. Size	Smaller than a 35 mm cinefilm container
5. Security	Storage should be reliable for at least 10 years.
6. Medium	The storage medium should be an industry standard
7. System specifications	Off-line viewing required; handling should be simple: A uniform protocol for data storage is to be used in all commercially available equipment. The hardware must be affordable.
8. Enhancement	The original data or processed image data may be archived. In case of processed images, the header must contain all informations necessary to restore the original images
9. Compression	Lossy compression should be avoided for archival storage. If used in image communication, it has to be shown that no loss of relevant medical information occurs at the compression ratio used
10. Data security	The data must be stored by techniques that minimize the practical risk of accidental or illegal changes of data.

Although some of these requirements are met by contemporary analog devices (e.g. laser optical video discs) it is likely, that storage will be digital in the future. Within the institution (on-site), this may be performed in a 'one-to-one way' (one medium for one investigation) or within the facilities of PACS or hospital information systems (HIS).

Off-site review and data exchange

This is a point of major importance and major concern. In contrast to the previous complexes, protocol standardization as well as a uniform exchange medium are absolute prerequisites. Requirements that have to be met by media that could replace the cinefilm for exchange alone or for exchange as well as intermediate storage are given on Tables 7.1 and 7.2. The ESC Task Force and the Task Force of the American College of Cardiology have similar views concerning these basic requirements. To avoid a 'tower of Babel' situation, it is of utmost importance to develop a protocol for data storage and exchange from the beginning, that will be uniformly accepted by cardiologists and the industry. For many reasons, this protocol will be most probably an addition to the DICOM-3–version of the ACR-NEMA protocol for radiologic data storage [4]. This protocol will be the basis for future developments of exchange media by the industrial companies.

Table 7.2. Requirements for storage media that could replace the cinefilm for exchange.

1. Quality	Image quality at least as good as with cinefilm
2. Capacity	Should be sufficient to store all images of one patient's investigation
3. Size	Smaller than a 35 mm cinefilm container
4. Medium	The storage medium should be an industry standard
5. System Specifications	Off-line viewing has to be simple; the hardware must be affordable; a uniform protocol for data storage is to be used in all commercially available equipment.

In this situation, the long term storage would take place in a data bank for the cathlab or in the hospital information system, that would provide long term reliability and quality.

Image quality

The Task Force realizes that the term 'quality' has to be defined more clearly by research into this important complex issue in the future. This will include:

- Promotion of instrumentation test procedures and development of phantoms for digital image acquisition in cardiology.
- Development and promotion of tests for cardiac image review workstations.
- Clinical assessment of image processing features such as data compression and decompression, enhancement by filtering and other processing routines.

The work of the ESC Task Force over 1 year has resulted in a proposal of basic recommendations for the field of digital angiocardiography, that has been submitted to the Board of the ESC. The Board has inbetween approved these recommendations and they will be published in the European Heart Journal in the near future.

Appendix

ESC task force members

R. Brennecke (Mainz)
O. Hess (Zürich)
B. Meier (Bern)
H. Reiber (Leiden)
R. Simon (Kiel, chairman)
C. Zeelenberg (Leiden)

ESC task force subcommittee members

I. Azancot (Paris)
P. de Feyter (Rotterdam)

P. Doriot (Geneva)
E. Fleck (Berlin)
P. Oriol (Barcelona)
O. Ratib (Geneva)
A. Rickards (London)
W. Rutishauser (Geneva)
J. Willems (Leiden)
T. Leclerque (CGR/Ge)
D. Heppe (Eigen)
P. Hellot (Hellige)
J. Könnigeit (Hewlett Packard)
G. Weiss (Kontron)
B. van Meurs (Philips)
G. Haufe (Siemens)
U. Stöcker (Toshiba)

References

1. Simon R. The filmless catheterization laboratory: when will it be reality? In Reiber JHC, Serruys PW (eds): Advances in quantitative coronary arteriography. Dordrecht: Kluwer Academic Publishers 1993: 113–22.
2. Simon RW. Interventional cardiology: the impact of digital imaging. Medica Mundi 1992; 37: 110–4.
3. Tobis JM. The future of digital angiography. Cathet Cardiovasc Diagn 1992; 27: 14–5.
4. Mattheus R. European standardization efforts: an important framework for medical imaging. Eur J Radiol 1993; 17: 28–37.

8. Which media are most likely to solve the archival problem?

JACK T. CUSMA & THOMAS M. BASHORE

Summary

Realization of the full potential of quantitative angiographic methods requires the replacement of cinefilm as the angiographic procedure record. The replacement must possess the same capabilities and functions which cinefilm presently provides: display, transport and archival. Potential replacement options should also provide portability between institutions and at low cost. A true digital solution would provide immediate access to the results of the angiographic procedure, transfer of image data over digital networks, multiple-user viewing capability, and quantitative analysis on a routine basis for all patients. If a single media cannot provide all the necessary functions, multiple media may need to be employed, i.e. the archival media may not be the portable patient record as well. Separation of the archival function from other functions reduces the demands on a single media and makes the replacement of cinefilm in the near future more probable. A number of archival options are available today: 1) magnetic disks; 2) analog laser optical disks; 3) digital laser optical disks; 4) digital file-based magnetic tape; 5) digital video magnetic tape. In evaluating each of these alternatives, an accounting is required of how each meets the archival requirements along with an approximate breakdown of cost and its readiness for implementation as a clinical solution today.

Introduction

The elimination of 35 mm cinearteriographic film as the recording and archiving medium for coronary arteriographic procedures has been long anticipated. It has become evident, however, that the introduction alone of digital angiographic technology [1, 2] does not justify replacing cinefilm as the permanent patient record. The first implementations of digital angiography did not possess the necessary acquisition and display requirements to replace cinefilm. While this has improved, the cost of providing the capabilities required to record the dynamic information produced in contrast arteriography and ventriculography continue to make replacement of cinefilm prohibitive. Nonetheless, the desire to find 'something better' than cinefilm has grown among cardiologists, technicians, hospital administrators, and researchers [3]. The replacement of cinefilm remains difficult, to a large

J.H.C. Reiber and P.W. Serruys (eds): Progress in quantitative coronary arteriography, 111–126.

degree, because the performance requirements are greater than those for other technology such as that used for storage of computer data. These requirements include high-speed acquisition and display capability, high storage capacity, portability of data, and low cost. The desire to utilize the data in a digital format, allowing for the integration of the patient angiographic record with the hospital information system (HIS), transport of images over computer networks, and the application of quantitative analytical methods complicates the task as well [4].

Replacement of cinefilm first requires the definition and separation of its functions, e.g. acquisition and/or display versus image archival. This analysis provides a way to possibly provide the functional requirements through the use of multiple media. Such an approach may increase the probability that these functions are provided in the near future and at an economical cost. For the purposes of this paper, therefore, the archival of cardiac angiographic data will be treated as a separate function from cinefilm's other capabilities. This issue will be emphasized below as each of the potential replacements are discussed in order to assess which media are most suitable for specific needs.

Requirements for a cine replacement

Performance requirements

The basic requirements that must be met by any media which replaces cinefilm as the patient record in the cardiac catheterization laboratory have been established through thirty years of use in a variety of clinical environments [5]:

- *High acquisition rate* – Images are acquired during a cardiac catheterization procedure at rates of 15 to 60 frames/s, with 25 and 30 frames/s being most common. Since most observers agree that the minimum equivalent resolution required corresponds to an image matrix of $512 \times 512 \times 8$ bits [6], this corresponds to an acquisition rate of 7.5 Mbytes/s but it may be as high as 60 Mbytes/s (if a matrix of 1024×1024 is found desirable).
- *Large storage capacity* – The total amount of data required to store a single procedure corresponds to 50–100 seconds of images or approximately 600 Mbytes of digital data (at the smallest matrix size). A patient volume of approximately 1500 examinations annually per laboratory would require 900 Gbytes of storage per laboratory per year. In a large institution with multiple labs, this number may be as high as 4000–5000 Gbytes of data per year. The requirement for ready access to patients' data for a period of 5–10 years means that a total of 3,000 Gbytes (for a small-volume laboratory) to 50,000 Gbytes of storage must be available.
- *Dynamic display of images* – Cinefilm provides a continuous real-time

display required for diagnosis of cardiovascular disease; the detection of abnormalities in ventricular function and detection of coronary artery stenoses require such display. In digital terms, this translates to the same value of 7.5–30 Mbytes/s as mentioned above. The cinefilm projectors and viewers currently used to provide this function also provide real-time direction changes, rapid magnification, and brightness adjustment.
- *Portability of images* – Arguably the most valuable capability possessed by cinefilm is its portability between institutions. The widespread availability and standardized use of cinefilm viewers make it straightforward to transfer angiographic data among institutions. The cinefilm record is also transferred from the acquisition laboratories to central analysis laboratories in multi-center clinical trials used to evaluate new technologies and therapies.
- *Low cost per patient* – The cost required to provide all the above functions is approximately $70–100 per patient. In digital terms, the 600 Mbyte digital equivalent of one patient's data translates to a cost of approximately $0.16 per Mbyte which typically includes the costs of short-term and long-term storage as well. The cost of any replacement should be approximately the same.

The increasing use of computer networks in and between hospitals requires a means for transporting patient demographic data and procedure results throughout a hospital and over inter-institution networks. A cine replacement will need to interface to these data networks, making it feasible to display angiographic data at multiple stations (simultaneously) within a hospital without the physical transport required for cinefilm. Since this may involve numerous repeated displays of the data, it is important that there be minimal loss or degradation of the angiographic data. A related requirement for the cine replacement is the ability to perform quantitative analysis of the angiographic images in order to provide an objective and reproducible method for diagnostic assessment [7, 8].

Reviewing the functions listed and described above, one can group them into the categories shown in Table 8.1: 1) acquisition; 2) display/review; 3) transfer; 4) archive. Such grouping is helpful in evaluating media options to determine their suitability as a cine replacement. While no single media choice will fall into all categories, some media may fall into multiple categories. For reference, Table 8.2 shows the characteristic value for cinefilm of each parameter listed in Table 8.1. In order to truly replace cine, one or more media must be used which deliver all categories of functions and which meet or exceed the parameter values provided by cinefilm.

Data format

The rapid advances in computer and imaging technologies which have taken place in the last decade have accustomed users to the availability of increasing

Table 8.1. Cine function groups.

Parameter	Acquisition	Display/Review	Transfer	Archive
Fast transfer speed	V	V	D	N
Large storage capacity	N	D	N	V
Standard format	N	N	V	D
High resolution	V	V	V	V
Low cost/patient	D	D	V	V
Random access	V	V	D	D
Unit record	N	N	V	D
Long lifetime	N	N	V	V
Digital data	V	D	D	D
Compatible with computer formats	N	D	D	D
Quantitative analysis	V	V	D	D

Key: V = very important, D = desirable, N = not important.

Table 8.2. Performance characteristics of Cinefilm.

Parameter	Measurement	Data equivalent
Transfer speed	60 frames/s	15 Mbytes/s
Storage capacity	100 seconds	1.5 Gbytes[1]
Standard format	Yes	–
Spatial resolution	2.5–3 1p/mm[2]	.18 mm pixel
Cost	$100	$.01/Mbyte
Random access	No	–
Unit record	Yes	–
Lifetime	10 years	–
Digital data format	No	–
Computer format	No	–
Quantitative analysis	Some – requires digitization	–

Notes

[1] Assuming 60 frames/sec at 1024 × 1024 × 8 bit.

[2] Typically achieved in patients, e.g. with 15 cm image intensifier mode.

levels of performance at ever decreasing cost. In addition, the many cited advantages of digital image data [9] have led to an increasing degree of acceptance and expectation that such capabilities will become available in the short-term. These advantages of digital angiographic data include: 1) immediate access to image data; 2) real-time image enhancement, such as zoom, pan, contrast and brightness enhancement, and edge enhancement; 3) application of automated quantitative analysis; 4) integration with other digital image modality data; 5) integration with digitized physiological data; 6) capability for data transfer via existing computer networks and phone lines.

Most catheterization laboratories have had experience with digital data and this has raised the expectations that, if film is to be eliminated, all of the above advantages will be available immediately and at a lesser cost than with film. Such expectations are as yet not justified so some laboratories have chosen an intermediate path. In this approach, a replacement for cinefilm has been utilized which stores data not in a digital format which can be directly input to digital processing and communications equipment but, instead, in an analog form which requires an additional conversion step to make the information available for such processing. Two examples are the use of standard analog videotape and the use of analog optical disks. The advantage of the analog approach is that the necessary acquisition and display rates, along with capacity, are available today at a reasonable cost. Issues which arise when discussing storage of image data in analog format are the degree of degradation of the data following repeated display and multiple copies and the degradation in image quality during the conversion process used to transfer the analog image data to a digital format. The amount of weighting accorded to such considerations depends on the needs of the individual laboratory and possible legal concerns. The unsuitability of standard analog videotape for providing multiple copies of adequate quality and for long-term data integrity make it a poor choice as the sole cine replacement [10]; the analog optical disk, however, does not suffer from the same disadvantages [11] and is discussed below along with other digital media choices.

Standardization efforts

Several efforts have been initiated to ensure that any media chosen to replace cinefilm delivers all of the functions listed above with no loss of performance. The intent of these efforts is also to assure that manufacturers of diagnostic imaging equipment do not force customers to select proprietary options for image storage which may not be compatible with equipment belonging to another institution. In this way, the portability of patient data will be assured as we enter the cine-less era. One example of these efforts underway in the United States is a collaboration between the American College of Cardiology (ACC) and the National Electronics Manufacturer's Association (NEMA). The ACC has joined a collaborative effort begun by NEMA and the American College of Radiology (ACR) to standardize the format and transmission protocols for digital medical images through a Digital Imaging and Communications in Medicine (DICOM) standard. Previous DICOM efforts, underway since 1982, did not address issues unique to cardiology and the ACC participation is intended to ensure that manufacturers of archival equipment for cardiac procedures have a standard set of requirements so that all future purchasers of such equipment can retain the same compatibility and exchange capability characteristic of cinefilm today. Similar efforts for the development of guidelines are underway under the auspices of the European Society for Cardiology (ESC).

The focus of the ACC/NEMA efforts, begun by Working Groups in early

1993, will be to extend the existing DICOM Standard to meet the needs of the cardiology community. In brief, these efforts have two major objectives:

- The selection (from existing technologies) of a physical media which can serve as a suitable *exchange* media for interchange of digital angiographic data between institutions;
- The definition of a library of cardiac angiographic data objects which serve to identify such data uniquely and which, combined with the chosen exchange media will ensure compatibility of image data between institutions.

It is evident from the description of these initial tasks that the Working Groups *will not* attempt to establish a *single* standard for an image archival media. This is in part because: (1) the technology itself is changing rapidly; (2) it is felt that manufacturers should not be restricted from developing alternative methods for archiving image data; (3) the issue of data exchange is considered a higher priority to the cardiology community. Establishment of a standard means of interchange will reassure purchasers of archiving equipment that, regardless of the vendor they choose or the specific archival media used by that vendor, there will be a means for translating from their archival system to a format and onto a media which can be interpreted at *any other* laboratory. The only remaining concern for the laboratory is that the archival system they use does possess such a translation capability; at this time the majority of vendors of such equipment are committed to supporting a standard once established.

Media options for image archival

There exists a variety of media choices available today which have the technical capability for providing archival of cardiac procedures. These choices can be grouped into three major categories as shown in Table 8.3: (1) Magnetic disks; (2) Optical disks; (3) Magnetic tape. Each of these categories is further subdivided in the following discussion of their relative advantages and disadvantages; in assessing each of the technologies, the extent to which they meet the technical requirements listed in Tables 8.1 and 8.2 is discussed.

Magnetic disks

Magnetic digital disks have been the media of choice for storage of computer data for decades and, as their costs have decreased and their data transfer rates have increased, they have become a common fixture in the cardiac catheterization laboratory. Most of the manufacturers of digital angiography equipment include a parallel transfer (Winchester) disk to acquire digital data at rates up to 30 Mbytes/s. As seen from the list of their technical

Table 8.3. Media choices for Cine replacement.

Magnetic disks	Optical disks	Magnetic tape
(1) Parallel transfer disks	(1) Analog optical disks	(1) Computer data
(2) RAIDS's	(2) Digital optical disks	3490
	WORM	8 mm, 4 mm
	Rewritable	(2) Digital video
		D2 D3
		DD2 DD3

Table 8.4. Characteristics of disk storage.

Parameter	Magnetic	Analog optical	Digital optical
Transfer speed	30 frames/s	30 frames/s	2 frames/s
Storage capacity	800 Mbytes	40 minutes	600 Mbytes
Standard format	No	No	No
Spatial resolution	>2.5 lp/mm	>2.5 lp/mm	>2.5 lp/mm
Cost per patient	$30,000	$10	$150
Random access	Yes	Yes	Yes
Unit record	Yes	Yes	Yes
Lifetime	>10 years	>10 years	>10 years
Digital data	Yes	No	Yes
Computer format	Yes	Requires conversion	Yes
Quantitative analysis	Yes	Requires conversion	Yes

capabilities (Table 8.4), magnetic disks meet many of the technical demands required for an archival cine-replacement, along with most of the requirements for dynamic display. Typical parallel transfer disks provide storage capacity for 1,600 to 24,000 angiographic frames, 400–6,000 Mbytes worth of data, or from less than one to as many as eight patients' worth of procedure data. A serious disadvantage of magnetic disks, however, is the high cost required to produce these capabilities – an approximate cost of $30,000 per Gbyte of data capacity is obviously unsuitable for an archive but is quite suitable for a temporary storage device from which the image data can be transferred to an interchange or archival device. One example of how magnetic disks might be utilized is shown in Figure 8.1 where Redundant Arrays of Interchangeable Disks (RAID) arrays are used to provide short-term storage and display of images which are downloaded to much more economical (and possibly slower) devices at the end of the case.

Optical disks

Driven by technical improvements in the entertainment and the computer industry, optical disk technology has recently begun to make its presence felt as well in the cardiac catheterization laboratory. There are two choices available for storage of angiographic data – analog optical and digital optical

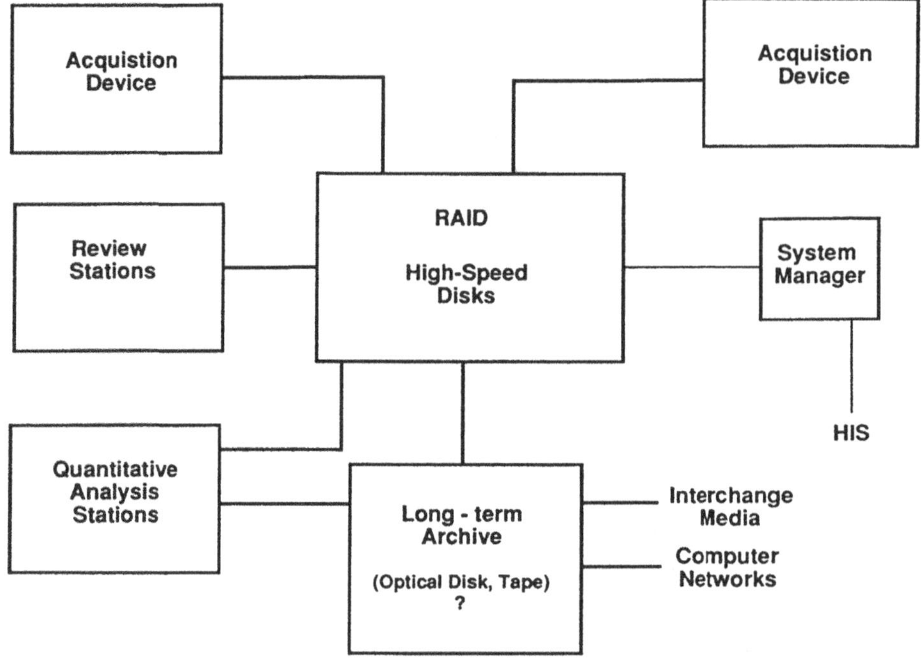

Figure 8.1. Schematic diagram of a modular approach for the replacement of cinefilm in the cardiac catheterization laboratory. In the scheme shown, high speed Redundant Arrays of Inexpensive Disks (RAID) provide acquisition and short-term storage and a separate archive system is utilized for long-term storage.

disks. The use of laser optical disks, or videodisks, which store standard video images by means of analog recording techniques dates back nearly two decades to the first introduction of pre-recorded media. In this type of recording an analog waveform, such as the voltage waveform displayed on a video monitor, is written to an optical platter with the use of a laser; the reversal of the process enables the image data on the disk to be displayed on standard video monitors. With current technology, summarized in Table 8.4, up to 40 minutes of video information can be stored on a single platter, corresponding to approximately 25 patients.

As shown in Table 8.4, analog optical disks provide real-time display at a relatively low cost, on the order of $10 per patient. Among the disadvantages to the technology are that, to keep the cost per patient that low, images for many patients have to reside on a single physical piece of media, restricting access to the piece to a single user. The optical disk itself, therefore, cannot serve as the patient unit record, suitable for interchange; instead, some type of additional duplication or transfer is required. Another potential disadvantage of this technology is the intrinsic analog format of the waveform stored on the optical disk. Even though the original image data may have been in a digital format on the acquisition device, the only way to record it onto the optical disk is to convert it to analog and, conversely, the only way to access the data from the optical disk is via analog means. Among the consequences of this limitation are the possibility that data stored on disk may include the effects of post-acquisition image enhancement techniques such as edge enhancement, contrast changes and zooming. In that regard, therefore, the data stored on optical disk may not be representative of the original data. In a related issue, performance of quantitative analysis requires the re-digitization of the image data, with the potential for the introduction of additional noise to the image. Since the output video will reflect the effects of the enhancement present at the input, quantitative analysis may produce results different from those which might be obtained from original or 'raw' data.

The more recent digital optical disk technology avoids the disadvantages listed above for the analog optical disk. As shown in Table 8.4, the capacity of a piece of media makes it feasible as an individual patient record, and the digital format of the data means that the original form of the angiographic data can be preserved. Similarly, existence of data in a digital format allows the transfer of data directly into computers and over networks for quantitative analysis. The disadvantages of digital optical disk technology at this time include acquisition and display rates which, without extensive data compression, do not meet the requirements in Table 8.2. Several applications use data compression to store more data on a single piece of media and/or to allow faster transfer rates to display devices [12]. At present, the issue of the degree of acceptable data compression for medical image storage remains unresolved. Some preliminary reports indicate that the use of lossy compression, i.e. where original data cannot be perfectly recovered, can be applied to coronary angiograms with minimal effects on either visual assessment or quantitative assessment [13, 14]. In one hybrid application, the original data is stored completely uncompressed and a second copy of the data is stored with a significant amount of compression to allow rapid viewing of the angiographic sequences. Major drawbacks to the digital optical disk at this time are its inability to acquire the original data without compression and a relatively high cost for the media – in the range of $100 per patient exam. It may be a viable choice if the media cost drops but it may find utility sooner in combination with one of the other available technologies.

Magnetic tape

The long-standing use of magnetic tape formats to store computer data and to record video images make them a contender for selection as a cine replacement. The wide array of implementations of magnetic tape storage also leads to a certain degree of confusion because it is difficult to separate and distinguish the different data formats, sizes, most common uses, etc. A

Table 8.5. Characteristics of magnetic tape storage.

	Computer		Broadcast	
Parameter	3490	8 mm	D2	DD3
Transfer speed	3 Mbytes/s	<1 Mbyte/s	15 Mbytes/s	15 Mbytes/s
Storage capacity	800 Mbytes	1.0 Gbyte	25 Gbytes	10 Gbytes
Standard format	No	No	Yes	?
Spatial resolution	>2.5 lp/mm	>2.5 lp/mm	>2.5 lp/mm	>2.5 lp/mm
Cost/patient	$10.00	$3.00	$2.00	$2.00
Random access	Yes	Yes	Yes	Yes
Unit record	Yes	Yes	No	No
Lifetime	>10 years	>10 years	>10 years	>10 years
Digital data	Yes	Yes	Yes	Yes
Computer format	Yes	Yes	?	?
Quantitative analysis	Yes	Yes	?	?

related characteristic of magnetic tape is that, since they have been originally intended for a purpose other than medical imaging, some degree of accommodation is required to adapt them to the medical application. As shown in Table 8.5, the tape choices can be grouped according to their original intended use, the two major categories being as a computer storage device and for digital recording in the television industry. The requirements of those two industries overlap to a degree with those necessary for cine replacement, i.e. low cost, high transfer rate and high capacity. In addition, both applications require that the data be available for retrieval for extended lengths of time, to as long as 15 years, similar to the need in medical imaging.

Among the storage media options which are heavily utilized for computer data storage, three which have achieved acceptance as a cine archive media are the 3490 1/2 inch tape format and the 8 mm and 4 mm tape formats used for data backup. As shown in Table 8.5, these formats provide a large storage capacity, from one up to 10 patients' worth of data, at an economical cost, on the order of less than $10 per patient. In addition to a low cost for media, the record/retrieve device is also inexpensive. None of these media, however, are capable of attaining the necessary acquisition and display rates listed in Table 8.2 in the absence of some degree of data compression. The digital computer data tape formats, therefore, may be a very appropriate long-term option for storage and/or transfer in combination with other media for acquisition and display. Several vendors are pursuing that development philosophy as either an interim or long-term solution.

A recent development from the broadcast television industry is that of digital videotape for storage, display, and editing of standard television video data [15]. As shown in the table, these tape formats, known as D2 and D3 possess a high acquisition and display rate, a large media capacity and a low price per patient. The digital formats assure that there is no degradation of data with multiple play and that multiple identical copies are possible. While the cost of the tapes is low enough to allow their use as an exchange media, this would require that both the sending and receiving lab possess a special D2 or D3 recorder. Despite the fact that these formats (especially the D2) have become accepted as standards in the television industry, the cost of a drive remains fairly high, on the order of $40–50,000 per drive. Similarly, a special interface is required to link with the often proprietary formats of digital acquisition devices if a direct digital transfer is desired, and a similar interface is required for transfer to a computer format for analysis or transport over computer networks. Like the computer storage tapes listed above, these media may be best utilized in combination with another interchange media which may establish itself as a standard.

A recent hybrid development combines the best attributes of the computer storage industry and the broadcast industry to develop a form of the D2 and D3 formats used for recording of digital video data to store data in a file format similar to that employed with the data backup tapes described above. While this technology, known as DD2 and DD3, remains several years away, it would combine the advantages of both including high transfer rate, high capacity, and low cost while not having the disadvantage of the digital video format of being restricted to a specific file format.

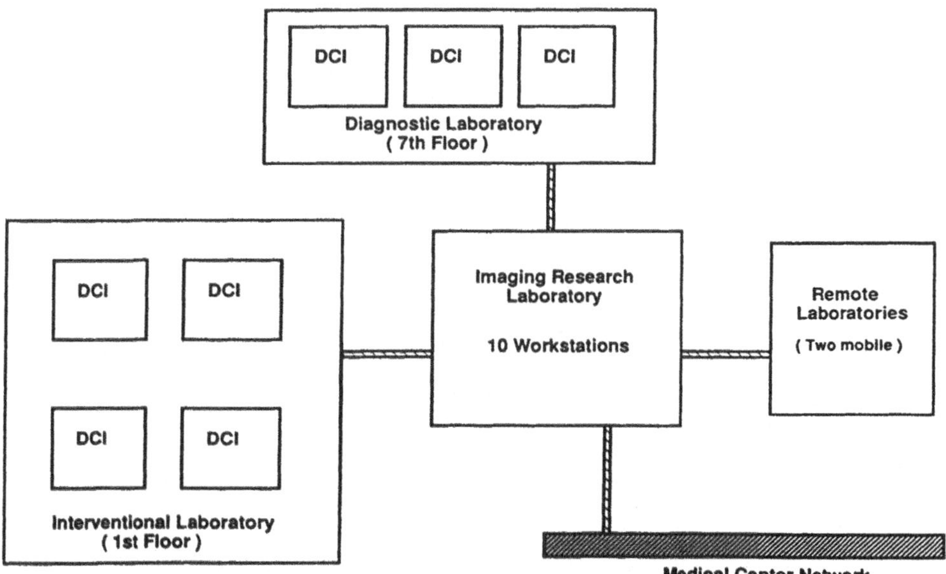

Figure 8.2. Schematic diagram of the existing environment in the Duke University Catheterization Laboratories depicting the relationship between the angiographic procedure laboratories and related clinical and research resources.

Implementation of a digital image network and library

One approach to the selection of a digital replacement for cine is demonstrated with a system being implemented at Duke University Medical Center. In making the media selection the factors considered were the number of catheterization laboratories and the capabilities of the existing angiographic equipment, the patient volume, and the future needs of our laboratory and institution. Following an analysis of such factors, available technology was evaluated and the D2 digital video format was selected for a digital archival system [16].

As shown in Figure 8.2, the necessary acquisition, display and short-term storage exist on digital angiography devices in each of seven laboratories. The patient volume of 7,000 patients per year meant a requirement for storage of 3500 Gbytes of data per year and access for up to 20,000 Gbytes. In addition, there was the need for interface to an extensive network of analysis workstations and to a long-standing patient database. A special interface was designed and constructed to transfer digital images into a digital Cardiac Acquisition Station (CAS) from which all of a patient's images are transferred to the central library (LMS) at real-time rates. The LMS has a total on-site storage capacity of 20,000 procedures of *uncompressed* image data. Multiple players in the LMS can be allocated to send images to remote cardiac review stations (CRS) for display or to analysis workstations for performance of quantitative analysis.

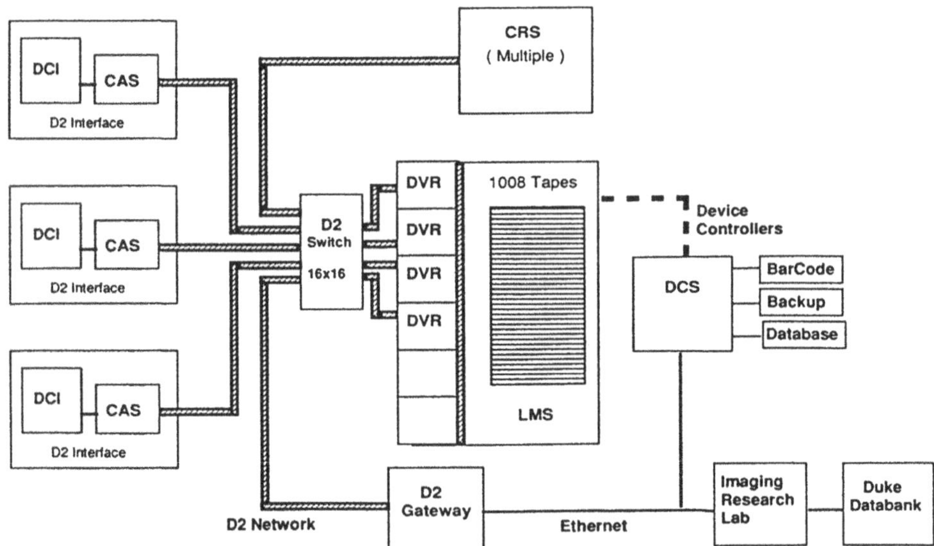

Figure 8.3. Initial phase in the implementation of a high speed, high capacity digital image archive and network at Duke University. Shown in the diagram are the interconnections between the central storage library and the acquisition and research laboratories.

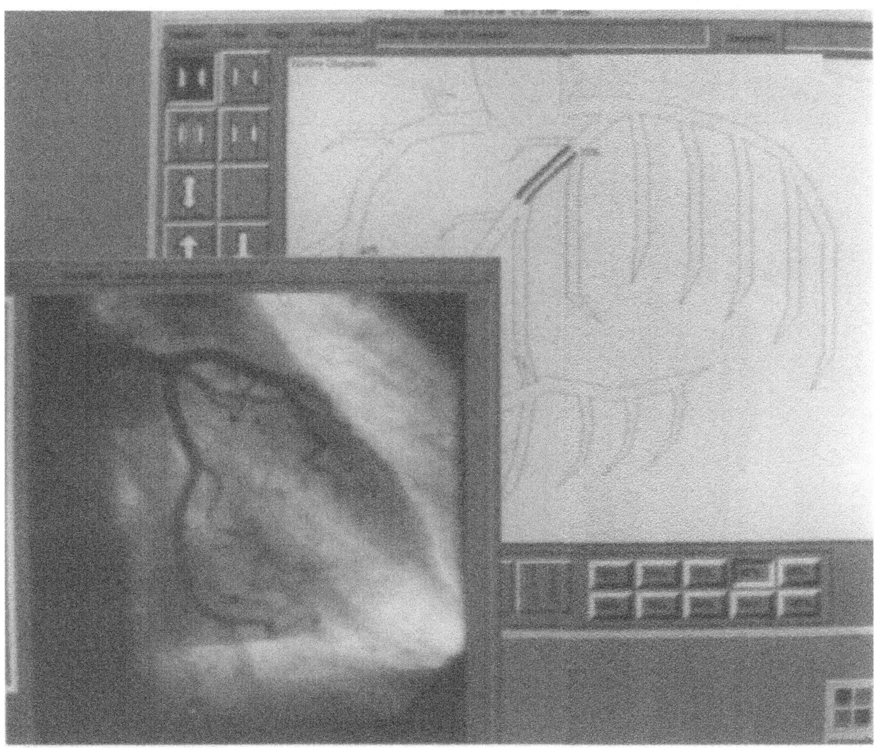

Figure 8.4. Coronary artery diagramming and reporting system used to depict the results of a catheterization procedure. Digital image files are viewed while the anatomical diagram is generated and can be retrieved via the diagram.

The first phase of the implementation, shown in Figure 8.3, includes three clinical catheterization laboratories and three remote CRS stations for diagnostic review. An image gateway provides a means for transfer of images into the network of existing analysis stations. An extensive effort has been underway in our laboratory to develop a system of computer hardware and software for application of image processing and analysis methods as well as the implementation of a relational database and an automated reporting system. Among the applications in clinical and research use, a Coronary Tree Diagramming and Reporting System [17] utilizes a graphical interface to generate a patient-specific diagram of the coronary anatomy. An interface links the laboratory database with the digital image database in the LMS, enabling users to access digital angiographic sequences from the LMS for viewing in parallel with the generation of a Tree (Figure 8.4). This, in turn, eliminates the need for cinefilm viewing prior to generation of the Tree diagram.

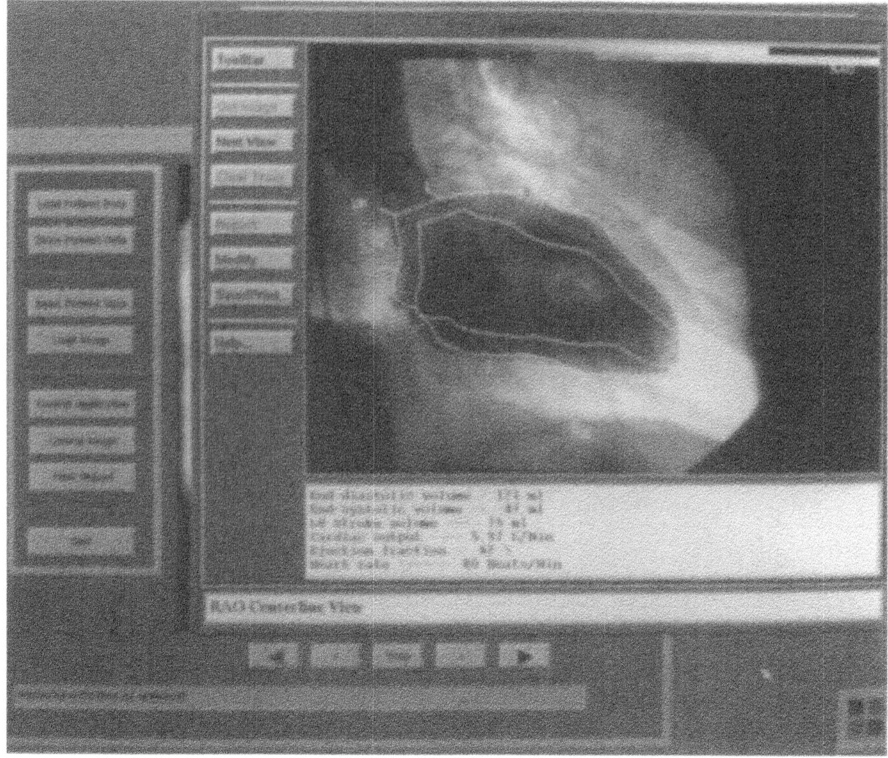

Figure 8.5. Example of a results screen from the left ventricular analysis program in use at Duke University. Results of volume and wall motion calculations are stored in a relational database for generation of reports and retrieval over a local area network (LAN).

Quantitative analysis methods applied to angiographic images in the research and clinical laboratory setting also include ventricular analysis (Figure 8.5) and quantitative coronary angiography (Figure 8.6). These algorithms will be applied to image sequences retrieved from the LMS by accessing the system database and, in turn, the analysis results will be included in the automated report. While the analysis methods have been used in a large number of research studies, their extension to routine use on clinical images for all patients requires fast and easy access to all coronary angiograms. The combination of the digital library, the image network, and the relational database provides the capability required to perform quantitative analysis on all patients on a routine basis, thus achieving the potential which has been promised for digital angiography and quantitative methods.

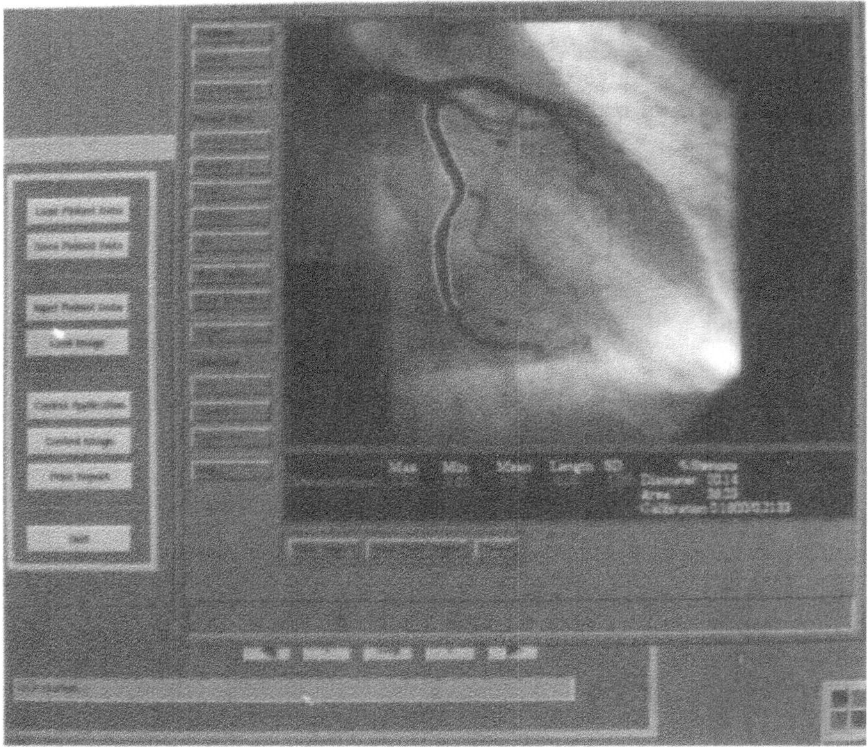

Figure 8.6. Quantitative coronary angiography (QCA) software interfaced to the image and patient database utilized for the analysis system.

Conclusions

The long awaited arrival of a single media as the replacement for cinefilm recording in coronary angiography remains an elusive goal. A number of options do exist, however, which in combination may be suitable for filling the multiple roles served by cinefilm. With an appropriate and thorough analysis of the needs of a specific laboratory or institution, an archival solution can be selected from one of these options. As a standard interchange format becomes established, purchasers of archival system today will be assured that the interchange of data among laboratories will continue unimpeded. For those users who continue to await the arrival of a single media which meets all their needs and desires, its arrival remains most likely several years away.

Acknowledgements

The authors acknowledge the assistance of Cathey Teater and Debbie Riley in the preparation of this manuscript.

References

1. Kruger RA, Mistretta CA, Houk TL *et al.* Computerized fluoroscopy in real time for noninvasive visualization of the cardiovascular system. Radiology 1979; 130: 49–57.
2. Brennecke R, Brown TK, Bürsch JH, Heintzen PH. Computerized video image preprocessing with applications to cardio-angiographic roentgen-image series. In Nagel HH (ed): Digitale Bildverarbeitung. Berlin: Springer 1977; 244–62.
3. Morris KG. A perspective: designing the all digital cardiac catheterization laboratory. Am J Card Imaging 1988; 2: 251–8.
4. Brennecke R, Lang M, Fritsch JP, Erbel R, Meyer J. A framework for PACS development in cardiology. Comput Cardiol 1992: 259–61.
5. Sones FM Jr, Shirey EK, Proudfit WL, Westcott RN. Cine-coronary arteriography [abstract]. Circulation 1959; 20: (Suppl): 773.
6. Mistretta CA, Peppler WW. Digital cardiac x-ray imaging: fundamental principles. Am J Card Imaging 1988; 2: 26–39.
7. Mancini GBJ. Digital coronary angiography: advantages and limitations. In Reiber JHC, Serruys PW (eds): Quantitative coronary arteriography. Dordrecht: Kluwer Academic Publishers 1991: 23–42.
8. Reiber JHC, Serruys PW. Quantitative coronary angiography. In Marcus ML, Skorton DJ, Schelbert HR, Wolf GL (eds): Cardiac imaging. Philadelphia: Saunders 1991: 211–80.
9. Whiting JS. Physical principles and instrumentation in digital angiography. In Marcus ML, Skorton DJ, Schelbert HR, Wolf GL (eds): Cardiac imaging. Philadelphia: Saunders 1991: 281–94.
10. Gray JE, Wondrow MA, Smith HC, Holmes DR Jr. Technical considerations for cardiac laboratory high-definition video systems. Cathet Cardiovasc Diagn 1984; 10: 73–86.
11. Browne J. The recordable laser videodisc: a technical perspective. SMPTE 1988; 97: 4–7.
12. Rabbani M, Jones PW. Image compression techniques for medical diagnostic imaging systems. J Digit Imaging 1991; 4: 65–78.
13. Whiting J, Eckstein M, Honig D, Gu S, Einav S, Eigler N. Effect of lossy image compression on observer performance in dynamically displayed digital coronary angiograms [abstract]. Circulation 1992; 86 (4 Suppl): I444.
14. Wondrow MA, Wegwerth PJ, Mitchell MP, Gilbert BK. A study of medical image data-compression. SMPTE 1993; 102: 9–13.
15. Engberg E, Brush R, Lemoine M *et al.* The composite digital format and its applications. SMPTE 1987; 96: 934–42.
16. Cusma JT, Spero LA, Groshong BR, Cho T, Bashore TM. Design and evaluation of a high capacity digital image archival library and high speed network for the replacement of cinefilm in the cardiac angiography environment. Proc SPIE, Medical Imaging VII. In press.
17. Hermiller JH, Cusma JT, Spero LA, Fortin DT, Harding MB, Bashore TM. Quantitative and qualitative coronary angiographic analysis: review of methods, utility, and limitations. Cathet Cardiovasc Diagn 1992; 25: 110–31.
18. Spero LA, Fortin DF, Cusma JT, Bashore TM. A distributed user-friendly coronary artery diagramming and reporting system [abstract]. J Am Coll Cardiol 1992; 19 (3 Suppl A): 6a.

PART THREE

Intracoronary pressure, coronary blood flow and flow reserve

9. Control and mechanics of the coronary circulation

JOS A.E. SPAAN

Summary

The determinants of coronary blood flow are coronary arterial pressure and coronary resistance. Coronary resistance is made up on the one hand by resistance of the small arteries and arterioles being subjected to local and nervous control mechanisms and on the other hand by the effect of contraction on the intramyocardial micro vessels. Normally there is much room for increasing blood flow, the so-called coronary reserve. Coronary flow is adjusted to the need of the myocardium. Increasing resistance by compression of micro vessels is also compensated by vasodilatation. However, when coronary flow is compromised by a stenosis the contraction impediment of flow may become a dominant factor. The interpretation of coronary hemodynamic data should be done with the recognition of its dynamic nature. Coronary vasomotor tone may change coronary flow in seconds. Additionally, the compliant nature of the myocardial microcirculation makes that pressure and flow in the coronary arteries are rarely in equilibrium also not in prolonged diastoles.

Introduction

With increasing miniaturization of instruments allowing the measurement of flow and pressure in human coronaries and progress in acquiring and processing images related to perfusion of the myocardium it becomes important for the cardiologist to understand the meaning of all this information. The perfusion of the heart has been studied for centuries [1]. However, the basic scientists are still struggling with the concepts by which mechanics, distribution and control of coronary flow are best explained. The major illness of the coronary system is arterial narrowing. Fortunately, not a lot of physics is needed to understand that such narrowing is detrimental for myocardial perfusion. The conclusion that one should be aiming to abolish this obstruction is obvious. However, with small vessel obstructions, interventions become more difficult and a physiological measure of the function of the coronary arterial tree is desired. This chapter will attempt to pinpoint to the physiological properties that are relevant to understand the measurements on myocardial perfusion.

In outlining the different phenomena important for the interpretation of

J.H.C. Reiber and P.W. Serruys (eds): Progress in quantitative coronary arteriography, 129–140.

data on coronary blood flow it is important to appreciate that most mechanisms interact. As will be explained below, heart contraction does impede myocardial perfusion, which is normally compensated for by a system that controls smooth muscle tone in the resistance vessels. The same holds for the addition of a coronary narrowing by atherosclerosis. However, if added resistance is too large, the control system will be exhausted and part of the myocardium perfused by the obstructed branch will be hampered in mechanical performance. This will have an indirect effect on the flow through the remaining part of the myocardium. Oxygen consumption there will increase, which is a stimulus to increase flow. However, most probably the mechanical impediment of flow will increase in this part of the muscle as well.

In this chapter we will outline the different mechanics of coronary blood flow separately as they are understood from basic research. In the end it will be attempted to indicate their interrelationships which form pitfalls for interpretation.

Coronary blood flow control

Static behavior

Under static behavior one understands the relationships between the variables under equilibrium conditions. In this case the dependent variable is coronary blood flow and the independent variables are myocardial oxygen consumption and coronary arterial pressure. In general, two characterizations of coronary flow control are distinguished; autoregulation and metabolic adaptation [2]. Autoregulation is the ability of the heart to maintain perfusion at a certain level independent of perfusion pressure. Metabolic adaptation refers to the ability of the heart to match flow to the oxygen of the heart at a constant perfusion pressure. It is sometimes suggested that these two phenomena are the result of separate control mechanisms. Especially the myogenic mechanism is held responsible for autoregulation since this response of single arterioles may reduce arteriolar diameter as a response to a pressure increase. Additionally, metabolic adaptation is regarded as a servo system. Some metabolic signal would then be telling the resistance vessels how much tone is needed to provide the myocardium with sufficient flow. However, autoregulation and metabolic adjustment can not be independent since the effector of flow control is the same for the two processes. Hence there must be interaction between the two.

Static control of blood flow can best be understood on the basis of a model by which tissue oxygen pressure is the controlled variable. In the model it is assumed that a decrease in tissue oxygen pressure provides a stimulus for vasodilatation. This stimulus should not be regarded as an anoxic stimulus since the control systems works under normoxic conditions. Moreover, it has been demonstrated in conscious animal experiments with trained dogs that coronary sinus PO2 may decrease below normal levels during exercise [4]. Metabolic adaptation is understood from the model. An increase in oxygen

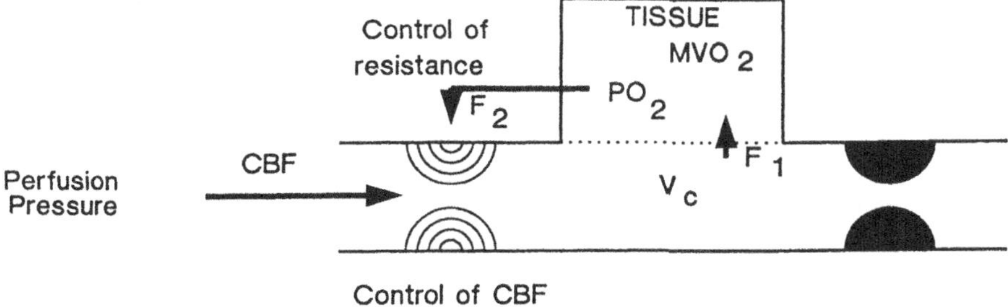

Figure 9.1. Tissue oxygen pressure model. The tissue is represented as one compartment. Tissue oygen pressure is determined by the balance of supply and demand. Control of coronary flow is assumed to be the result of tissue oxygen pressure and resistance vessels. A decrease in tissue oxygen pressure as a result of increase in MVO_2 or decrease in perfusion pressure results in vasodilation. The model predicts the steady state control behavior of coronary flow discussed in relation to Figure 9.2 (redrawn from [3]).

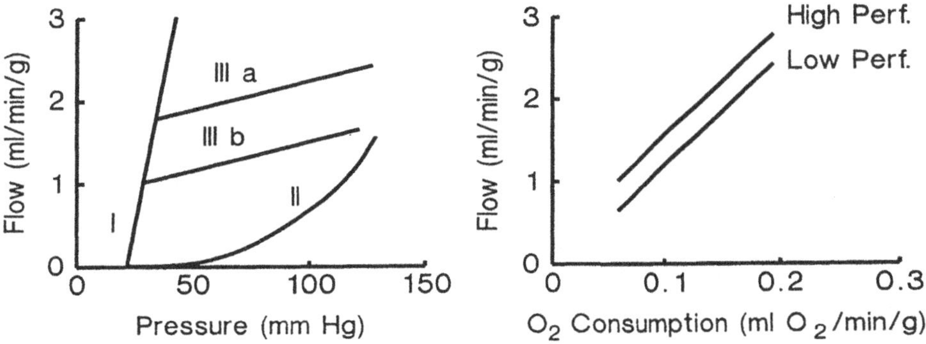

Figure 9.2. Left panel: different modi of coronary pressure flow relations; I symbolizes complete vasodilation when flow depends linearly on pressure. II Maximal constriction. This is a hypothetical curve since metabolism of the myocardium is always such that the bed is in some vasodilated state. III a and IIIb symbolize autoregulation curves at different levels of oxygen consumption. Right panel: relationships between flow and oxygen consumption. Note that these relationships depend on the level of perfusion pressure (redrawn from [5]).

consumption will first result in a decrease of tissue oxygen pressure. As a response the arterioles will dilate and blood flow will increase until the decrease in tissue oxygen pressure is compensated for. A similar reasoning holds for the response to a decrease in arterial pressure. This will first reduce coronary blood flow and consequently tissue oxygen pressure. Hence, a reduction of arterial pressure will also result in vasodilatation and an increase of flow

It should be appreciated that restoration of tissue oxygen pressure will never be perfect since, as is often the case with feedback systems, a so-called error signal is required as driving force for the controller, in this case the arteriolar resistance. The predictions of the model are for normal metabolic circumstances in good agreement with experimental findings on goat, dog and man. The predictions are schematically depicted in Figure 9.2.

Later work of Feigl and coworkers [6, 7] has demonstrated modulating effects of tissue CO_2 and pH. However, under normal circumstances tissue oxygen pressure is the main predictor for coronary blood flow.

Dynamic behavior

Under dynamic behavior is understood the relationships between variables when the system under study is not in equilibrium. In general, the dependent variable will not be steady but vary in time. However, sometimes it happens that the dependent variable seems to be steady under conditions in which the independent variable(s) are varying. Hence, as long as one of the variables, dependent or independent, is not stationary the system behaves dynamically [2].

A dynamic response of the coronary regulatory system is seen when, in an experimental model where the left main coronary artery is perfused artificially, the perfusion pressure or heart rate changes instantaneously [3, 8, 9]. Results of these interventions are shown in Figure 9.3. On the vertical axis the conductance (flow/pressure; the inverse of resistance) is plotted normalized to the static difference between conductance before the intervention, control, and after the new steady state has been established. Pressure and flow were averaged over each heart beat before calculating the conductance.

Both interventions invoke vasodilatory responses. Note, however, that with both interventions a response is seen in opposite direction. This initial response should be interpreted as vasoconstriction since it is the result of mechanical cause. If heart rate is increased the squeeze on the intramyocardial vessels increases, which under some circumstances may result in retrograde arterial flow [10]. With regard to the decrease in perfusion pressure a similar event takes place. The sudden reduction in arterial pressure may result in a temporally back flow but also in an increased resistance, since the vascular diameter will decrease at lower vascular pressure, thereby increasing resistance. These effects on resistance, especially with heart rate changes, are permanent, at least as long as the HR remains elevated. However, vasodilatation will compensate for this effect. Hence, the vasodilation at increased heart rate does not only compensate for the increased oxygen demand but also for this added resistance.

The response to a decreased perfusion pressure exhibits an overshoot which is evidence for a very rapid responding subsystem within the coronary flow control system especially active when pressure is reduced. In the end the dominating subsystem, probably linking the arteriolar resistance to tissue oxygen pressure, dominates and the overshoot is regulated away.

The dynamic responses of coronary conductance is not always the same.

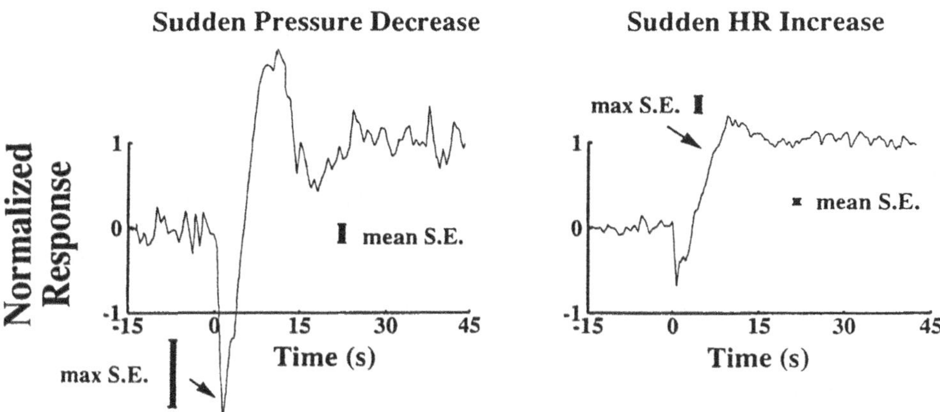

Figure 9.3. Dynamic responses of coronary conductance to an increase in heart rate (right panel) and a decrease in perfusion pressure (left panel) in the dog. The conductance is normalized and as a result they vary from 0 to 1 per definition. The conductances were calculated from pressure and flow signals averaged per beat. The curves are the average responses obtained from 6 dogs.The initial reversed direction of conductance is the consequence of mechanical effects (data from [9]).

Experiments similar to the one from which the results are shown in Figure 9.3 but performed in goats showed slower responses [3, 8]. Moreover, it appeared that the responses to interventions eliciting vasoconstriction were 3 to 4 times slower as those eliciting vasodilatation. Moreover, the rate of response was different when coronary flow was controlled in stead of coronary pressure. The differences between constant flow and constant pressure perfusion can very well be explained by the oxygen control model of Figure 9.1. However, the difference in response to constricting and vasodilatory responses point to control subsystems sensitive to the direction in which the stimulus is changing, inducing constriction or dilation. Moreover, it was shown in the dog that with deteriorating condition because of the duration of the perfusion period the rate of response of the coronary conductance could be reduced by a factor of 4.

Factors involved in coronary flow control

Many factors are known to affect coronary resistance. *Nitrus-oxyde* is released from endothelial cells when coronary flow is increased resulting in vasodilatation. A role for flow induced vasodilatation is not very obvious. If by an error signal flow would increase, vessels would dilate in response and vessels would dilate further, again increasing flow. Hence if flow dependent vasodilatation would be the dominant factor in coronary blood flow control the coronary vessel would always be maximally dilated. It has been suggested that the *myogenic response* plays a role in coronary autoregulation. In case intra-luminal pressure increases a resistance vessel will respond by a decrease in diameter. This indeed is consistent with a contribution to autoregulation since resistance increases with increasing perfusion pressure. However, it is not allowed to extrapolate the behavior of a single vessel segment to that of the coronary arterial tree as a whole. It can be shown that if more than one vessel segment with a myogenic response are put in series the combination of those segments does not exhibit autoregulation [11]. The simple reason for this is that constriction of the first vessel segment will reduce the stimulus for the myogenic response of the more distal segments. *ATP dependent potassium channels* have been put forward as playing an important role in the control of coronary blood flow. However, we recently demonstrated that blockage of these channels by glibenclamide diminishes the rate of response of coronary blood flow by about a factor of 4 to 5, but does not affect the static coronary flow control behavior. *Adenosine* is a potent vasodilatator and endogenously produced. However, when interstitial adenosine is diminished by administering adenosine deaminase control behavior of coronary flow is hardly influenced. *Interstitial free potassium* has only a transient effect on coronary blood flow [12].

The above mentioned mechanisms are all functional in the coronary circulation but cannot be responsible for the final link between tissue oxygen pressure and/or metabolism and coronary vascular tone. However, these mechanisms should work in concert with this yet undefined link. The myogenic response may play an important role in stabilizing the mechanical behavior of blood vessels. For an elastic tube it is impossible to maintain a diameter at constant pressure. The law of Laplace predicts that with increasing pressure the vessel diameter will increase. This effect is known to everyone who has, at one time or another, inflated a balloon. The experience is that it becomes easier and easier to add volume to the balloon as it becomes larger. This normally does not happen to a physiological container without active muscle in the wall, because these walls are reinforced with collagen structures and hence become more stiff when inflated. This reinforcement, however, is of no use when smooth muscle is active. However, the myogenic response compensates for that effect. Hence, the myogenic mechanism in itself does not need to be involved in feedback for control of blood flow.

Flow dependent dilation may play a role in the transmission of the feedback signal from the smallest arterioles to the larger resistance vessels. It is known that coronary resistance is controlled from the smaller arteries in the order of 350 μm down to arterioles of 10 μm [13]. From this array, the smallest arterioles will be best under the influence of local metabolism via the yet unknown factor. Dilation of these smallest vessels will increase flow which induces flow dependent dilation at the larger resistance vessels. Hence, although the larger resistances vessels may be less under the control of tissue factors because of larger diffusion distances, their response will still be determined by these factors

Heart contraction and coronary flow

Another factor important for understanding coronary flow distribution in the myocardium is the effect of heart contraction on flow. Contraction of the heart does impede perfusion which under normal circumstances is compensated for by the control mechanisms described above. However, when the compensating mechanisms are exhausted for compensation of pressure loss over a stenosis in one of the larger arteries, perfusion to a local area is completely dependent on the interplay of perfusion pressure and mechanical impediment. At complete vasodilatation, subendocardial perfusion is strongly heart rate dependent but not supepicardial perfusion. If the heart is arrested, but perfusion pressure maintained, subendocardial flow is 50% higher [14, 15] than subepicardial flow. At a HR = 100 beats/min., the distribution is about even and at HR = 200 beats/min. subendocardial flow has reduced to about 50% of subepicardial flow [16]. Hence, beating of the heart may increase subendocardial resistance by a factor of three. This is seen as the reason why the subendocardium is most vulnerable for ishemia.

The effect of contraction on coronary flow is also apparent from arterial and venous flow being pulsatile. Arterial flow is low in systole an high in diastole. Venous flow is high in systole and low in diastole. Based on observation of arterial flow diastole has been considered as the period in which the myocardium is perfused since arterial flow is high in that phase. The coincidence of high flow and relaxed state of the myocardium was interpreted such that in end-diastole coronary flow would be determined by the vascular bed alone without effect of contraction [17]. However, since coronary venous flow is predominantly systolic, one could also have concluded that systole is the phase of perfusion. In reality diastole and systole cannot be separated. The squeeze of the intramyocardial vascular bed by the contraction results in a periodic changing intramyocardial blood volume. The time constant for changing this volume is in the order of 1.5 s., hence longer than the duration of a heart beat [18].

With respect to the mechanism underlying this impeding effect of cardiac contraction on perfusion there are still uncertainties. The classical concept was based on the idea that tissue pressure within the left ventricular wall would decrease linearly from left ventricular pressure at the endocardium to atmospheric in the subepicardium (e.g. [19, 20]). However, coronary arterial flow is still pulsatile when the heart beats empty [21, 22] and, moreover, the subendocardium is still underperfused when left ventricular pressure is kept zero in a beating heart [23]. The alternative mechanism is the direct effect of myocyte contraction on the intramural vessels. The myocardium is exerting pressure on the filled left ventricular cavity by increasing its elastance [24], so why would this increased stiffness of myocytes in systole not exert a force on the vessels submersed between them. Indeed, Krams [21, 22] and Westerhof [25] demonstrated in series of papers that many observations on coronary flow mechanics can be explained in a way similar to the pump function of the ventricles. However, the main challenge of the elastance concept applied to the coronary circulation is the explanation of the subendo-subepicardial differences. If the effect of contraction on vessels is only determined by local elastance, why would there be a difference? The local mechanical properties of myocytes are not known to be so different.

Recent studies on arterial blood flow patterns and epicardial lymphatic pressure revealed that both pressure transmission and time varying elastance do play a role. In the beginning of systole and diastole the transmission of left ventricular pressure to intramyocardial fluid spaces is good. However, in mid systole the myocardial wall is so stiff that pressure is hardly transmitted and local contraction patterns are dominating the squeeze of the local vessels. [26–28]

It also has been demonstrated that when contractility is diminished locally, blood flow is reduced by an increase of left ventricular pressure. Therefore, under conditions where the myocardium is underperfused at some parts but not at others, the underperfused areas may have a reduced contractility and become very sensitive to the pressure generated by the part of the muscle that is still functioning properly. It was postulated that the stiffer myocardium protects the intramural vessels from collapsing through left ventricular pressure in case the ventricle would not stiffen through increasing elastance. Understanding of this interplay between pressure transmission and myocardial stiffness is important for the perfusion of the heart with local dysfunction.

Diastolic pressure flow lines

As was already touched upon, the classical concept was that in diastole coronary flow would not be influenced by cardiac contraction. Based on this idea the concept of end-diastolic resistance was formulated. The ratio between arterial pressure and flow at the end of diastole would reflect the resistance of the coronary vascular bed not affected by cardiac contraction. However, in the late seventies Belamy [29] discovered that coronary arterial flow in diastole could stop at an arterial pressure as high as 45 mm Hg. Furthermore, when he plotted pressure versus flow an almost linear curve was obtained which after some extrapolation intercepted the pressure axis at a value denoted as P_{zf}. This high intercept pressure was thought to be explained by collapse of arterioles. This collapse would be the result of the summation of vessel wall forces due to smooth muscle tone and surrounding tissue pressure [30]. This idea was further supported by the finding that P_{zf} was higher at higher levels of smooth muscle tone [31]. The idea was formulated that diastolic coronary blood flow could be calculated by the ratio between $(P_{art}\text{-}P_{zf})/R_{cor}$. The inverse of the tangent of the pressure-flow relation would equal R_{cor} and represent the resistance proximal of the point of closure where pressure would stay equal to P_{zf}. This would imply that e.g. the effect of pharmaca should be studied on both R_{cor} and P_{zf}.

The interpretation of diastolic pressure flow lines is, however, more difficult than the simple model with vascular collapse [32, 33]. It has been shown that venous outflow continues after the arterial flow has ceased [34]. Moreover, if arterial pressure is reduced to very low values in a gradual manner, coronary arterial flow can become retrograde. This retrograde flow is difficult to observe in an intact preparation like the chronically instrumented dog or for that matter in patients with induced long diastoles. An example of pressure and flow tracings obtained from an acute experiment in which arterial pressure was reduced gradually, is demonstrated in Figure 9.3. From this figure it is clear that the intercept of the pressure flow relation with the pressure axis is just an arbitrary point on the curve. When the decay of pressure should have been halted when flow ceased, P_{zf} would have been high indeed.

The explanation presenting an alternative to the arteriolar collapse is that of intramyocardial compliance [20]. The intramyocardial vessels form a windkessel analogous to the aorta. If the aortic valve is patent there is now flow through it and the pressure in the aortic root can be considered as a zero flow pressure decaying when aortic volume is flowing through the peripheral resistance. In fact, when the coronary artery is occluded a similar decay of coronary peripheral pressure can be measured as well. Such a decay in peripheral pressure is measured also during coronary arterial occlusion applying balloon dilatation in patient. If the aortic valve is leaky and ventricular pressure is below aortic pressure, blood would flow retrogradely into the ventricle. This again is possible in the coronary arteries when arterial pressure drops below the blood pressure within the intramural microcirculation.

It should not be understood that micro vessels cannot collapse when their luminal pressure is decreasing. There are studies in mesenteric preparations showing collapse of micro vessels when flow stopped by reducing arterial pressure [35]. However, these same vessels were open when blood was flowing. Hence, with open arterioles there should be free communication between the larger arteries and the microcirculation. Consequently, P_{zf}, when it is measured in a steady state, has no direct meaning as a determinant for blood flow when blood actually flows. Apart from these theoretical grounds it should also be noted that micro vessels were not noticed to collapse when looking for this phenomena by a floating microscope technique in the epicardium [36].

Transients in the coronary arterial and venous signals

Analysis of transient signals is always more complicated than steady signals since the relations between independent and dependent variables are not unique but depend on history. A simple example of a system with memory is, again, the windkessel function of the aorta. The time course of aortic pressure is dependent on the systolic inflow through the aortic valve. Coronary venous outflow and arterial inflow differ considerably in periods were circumstances are changing, e.g. change in heart rate, change in perfusion pressure, force of contraction etc. In general it seems that coronary arterial flow is more rapidly in equilibrium with pressure after either a pressure

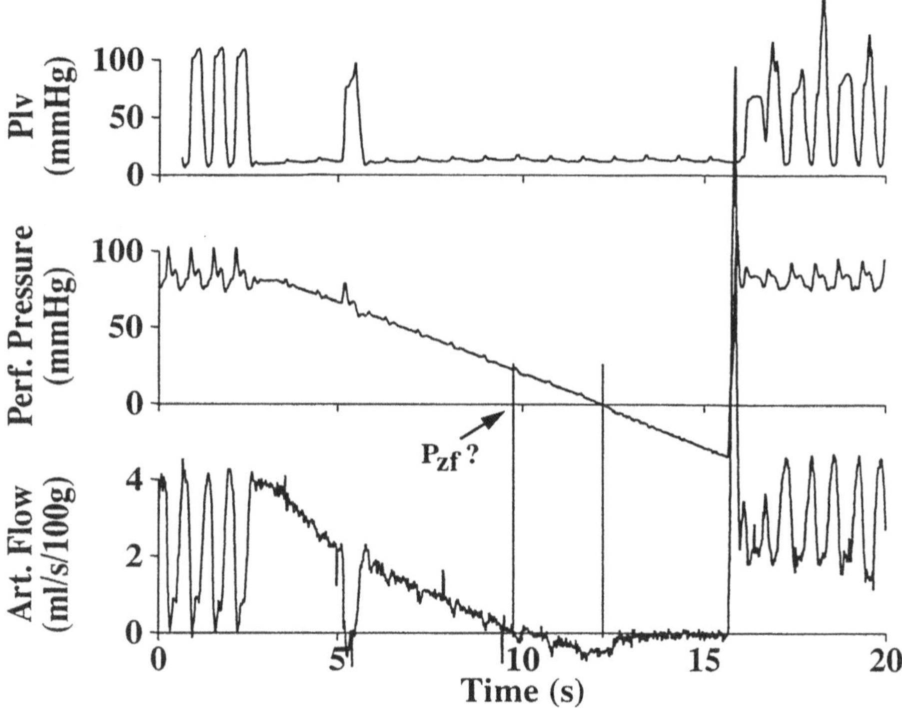

Figure 9.4. Response of flow on a decay of perfusion pressure to values below P_{zf}. The experiment was performed in an anesthetized goat with cannulated left main coronary artery. Note the vertical line drawn at the moment flow reaches zero. If pressure were halted at this level a high P_{zf} would have been concluded to. Note that flow remains negative until pressure decays to negative values. Collapse of vessels at such a low pressure is not unlikely.

step or transition to cardiac arrest [32, 37]. These observations have been interpreted as evidence for a site of uncoupling between the arteries and venous parts of the coronary circulation; i.e. the arteriolar waterfall discussed above. However, the arguments are intuitive and based on the analysis of linear systems. In a linear system time constants are exponential decay times of simple first order processes such as the decay of diastolic aortic pressure. However, the coronary system is highly non-linear. Compliance of the vessels, small and large, as well as resistance, is dependent on pressure. At a higher pressure the vessels become more stiff and hence less compliant while the increased diameter lowers the resistance. If all these processes are occurring at the same time, the simple interpretation of pressure and flow relations by linear models are quite dangerous [2, 38]. Taking into account the pressure dependency of the coronary resistance the rapid arterial and slow venous responses occurring at the same time can readily be explained.

Conclusions

In this chapter some basic physiological information was provided on phenomena and mechanisms relevant to the coronary circulation. The other studies in this book will demonstrate that progress in clinical instrumentation is rapid and that we are able to measure signals, which until today, were only obtainable in animal experimentation. However, due to the limitations of the patient model the interventions which can be performed have their ethical limitations. The challenge is to couple clinical and basic animal research in order to come to a better understanding of the disease processes in the human and to further develop the rational basis of patient treatment.

References

1. Scaramucci J. De motu cordis, theorema sextum. In Anonymous. Theoremata familiaria de physico-medicus lucubrationibus Iucta leges mecanicas. 1695.
2. Hoffman JIE, Spaan JAE. Pressure-flow relations in coronary circulation. Physiol Rev 1990; 70: 331–89.
3. Dankelman J, Spaan JAE, Stassen HG, Vergroesen I. Dynamics of coronary adjustment to a change in heart rate in the anaesthetized goat. J Physiol (Lond) 1989; 408: 295–312.
4. Von Restorff W, Holtz J, Bassenge E. Exersize induced augmentation of myocardial oxygen extraction in spite of normal coronary dilatory capacity in dogs. Pflugers Arch 1977; 372: 181–5.
5. Dankelman J, Vergroesen I, Spaan JAE. Static and dynamic analysis of local control of coronary flow. In Spaan JAE (ed): Coronary blood flow: mechanics, distribution, and control. Dordrecht: Kluwer Academic Publishers 1991: 219–60.
6. Broten TP, Feigl EO. Role of myocardial oxygen and carbon dioxide in coronary autoregulation. Am J Physiol 1992; 262: H1231–7.
7. Broten TP, Romson JL, Fullerton DA, Van Winkle DM, Feigl EO. Synergistic action of myocardial oxygen and carbon dioxide in controlling coronary blood flow. Circ Res 1991; 68: 531–42.
8. Dankelman J, Spaan JAE, Van der Ploeg CPB, Vergroesen I. Dynamic response of the coronary circulation to a rapid change in its perfusion in the aneasthetized goat. J Physiol (Lond) 1989; 419: 703–15.
9. Dankelman J, Vergroesen I, Han Y, Spaan JAE. Dynamic response of coronary regulation to heart rate and perfusion changes in dogs. Am J Physiol 1992; 263: H447–52.
10. Spaan JAE, Breuls NPW, Laird JD. Forward coronary flow normally seen in systole is the result of both forward and concealed back flow. Basic Res Cardiol 1981; 76: 582–6.
11. Van Bavel E, Giezeman MJMM, Spaan JAE. Arteriolar mechanics and coronary flow. In Spaan JAE (ed): Coronary blood flow; mechanics, distribution, and control. Dordrecht: Kluwer Academic Publishers 1991: 193–218.
12. Murray PA, Belloni FL, Sparks HV. The role of potassium in the metabolic control of coronary vascular resistance of the dog. Circ Res 1979; 44: 767–80.
13. Chilian WM, Layne SM, Klausner EC, Eastham CL, Marcus ML. Redistribution of coronary microvascular resistance produced by dipyridamole. Am J Physiol 1989; 256: H383–90.
14. Domenech RJ. Regional diastolic coronary blood flow during diastolic ventricular hypertension. Cardiovasc Res 1978; 12: 639–45.
15. Wusten B, Buss DD, Deist H, Schaper W. Dilatory capacity of the coronary circulation and its correlation to the arterial vasculature in the canine left ventricle. Basic Res Cardiol 1977; 72: 636–50.

16. Bache RJ, Cobb FR. Effect of maximal coronary vasodilation on transmural myocardial perfusion during tachycardia in the awake dog. Circ Res 1977; 41: 648–53.
17. Green HD, Gregg DD, Wiggers CJ. The phasic changes in coronary flow established by differential pressure curves. Am J Physiol 1935; 112: 627–39.
18. Vergroesen I, Noble MIM, Spaan JAE. Intramyocardial blood volume change in first moments of cardiac arrest in anesthetized goats. Am J Physiol 1987; 253: H307–16.
19. Downey JM, Kirk ES. Inhibition of coronary blood flow by a vascular waterfall mechanism. Circ Res 1975; 36: 753–60.
20. Spaan JAE, Breuls NPW, Laird JD. Diastolic-systolic coronary flow differences are caused by intramyocardial pump action in the anesthetized dog. Circ Res 1981; 49: 584–93.
21. Krams R, Zegers J, Sipkema P, Westerhof N. Contractility is the main determinant of coronary systolic flow impediment. Am J Physiol 1989; 257: H1936–44.
22. Krams R, Sipkema P, Westerhof N. Varying elastance concept may explain coronary systolic flow impediment. Am J Physiol 1989; 257: H1471–9.
23. Van Winkle DM, Swafford AN Jr, Downey JM. Subendocardial coronary compression in beating dog hearts is independent of pressure in the ventricular lumen. Am J Physiol 1991; 261: H500–5.
24. Suga H, Sagawa K, Shoukas AA. Load independence of the instanteneous pressure-volume ratio of the canine left ventricle and effects of epiniphrine and heart rate on the ratio. Circ Res 1973; 32: 314–22.
25. Westerhof N. Physiological hypotheses – intramyocardial pressure. A new concept, suggestions for measurements. Basic Res Cardiol 1990; 85: 105–19.
26. Han Y, Vergroesen I, Spaan JAE. Stopped-flow epicardial lymph pressure is affected by left ventricular pressure in anesthetized goats. Am J Physiol 1993; 264: H1624–8.
27. Han Y, Vergroesen I, Goto M, Dankelman J, Vanderploeg CPB, Spaan JAE. Left ventricular pressure transmission to myocardial lymph vessels is different during systole and diastole. Pflugers Arch 1993; 423: 448–54.
28. Kouwenhoven E, Vergroesen I, Han Y, Spaan JAE. Retrograde coronary flow is limited by time-varying elastance. Am J Physiol Heart 1992; 263: H484–90.
29. Bellamy RF. Diastolic coronary artery pressure-flow relations in the dog. Circ Res 1978; 43: 92–101.
30. Farhi ER, Klocke FJ, Mates RE *et al.* Tone-dependent waterfall behavior during venous pressure elevation in isolated canine hearts. Circ Res 1991; 68: 392–401.
31. Dole WP, Bishop VS. Influence of autoregulation and capacitance on diastolic coronary artery pressure-flow relationships in the dog. Circ Res 1982; 51: 261–70.
32. Klocke FJ, Mates RE, Canty JM Jr, Ellis AK. Coronary pressure-flow relationships. Controversial issues and probable implications. Circ Res 1985; 56: 310–23.
33. Spaan JAE. Coronary diastolic pressure-flow relation and zero flow pressure explained on the basis of intramyocardial compliance. Circ Res 1985; 56: 293–309.
34. Chilian WM, Marcus ML. Coronary venous outflow persists after cessation of coronary arterial inflow. Am J Physiol 1984; 247: H948–90.
35. Baez S. Response characteristics of perfused microvessels to pressure and vasoactive stimuli. Angiology 1961; 12: 452–61.
36. Kanatsuka H, Ashikawa K, Komaru T, Suzuki T, Takishima T. Diameter change and pressure-red blood cell velocity relations in coronary microvessels during long diastoles in the canine left ventricle. Circ Res 1990; 66: 503–10.
37. Katz SA, Feigl EO. Systole has little effect on diastolic coronary artery blood flow. Circ Res 1988; 62: 443–51.
38. Spaan JAE. Linear system analysis applied to the coronary circulation. In Spaan JAE (ed): Coronary blood flow: mechanics, distribution, and control. Dordrecht: Kluwer Academic Publishers 1991: 99–130.

10. Possibilities and limitations of myocardial flow reserve

FELIX ZIJLSTRA, PETR WIDIMSKY & HARRY SURYAPRANATA

Summary

The concept of coronary flow reserve is important for the understanding of the physiological significance of obstructive coronary artery disease. The recent development of an angiographic method has made the measurement of coronary or myocardial flow reserve possible during routine coronary angiography. The technical aspects, variability and limitations of this technique are discussed. Several clinical and investigational applications are presented: 1) functional assessment of stenosis severity, 2) assessment of the functional results of coronary angioplasty, 3) myocardial flow reserve in acute myocardial infarction, 4) the use of myocardial flow reserve in a model for pharmacological research.

Introduction

Visual interpretation of the coronary angiogram inadequately predicts the physiologic importance of obstructive coronary artery disease [1]. Computer-based quantitative analysis has helped to minimize the problems of high interobserver and intraobserver variability in the interpretation of the coronary angiogram. In addition, it allows the assessment of the pressure-flow characteristics of the coronary artery lesion, that are correlated with the translesional pressure gradient and with the results from exercise thallium perfusion scintigraphy [2–7]. However, the relationship between the quantitatively analyzed dimensions of an obstructive coronary artery lesion and the consequent limitation in coronary blood flow is not yet fully understood. The recent description of several techniques for the measurement of relative coronary blood flow has rendered the assessment of regional myocardial flow reserve possible by use of the ratio of maximal coronary blood flow to resting flow as a measurement of this variable [8–15]. Initial studies from our hand were based on cinefilm analyses of coronary perfusion images [12]. However, this angiographic method has now also been adapted for digital images on the Philips DCI system under the name Myocardial Flow Reserve (MFR) analytical package [18]. We will discuss here technical aspects, variability, limitations and finally several applications of this technique.

J.H.C. Reiber and P.W. Serruys (eds): Progress in quantitative coronary arteriography, 141–159.

Technical characteristics

The procedure for the myocardial flow reserve measurement from digitized coronary cineangiograms recorded on 35 mm cinefilm was first implemented on the research version of the Cardiovascular Angiography Analysis System [12]. The film speed was always chosen at 25 frames/s with a pulse time of 4 ms. For the right coronary artery a left or right anterior oblique projection was used, for the left coronary artery a left anterior oblique projection. The X-ray gantry settings were standardized in the short- and medium-term variability studies, which will be defined later on in this chapter. The heart was atrially paced at a rate just above the spontaneous heart rate, ranging from 70 to 90 beats/min. An ECG-triggered injection into the coronary artery was performed with a Medrad Mark IV infusion pump. The injection rate and volume of the contrast medium were judged to be adequate when back flow of contrast medium into the aorta occurred. The injection rate ranged from 3 to 7 ml/s and the injection volume ranged from 5 to 9 ml, depending on the size of the coronary artery. The angiogram was repeated with identical patient position and X-ray gantry settings, 30 s after pharmacologically induced hyperemia by a bolus injection of 12.5 mg papaverine into the coronary artery.

For the quantitative analysis of the image series five or six end-diastolic cineframes were selected from successive cardiac cycles and digitized at a resolution of $512 \times 512 \times 8$ bits. Logarithmic non-magnified mask-mode background subtraction was applied to the image subset, to eliminate non-contrast medium densities. The last end-diastolic frame prior to contrast administration was chosen as the mask. From the sequence of background-subtracted images, a contrast arrival time image was determined, using an empirically derived fixed density threshold. Each pixel was labeled with the sequence number of the cardiac cycle in which the pixel intensity level for the first time exceeded the threshold, starting from the beginning of the ECG-triggered contrast injection. In addition to the contrast arrival time image, a density image was computed with each pixel intensity value being representative for the maximal local contrast medium accumulation. The myocardial flow reserve was defined as the ratio of the relative regional flow computed from a hyperemic image (Q(h)) divided by the relative regional flow of the corresponding baseline image (Q(b)). Relative regional flow values were quantitatively determined from the relationship that relative regional blood flow equals regional vascular volume divided by the transit time. Regional vascular volume was assessed from the logarithmic mask-mode subtraction images using the Lambert-Beer relationship. Myocardial flow reserve (FR) can then be calculated as:

$$FR = Q(h)/Q(b) = D(h)/D(b): T(h)/T(b)$$

where D is the mean contrast density and T the mean appearance time at baseline (b) and hyperemia (h). Mean contrast medium appearance time and density were computed within user-defined regions of interest that were chosen in such a way that the epicardial coronary arteries visible on the angiogram, the coronary sinus and the great cardiac vein were excluded from the analysis. For each of the 3 major coronary arteries (right coronary artery, left anterior descending coronary artery, and circumflex artery) only one region of interest was chosen and analyzed. Normal values for myocardial flow reserve as measured with this technique have previously been established [17]. The mean myocardial flow reserve of 24 angiographically normal coronary arteries was 5.0 (SD: ± 0.6). The lower limit of a normal myocardial flow reserve is therefore 3.4 (2 SD below 5.0). This is comparable to the values for normal coronary flow reserve measured with intracoronary Doppler catheters as reported by Wilson *et al.* [9, 10].

It should be noted that the definitions for appearance time, mask-mode background subtraction, etc. for the modern digital version on the Philips DCI are slightly different from those described before for the cinefilm approach. Details are given in [18]. In addition, the digital MFR allows digital frame matching, additional subtraction for background densities and the generation of a MFR functional image, in which each pixel represents the local MFR value.

Variability

The X-ray gantry settings were standardised in the short- and medium-term variability studies. This resulted in a good reproducibility of isocenter-image intensifier distance, focus-isocenter distance and object-isocenter distance (see Table 10.1). Voltage (kV) and current (mA) of the X-ray generator were adjusted automatically in the catheterization laboratory by a microprocessor system during the first 3 or 4 cineframes of each cinerun. The on-line recorded voltage and current subsequently remained constant during the rest of the cinerun. This microprocessor based technique results in good reproducibility of both voltage and current of the X-ray generator [16].

Patient selection

Twenty-five patients underwent PTCA for disabling angina pectoris despite optimal pharmacological therapy. The right coronary artery was dilated in 5 patients, the circumflex artery in 5 patients and the left anterior descending artery in 15 patients. Their mean age (±SD) was 54 (±9) years. Twenty-four patients were male. Recatheterization was performed 3 to 5 months later as part of an ongoing study on restenosis after PTCA. Informed consent was obtained for the additional investigations. Patients were selected on the basis of the following criteria: primary successful PTCA for single vessel coronary artery disease (residual diameter stenosis less than 50%), normal blood pressure (mean aortic pressure ranged from 85 to 105 mmHg), normal

Table 10.1. Variability in X-ray gantry setings and voltage and current of the X-ray generator, with repeated cineangiographic studies (n = 20).

	Overall mean value	Mean difference	p-value	SD diff
LAO (degrees)	53	0.1	NS	0.2
IID (cm)	23.6	−0.1	NS	2.0
FID (cm)	72.3	0.0	NS	0.1
OID (cm)	5.4	0.0	NS	0.1
Voltage (kV)	71.2	0.1	NS	2.9
Current (mA)	717	−5.5	NS	16.1

Abbreviations: IID = image intensifier-isocenter distance, FID = focus-isocenter distance, OID = object-isocenter distance.

left ventricular wall motion with an ejection fraction of more than 55%, normal left ventricular end-diastolic pressure, no angiographic evidence of collateral circulation, cardiac hypertrophy, anemia, polycythemia, documented previous myocardial infarction, or valvular heart disease.

Intraobserver variability

Intraobserver variability was assessed by measuring the myocardial flow reserve in 11 regions of interest in 6 patients twice from the same cineangiograms by the same observer. In 5 patients two regions of interest in the myocardium supplied by the left coronary artery were analyzed, and in one patient a region of interest was analyzed in the myocardium supplied by the right coronary artery. Care was taken to ensure that the regions of interest in the duplicate determinations were identical. Figure 10.1 shows the results of measuring twice the myocardial flow reserve in 11 regions of interest in 6 patients by the same observer from the same coronary cineangiograms. No significant differences were found between the first and second measurements.

Interobserver variability

Interobserver variability was assessed by measuring the myocardial flow reserve in 12 regions of interest in 7 patients from the same coronary cineangiograms by two observers. In 5 patients two regions of interest in the myocardium supplied by the left coronary artery were analyzed, and in 2 patients one region of interest was analyzed in the myocardium supplied by the right coronary artery. The selected boundaries of the regions of interest were unknown to the other observer. Myocardial flow reserve measurements by two observers without the knowledge of each others selected regions of interest using the same coronary cineangiograms is shown in Figure 10.2.

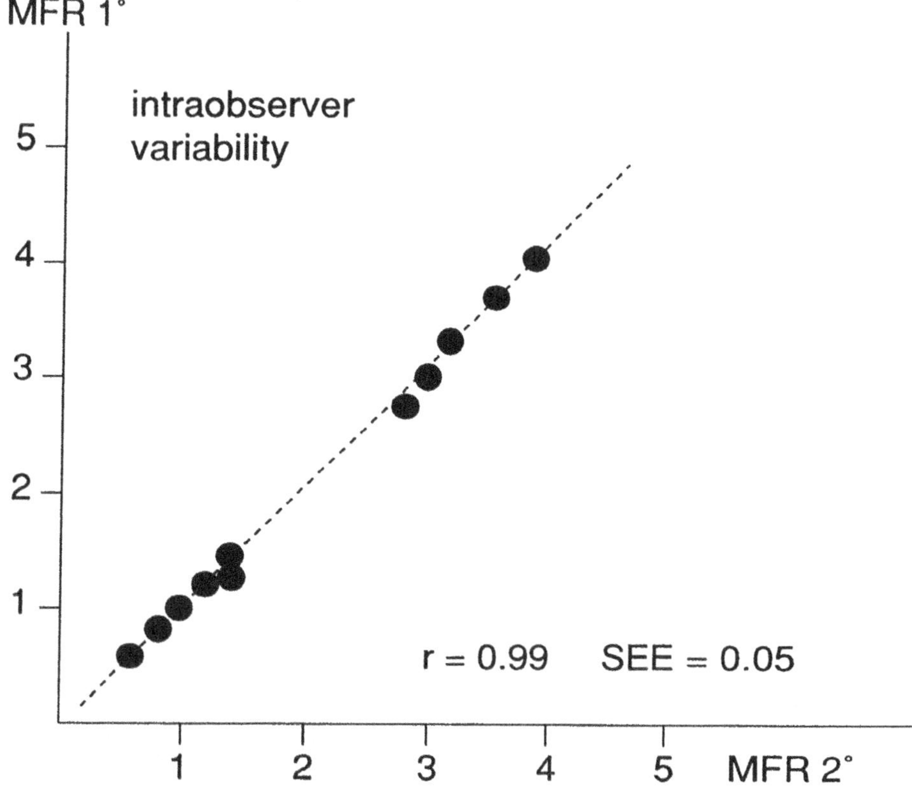

Figure 10.1. MFR 1 = first determination of myocardial flow reserve, MFR 2 = second determination of myocardial flow reserve, r = linear regression correlation coefficient, SEE = standard error of the estimate.

Again no significant differences were found in the measurements between the two observers.

Short-term variability (5 *min.*)

The short-term variability was defined as the variation in measured myocardial flow reserve from two coronary cineangiograms taken 5 min. apart with identical position of patient, X-ray source and image intensifier. Myocardial flow reserve was measured in 13 regions of interest in 7 patients. In 6 patients two regions of interest in the myocardium supplied by the left coronary artery were analyzed, and in one patient one region of interest was analyzed in the myocardium supplied by the right coronary artery. Care was taken to ensure that the selected regions of interest in the duplicate determinations were identical. Figure 10.3 presents the myocardial flow reserve in these

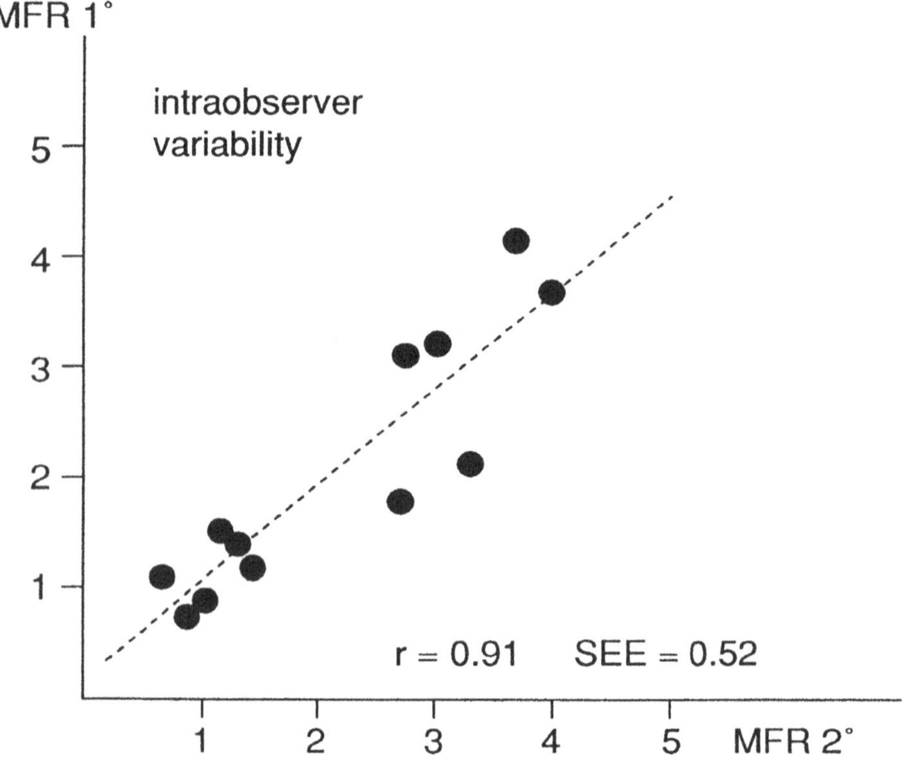

Figure 10.2. MFR 1 = first determination of myocardial flow reserve, MFR 2 = second determination of myocardial flow reserve, r = linear regression correlation coefficient, SEE = standard error of the estimate.

13 regions of interest from repeated acquisition and analysis of coronary cineangiograms taken 5 min. apart. No significant differences between the two measurements were found.

Medium-term variability (1–3 *hours*)

In this study myocardial flow reserve was measured before and immediately after PTCA in 25 patients. In 5 patients the right coronary artery was dilated. In 20 patients undergoing PTCA of the left anterior descending coronary artery or the circumflex artery, coronary flow reserve was measured in both myocardial regions. To calculate the medium-term variability, regions of interest (n = 20) were chosen in the myocardium supplied by the non-dilated coronary arteries. During the PTCA procedure various vasoactive drugs were administered (nitrates, Ca-antagonists) as clinically indicated, probably

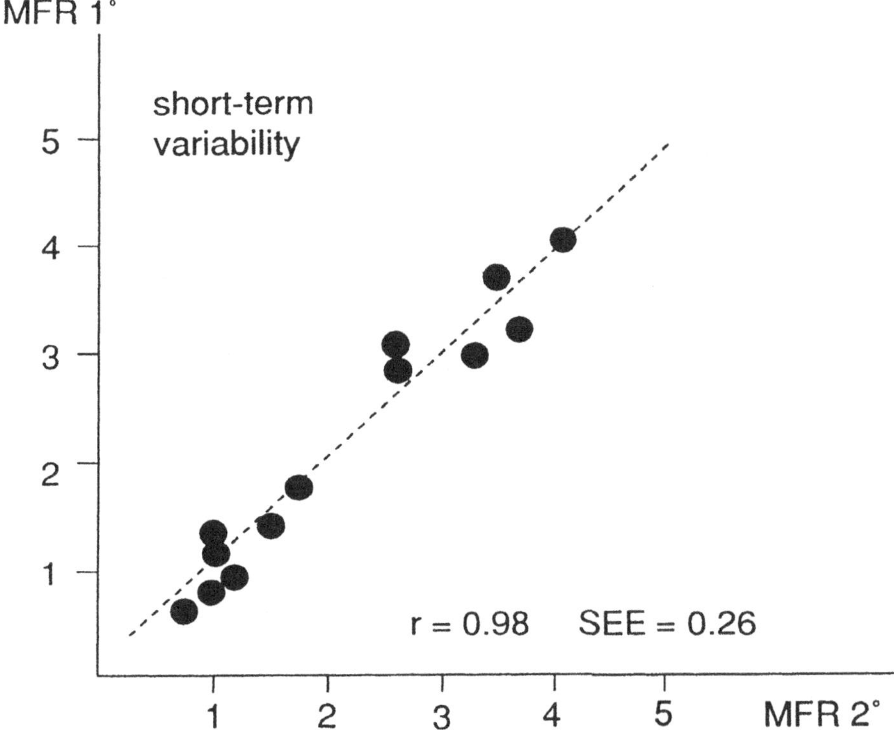

Figure 10.3. MFR 1 = first determination of myocardial flow reserve, MFR 2 = second determination of myocardial flow reserve, r = linear regression correlation coefficient, SEE = standard error of the estimate.

resulting in changes in vasomotor tone. Care was taken to ensure that cineangiographic projection and X-ray gantry settings as well as the analyzed regions of interest were identical before and after the PTCA. Figure 10.4 provides the data on the myocardial flow reserve measurements for myocardial regions supplied by coronary arteries which had not been involved in the dilatation process in 20 patients immediately before and after angioplasty. No significant differences were found between the measurements obtained before and after angioplasty.

Long-term variability (3–5 *months*)

During follow-up coronary cineangiography 3 to 5 months (mean 4,2 months) later myocardial flow reserve was measured again in these 25 patients. To calculate the long-term variability regions of interest (n = 20) were chosen in the myocardium supplied by the non-dilated coronary arteries. The follow-up investigation was always performed in a second cineangiographic room

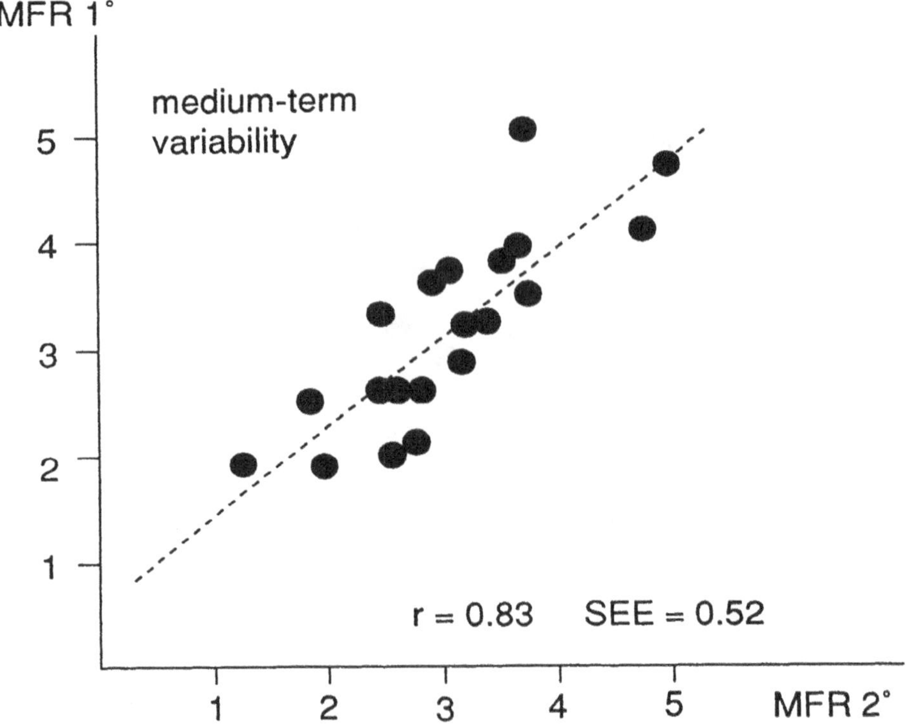

Figure 10.4. MFR 1 = first determination of myocardial flow reserve, MFR 2 = second determination of myocardial flow reserve, r = linear regression correlation coefficient, SEE = standard error of the estimate.

with different X-ray equipment. There was no standardized protocol for the administration of vasoactive medication before data acquisition; therefore, vasomotor tone in both conditions was unknown and ignored. Care was taken to ensure that identical regions of interest were analyzed. Figure 10.5 gives the myocardial flow reserve as measured in a myocardial region supplied by a non-dilated coronary artery, immediately following angioplasty as well as 3 to 5 months later. No significant differences were found between the two measurements.

Discussion

The concept of coronary flow reserve is complex, as it is a physiologic variable that might be influenced by a great number of factors, that cannot always be controlled completely in the clinical setting. Furthermore, all methods to measure flow reserve have their inherent limitations. A thorough

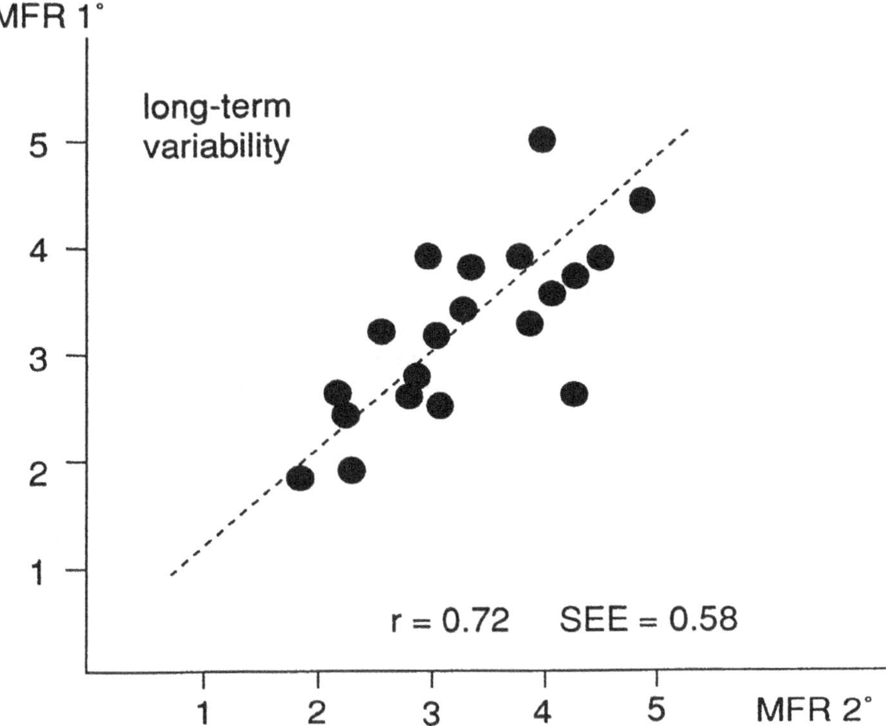

Figure 10.5. MFR 1 = first determination of myocardial flow reserve, MFR 2 = second determination of myocardial flow reserve, r = linear regression correlation coefficient, SEE = standard error of the estimate.

understanding of these aspects is essential before this technology can be applied with reliable results.

First, X-ray gantry settings and voltage and current of the X-ray generator must be identical to permit a valid comparison of the myocardial contrast density measurements on both the baseline and hyperemic cineangiograms. This is also a prerequisite if a comparison of two or more myocardial flow reserve acquisitions at different times is to be made. The X-ray equipment used in these studies seems adequate in this regard (Table 10.1).

Second, cinefilm development must be very stable. In our laboratories a 21 step (log 1.5 increment) sensitometric full frame strip was generated on each cinefilm with a dummy camera prior to the angiographic investigation. This strip was developed together with the angiographic data and was used to control the chemical process. The replenishment of developer was done per meter cinefilm instead of per unit of time and therefore independent of the speed of the machine. Together with accurate temperature control and the use of a medium grain developer, this resulted in a reliable chemical process characterized by a mean density of 0.82 and a gradient of 1.25. Fortunately, this problem does not play a role anymore with the latest digital version of the program that runs on the DCI equipment.

Third, many patient related factors are important determinators of the measured myocardial flow reserve and contribute to the variability of this radiographic method. Changes in heart rate may influence the myocardial flow reserve. Furthermore, subtraction in the selected end-diastolic frames is only possible when a strictly regular rhythm is present. Therefore, atrial pacing is sometimes necessary, although some patients have a regular spontaneous heart rate and do not require pacing. Changes in blood pressure can influence myocardial flow reserve in two ways. Firstly, myocardial oxygen consumption and therefore baseline coronary blood flow is to a large degree determined by the systemic arterial pressure. Since myocardial flow reserve is defined by the ratio of maximal to resting coronary blood flow, an increase in resting coronary blood flow as result of an increase in myocardial oxygen consumption results in a decrease of this ratio. Secondly, the coronary blood flow during maximal coronary vasodilation is linearly related to the coronary driving pressure. Angiograms that are used for the calculation of flow reserve during baseline and hyperemic conditions, or repeated radiographic myocardial flow reserve measurements should thus be obtained at the same blood pressure. Myocardial flow reserve measured in the animal laboratory can be reduced by a large increase in left ventricular diastolic pressure or a marked change in contractility and systolic function. As all patients in the present study had a normal left ventricular function, it seems unlikely that these factors played a significant role in the variabilities described in this report. Medium-, and long-term variabilities were certainly affected by changes in vasomotor tone. Alterations in collateral channel filling patterns during and after angioplasty may also play a role. Although we excluded patients with angiographically visible collaterals, collateral vessels not visible by standard angiographic techniques are often present. Especially the long-term study may have been influenced by changes in neurohumeral factors. Endothelium derived relaxing factor has a physiological dilator role by acting as a local autocoid on subjacent smooth muscle and may be an important controlling variable in coronary flow and myocardial flow reserve.

Fourth, a prerequisite of this radiographic technique is the use of an ECG triggered pump to inject a fixed volume at a fixed contrast injection rate. Although injection of a radiographic contrast agent induces profound alterations in coronary blood flow, the ratio of hyperemic coronary blood flow to baseline flow is unaffected by the contrast agent during the first 5 s after injection when injection rate and volume are identical under hyperemic and baseline conditions [14]. The injection rate and volume should be sufficient to ensure complete filling of the epicardial coronary arteries with contrast during pharmacologically induced hyperemia. The disturbance in coronary blood flow due to the radiographic contrast agent lasts for less than 20 s, and sequential injections of contrast agent in doses as used in this investigation will not result in persisting changes in coronary blood flow.

Fifth, the method of induction of an hyperemic response in the coronary circulation should be reproducible. Intracoronary papaverine induces a strong and short-lasting hyperemia that is reasonably reproducible in magnitude as well as in timing [9]. Wilson and White investigated the dose of intracoronary papaverine needed to produce maximal coronary vasodilation and reported a maximal hyperemic response after 8 mg in most coronary arteries and after 12 mg in all coronary arteries [13].

Sixth, the analysis of the angiogram to permit calculation of myocardial flow reserve from measured myocardial contrast appearance time and density involves the selection of end-diastolic frames and the selection of regions of interest. The boundaries of the regions of interest are drawn by the observer with a writing tablet or mouse which is interfaced with the computer. Although the entire analysis procedure can be performed with high reproducibility, the observer-dependent selection of the boundaries of the regions of interest introduces interobserver variability. Consequently, rigid criteria should be applied to the selection of the boundaries of the regions of interest, preferably in an automated manner, not dependent upon the user.

Applications

It is our belief that the radiographic assessment of myocardial flow reserve as described above is applicable under the following circumstances. For each of these applications we will present measurement data.

A: Functional assessment of stenosis severity

The correlation between quantitatively determined coronary artery dimensions and the myocardial flow reserve was analyzed in 81 patients. These patients were selected with great care to ensure that no known factors other than the coronary anatomy were present that have influence on the myocardial flow reserve [13].

Results

The minimal cross-sectional area of the 81 coronary arteries ranged from 0.4 to 10.3 mm^2, the percentage area stenosis ranged from 0 to 93%. The measured myocardial flow reserve ranged from 0.4 to 5.5 in the 57 patients with single vessel disease. The 24 patients with angiographically normal coronary arteries had a measured coronary flow reserve ranging from 3.4 to 6.5 with a mean value ($\pm$SD) of 5.0 ($\pm$0.8). The relationship between myocardial flow reserve (MFR) and absolute cross-sectional area (mm^2) at the site of obstruction (OA) was best described by the equation:

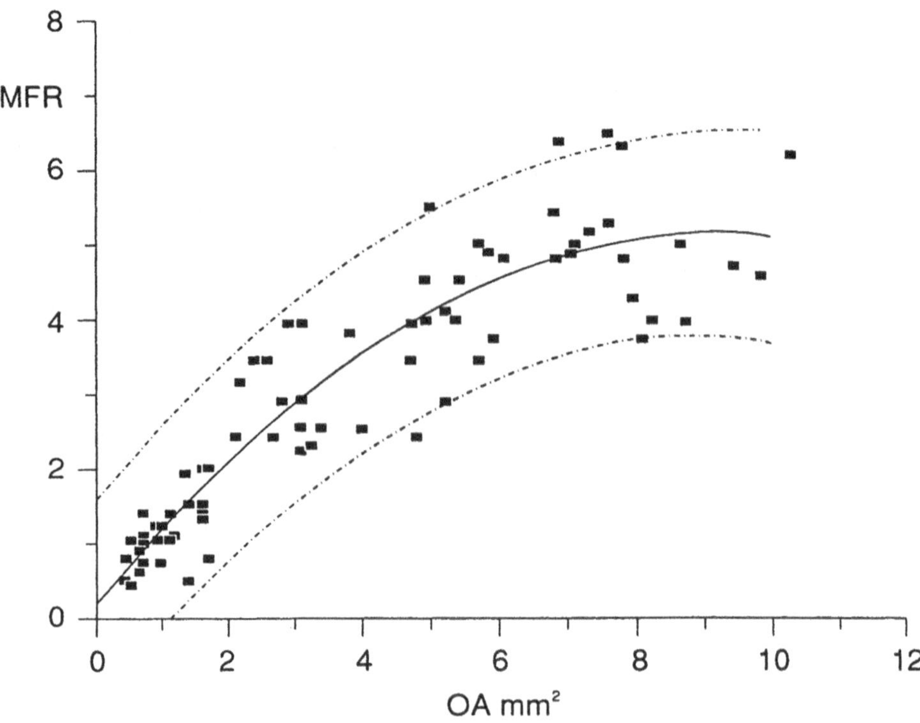

Figure 10.6. Correlation between myocardial flow reserve (MFR) and cross-sectional area at the site of obstruction. MFR = myocardial flow reserve, OA = cross-sectional area (mm^2) at the site of obstruction. The best curve fit and the 95% confidence limits (dashed lines) are shown.

$$\text{MFR} = 0.18 + 1.07\ \text{OA} - 0.058\ \text{OA}^2,\ r = 0.98,\ \text{SEE} = 0.66,$$

and is shown is Figure 10.6. The relationship between MFR and percentage area stenosis (AS) was best described by the equation:

$$\text{MFR} = 4.8 - 0.024\ \text{AS} - 0.00022\ \text{AS}^2,\ r = 0.98,\ \text{SEE} = 0.73,$$

and is shown in Figure 10.7.

B: Assessment of the functional results of coronary angioplasty

Patients

The study population consisted of 24 patients with angiographically normal coronary arteries and 15 patients with single vessel coronary artery disease. These 15 patients had undergone successful PTCA for disabling angina refractory to intensive pharmacological treatment. They were selected on the basis of a normal exercise thallium scintigram and complete relief of chest

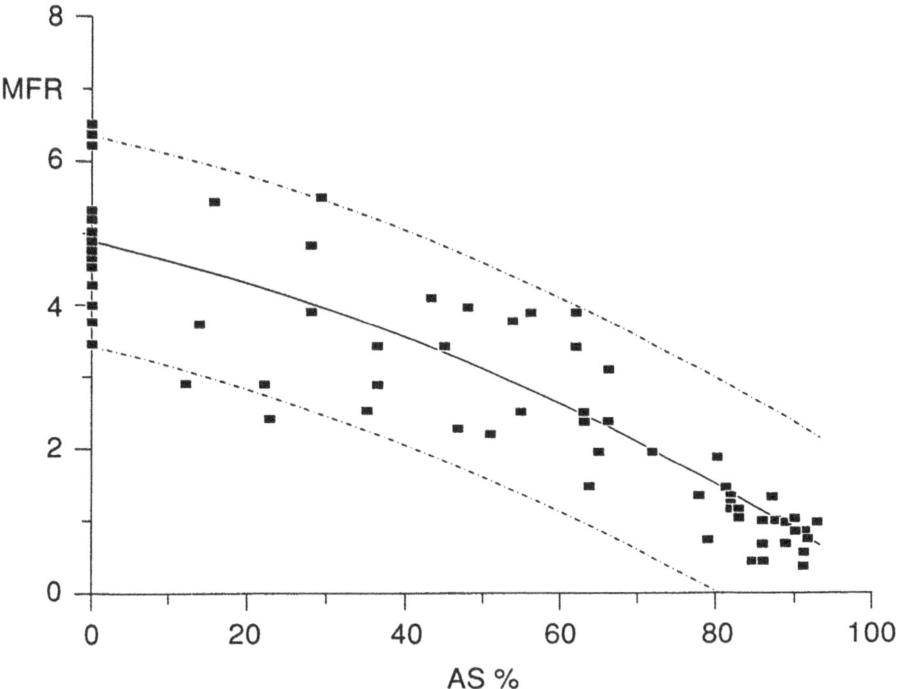

Figure 10.7. Correlation between myocardial flow reserve and percentage area stenosis. MFR = myocardial flow reserve, AS = percentage area stenosis. The best curve fit and the 95% confidence limits (dashed lines) are shown.

pain 5 months after PTCA, when coronary angiography and left ventriculography were performed as part of an ongoing study on restenosis after PTCA. Informed consent was obtained for all investigations. Before PTCA pharmacologic treatment consisted of nitrates, calcium antagonists and beta-blockers, and during the 5 months after PTCA the patients were treated with aspirin 500 mg/day and nifedipine 60 mg/day which medication was continued on the day of the cardiac catheterization. All 39 patients had normal systolic and diastolic wall motion and an ejection fraction greater than 55%. Patients with left ventricular hypertrophy, valvular heart disease, angiographic evidence of collateral circulation, anemia, polycythemia or hypertension were excluded because these conditions may influence myocardial flow reserve [17].

Quantitative cineangiography

The changes in minimal cross-sectional obstruction area (mm^2) are shown in Figure 10.8, the changes in percentage diameter stenosis in Figure 10.9. Percentage area stenosis (mean ± SD) decreased from 89 ± 7% to 51 ± 11%

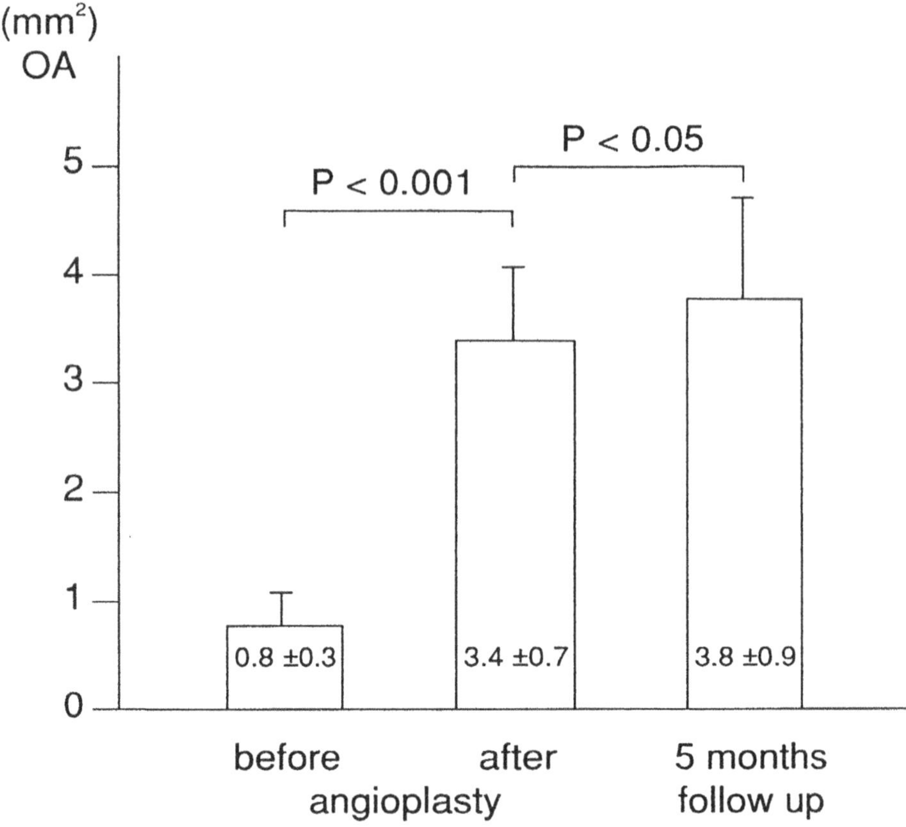

Figure 10.8. Results of quantitative analyses of coronary angiograms, before, immediately after and 5 months after percutaneous transluminal coronary angioplasty. OA = minimal cross-sectional area (mm^2) at the site of obstruction.

immediately following PTCA. Five months later percentage area stenosis was further decreased to 42 ± 14% ($p < 0.05$).

Myocardial flow reserve

Myocardial flow reserve was measured in the myocardial region supplied by the dilated coronary artery before PTCA, immediately following PTCA as well as 5 months later. Consecutive measurements were also obtained in 12 adjacent myocardial regions supplies by a non-dilated coronary artery (Figure 10.10). The myocardial flow reserve of these adjacent myocardial regions remained unchanged over the period between PTCA and the 5 months follow-up. Myocardial flow reserve (mean ± SD) in the myocardial region supplied by the dilated coronary artery increased from 1.0 ± 0.3 to 2.5 ± 0.6 immediately following PTCA ($p < 0.001$). In none of these patients myocardial flow reserve was restored to a normal level immediately following PTCA.

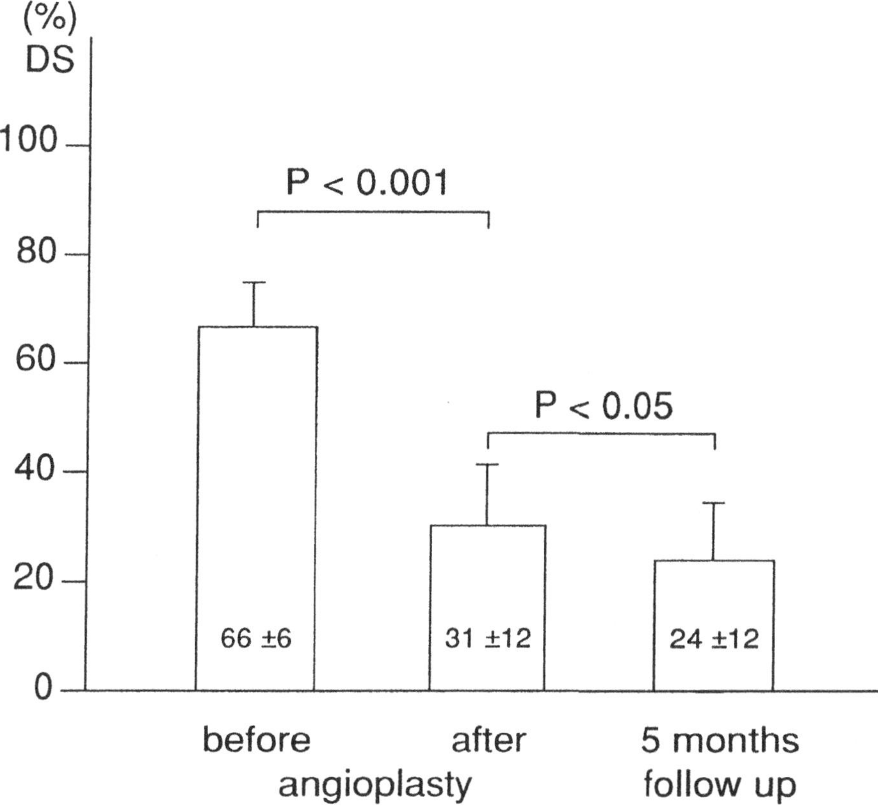

Figure 10.9. Results of quantitative analyses of coronary angiograms, before, immediately after and 5 months after percutaneous transluminal coronary angioplasty. DS = percentage diameter stenosis (%).

A substantial late improvement ($p < 0.01$) in myocardial flow reserve had occurred 5 months later. Myocardial flow reserve in the myocardial region supplied by the dilated coronary artery 5 months after PTCA was of the same magnitude as the flow reserve in the myocardial region supplied by a non-dilated and angiographically not diseased coronary artery. In 11 of the 15 patients (73%) flow reserve of the dilated coronary artery was restored to a normal level beyond the lower limit of 3.4, whereas in 4 of 15 patients (27%) flow reserve was still abnormal.

C: Myocardial flow reserve in acute myocardial infarction

Reactive hyperemic response during reperfusion and its impact on the recovery of regional myocardial function were investigated in 22 patients undergoing successful coronary angioplasty within 4 hours of acute myocardial

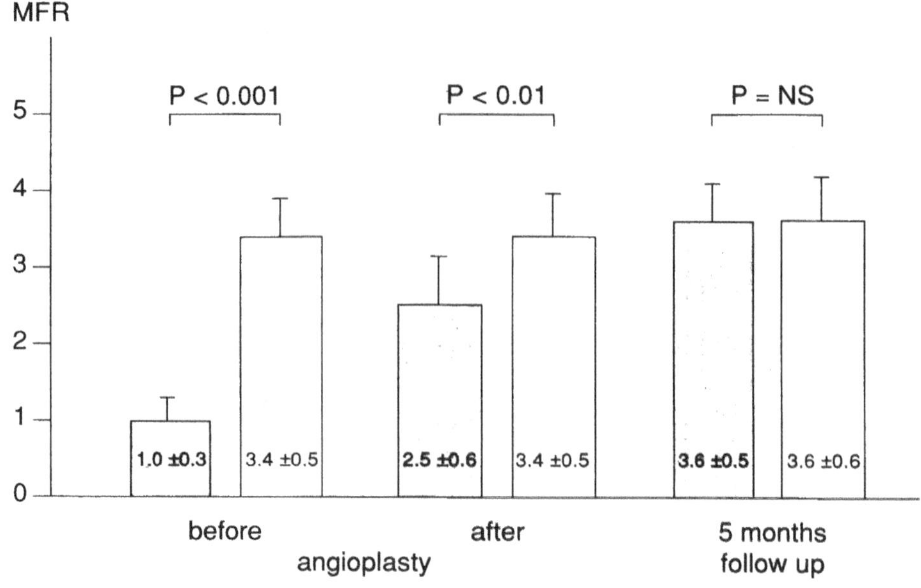

Figure 10.10. Myocardial flow reserve (MFR) measured before, immediately after and 5 months after percutaneous transluminal coronary angioplasty. The shaded bars represent the MFR of the myocardial region supplied by the dilated coronary artery. The open bars represent the MFR of an adjacent myocardial region supplied by a non-dilated and angiographically normal coronary artery.

infarction [19]. Papaverine-induced hyperemia was determined quantitatively, using computer-assisted digital subtraction cine-angiography, immediately after angioplasty and at follow-up angiography before hospital discharge.

Following papaverine, the mean contrast medium appearance time decreased significantly from 3.5 ± 0.7 to 2.7 ± 0.7 cardiac cycles ($p < 0.001$) immediately after successful coronary angioplasty, and from 3.8 ± 0.7 to 2.7 ± 0.9 ($p < 0.001$) at angiography prior to hospital discharge. The mean contrast medium density increased significantly from 48.7 ± 13.8 to 61.0 ± 19.0 ($p < 0.003$) and from 49.6 ± 19.7 to 80.3 ± 29.6 ($p < 0.001$), respectively. As a consequence, the calculated myocardial flow reserve increased significantly from 1.8 ± 0.7 to 2.6 ± 1.0 ($p < 0.001$). Furthermore, myocardial flow reserve correlated significantly with regional myocardial function of the infarct zone both during the acute stage ($r = 0.79$; $p < 0.002$) and at follow-up angiography ($r = 0.82$; $p < 0.001$). More importantly, flow reserve measurement upon reperfusion, immediately after angioplasty, correlated strongly with regional myocardial function at follow-up angiography ($r = 0.81$; $p < 0.001$), as shown in Figure 10.11.

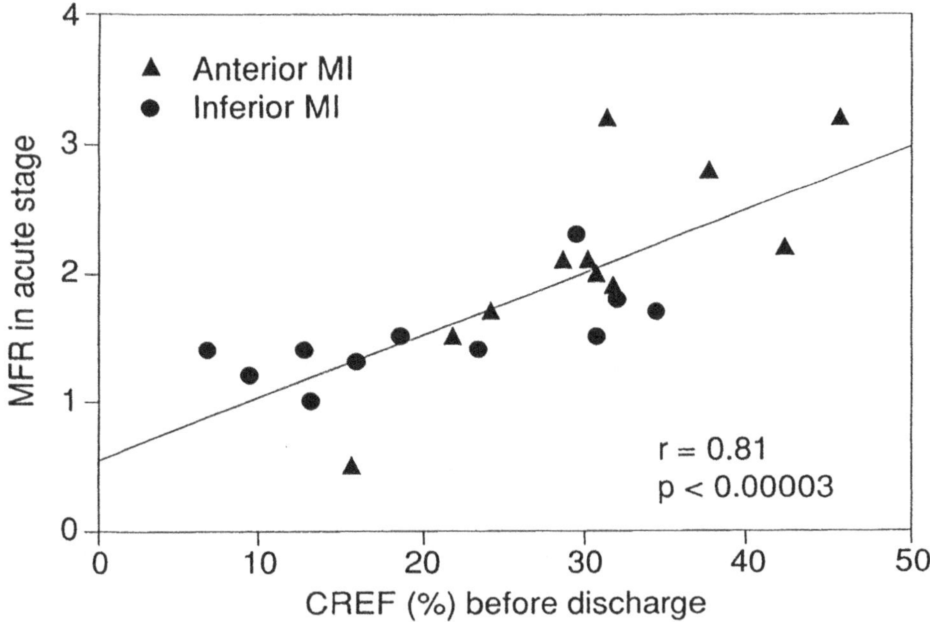

Figure 10.11. MFR in acute stage = myocardial flow reserve immediately following successful reperfusion by coronary angioplasty in patients with an acute myocardial infarction (MI). CREF (%) before discharge = regional ejection fraction measured from the left ventriculograms taken during cardiac catheterization before hospital discharge, r = regression correlation coefficient.

In view of these results, it can be concluded that there is a pharmacologically inducible vasodilatory reserve in reperfused ischemic myocardium after successful coronary angioplasty in patients with acute myocardial infarction, and that this further improves at 10 day follow-up angiography. More interestingly, the degree of reactive hyperemic response upon reperfusion has a predictive value regarding the ultimate degree of recovery of regional myocardial function.

D: The use of myocardial flow reserve in a model for pharmacological research

The objective of this study was to investigate the cardioprotective effect of aprikalim, a potassium channel activator, on myocardial ischemia during coronary angioplasty in patients with stable angina, normal left ventricular function, and single left anterior descending coronary artery stenosis without angiographic evidence of collaterals [20]. Twenty-four patients were enrolled and randomized into placebo or aprikalim infusion. The Cardiometrics intracoronary Doppler guide wire was used to assess blood flow velocity distal to the stenotic lesion. On-line intracoronary velocity was measured and recorded continuously before, during and after balloon inflation. Myocardial flow reserve was measured on-line with the Philips DCI, before and after the pharmacological intervention as well as the angioplasty using either ischemia or intracoronary papaverine to induce a hyperemic response. Left ventricular wall motion was analyzed qualitatively and quantitatively with echocardiography. This model allows the assessment of coronary flow, myocardial perfusion as well as wall motion simultaneously and has therefore great promise in pharmacological investigations. The flow reserve measurements were made simultaneously with the Doppler wire and the angiographic technique, using the same intracoronary papaverine injection for the induction of a hyperemic response. Before the angioplasty procedure a reliable flow reserve measurement could be obtained by both techniques in 22 of the 24 patients (92%), and after the angioplasty procedure both techniques were applied successfully in 23 of the 24 patients (96%). Atrial pacing was not required in any of these patients as the quality of the subtraction images was excellent during a spontaneous heart rate. The addition in this new program that allows for perfect matching of the digitized frames is very important in this regard. Flow reserve increased immediately after angioplasty by both methods: MFR from 1.8 ± 0.9 to 2.6 ± 1.4 ($p < 0.05$) and by intracoronary Doppler from 1.7 ± 0.6 to 2.2 ± 0.7 ($p < 0.05$).

References

1. White CW, Wright CB, Doty DB *et al.* Does visual interpretation of the coronary arteriogram predict the physiologic importance of a coronary stenosis? N Engl J Med 1984; 310: 819–24.
2. Zir LM, Miller SW, Dinsmore RE, Gilbert JP, Harthorne JW. Interobserver variability in coronary angiography. Circulation 1976; 53: 627–32.
3. Detre KM, Wright E, Murphy ML, Takaro T. Observer agreement in evaluating coronary angiograms. Circulation 1975; 52: 979–86.
4. Reiber JHC, Serruys PW, Kooijman CJ *et al.* Assessment of short-, medium-, and long-term variations in arterial dimensions from computer-assisted quantitation of coronary cineangiograms. Circulation 1985; 71: 280–8.
5. Gould KL, Kelley KO, Bolson EL. Experimental validation of quantitative coronary arteriography for determining pressure flow characteristics of coronary stenosis. Circulation 1982; 66: 930–7.
6. Serruys PW, Wijns W, Reiber JHC *et al.* Values and limitations of transstenotic pressure gradients measured during percutaneous coronary angioplasty. Herz 1985; 6: 337–42.
7. Wijns W, Serruys PW, Reiber JHC *et al.* Quantitative angiography of the left anterior descending coronary artery: correlations with pressure gradient and results of exercise thallium scintigraphy. Circulation 1985; 71: 273–9.
8. Hodgson JM, Legrand V, Bates ER *et al.* Validation in dogs of a rapid digital angiographic technique to measure relative coronary blood flow during routine cardiac catheterization. Am J Cardiol 1985; 55: 188–93.
9. Wilson RF, Laughlin DE, Ackell PH *et al.* Transluminal, subselective measurement of coronary artery blood flow velocity and vasodilator reserve in man. Circulation 1985; 72: 82–92.
10. Wilson RF, Marcus ML, White CW. Prediction of the physiologic significance of coronary

arterial lesions by quantitative lesion geometry in patients with limited coronary artery disease. Circulation 1987; 75: 723–32.

11. Vogel RA. Friedman HZ, Beauman GJ, Virano GR, Grines CL. Measurement of absolute coronary blood flow using a standard angioplasty catheter [abstract]. J Am Coll Cardiol 1987; 9 (2 Suppl A): 69A.
12. van Ommeren J, Zijlstra F, Serruys PW, Reiber JHC. A rapid Angiographic technique to measure relative coronary blood flow. In Young IT, Duin RPW, Biemond J, Gerbrands JJ (eds): Signal processing III: theories and applications. Amsterdam: Elsevier 1986: 1375–8.
13. Zijlstra F, van Ommeren J, Reiber JHC, Serruys PW. Does the quantitative assessment of coronary artery dimensions predict the physiological significance of a coronary stenosis? Circulation 1987; 75: 1154–61.
14. Hogdson JM, Mancini GBJ, LeGrand V, Vogel RA. Characterization of changes in coronary blood flow during the first six seconds after intracoronary contrast injection. Invest Radiol 1985; 20: 246–52.
15. Cusma JT, Toggart EJ, Folts JD *et al.* Digital subtraction angiographic imaging of coronary flow reserve. Circulation 1987; 75: 461–72.
16. den Boer A. A microprocessor system for on-line registration of the X-ray system settings. Rotterdam: Thoraxcenter 1982.
17. Zijlstra F, Reiber JHC, Juillière Y, Serruys PW. Normalization of coronary flow reserve by percutaneous transluminal coronary angioplasty. Am J Cardiol 1988; 61: 55–60.
18. Reiber JHC, Koning G, van der Zwet PMJ *et al.* Assessment of myocardial flow reserve with the DCI. Medica Mundi 1993; 38(2): 81–8.
19. Suryapranata H, Zijlstra F, MacLeod DC, van den Brand M, de Feyter PJ, Serruys PW. Predictive value of reactive hyperemic response upon reperfusion on recovery of regional myocardial function following coronary angioplasty in acute myocardial infarction. Accepted for publication in Circulation.
20. Widimsky P, Suryapranata H, Zijlstra F, Gregor P. Simultaneous angiographic and intracoronary Doppler guide wire assessment of flow reserve during coronary angioplasty. Submitted for publication.

11. Myocardial flow reserve: On-line versus off-line assessment techniques

MARC M.J.M. VAN DER LINDEN, JÜRGEN HAASE & PATRICK W. SERRUYS

Summary

Various methods can be applied to measure Myocardial Flow Reserve (MFR) as a functional parameter of the severity of coronary artery disease. Angiographic assessment of MFR was originally performed on-line, but the off-line implementation of the method to cinefilm is feasible. In 18 cardiac transplant recipients off-line assessment of MFR, based on time-density analysis of digital subtraction cineangiographic images on the Cardiovascular Angiography Analysis System (CAAS), was compared with the respective on-line technique on the Philips Digital Cardiac Imaging System (DCI), which has been recently validated using Doppler flow velocity measurements.

Introduction

Although coronary arteriography can be used for the location and description of coronary artery stenoses, information about their functional significance cannot always be obtained from the arteriogram alone [1–3]. The concept of myocardial flow reserve (MFR) describes the relationship between the angiographic severity of coronary artery disease and the resulting reduction or limitation in maximal coronary blood flow [2–6]. Moreover, MFR measurements can be used to evaluate dysfunction of the microcirculation.

Different techniques of myocardial flow reserve measurement have been developed for use during the catheterization procedure, such as thermodilution to measure coronary sinus flow, intracoronary Doppler measurements and digital substraction angiography. The thermodilution method requires the insertion of an additional coronary sinus catheter. The ultrasonic recording of phasic coronary blood flow by Doppler requires the insertion of hardware in the coronary artery tree, and is extremely 'space dependent' [7]. Compared with these techniques to measure MFR, the digital substraction angiography has the advantage that no additional catheter or intracoronary device needs to be used. Therefore, it is more easily applicable during routine catheterization, safer, less time consuming and less expensive. Moreover, this technique provides flow information from various subsegments of the coronary artery tree since multiple regions of interest (ROI's) are analyzed.

Since the introduction of digital facilities in the catheterization labora-

J.H.C. Reiber and P.W. Serruys (eds): Progress in quantitative coronary arteriography, 161–171.

tories, both on- and off-line systems for assessment of MFR by digital substraction are available. The on-line assessment of myocardial flow reserve can be very useful in the setting of pharmacological or mechanical interventions, where the results have to be estimated directly after the catheterization [4]. The off-line assessment of MFR, on the other hand, allows objective evaluation of multicenter trials in core laboratories, because the selection of ROI's can be carried out, non-biased by the investigator.

On-line and off-line assessment of myocardial flow reserve

The technique to assess myocardial flow reserve by digital substraction angiography has been extensively described [8–15]. A fixed amount of non-ionic contrast medium is injected at 37°C into the coronary artery using an ECG-triggered infusion pump. The injection rate of the contrast medium is judged to be adequate when back flow of contrast medium into the aorta occurs. The X-ray exposure per frame is kept constant by selecting the lock-in mode on the X-ray generator. Basal coronary angiography is performed after intracoronary administration of 2 mg isosorbide dinitrate. This angiogram is repeated, 30 seconds after pharmacologically induced maximal hyperemia, using an intracoronary bolus injection of 12.5 mg papaverine.

Off-line

Myocardial flow reserve measurement with digital subtraction cineangiography from 35 mm cinefilm has been implemented in the Thoraxcenter research version of the Cardiovascular Angiography Analysis System (CAAS) [16]. Thereby, five end-diastolic cineframes are selected from successive cardiac cycles. Using the last end-diastolic frame prior to contrast administration as a mask, logarithmic non-magnified mask-mode background subtraction is applied to the image subset to eliminate non-contrast medium densities. In the CAAS system at the Thoraxcenter, the appearance-time-contrast density approach, according to Vogel *et al.* [12], is used. From the sequence of background subtracted images, a contrast arrival time image is automatically determined, using an empirically derived fixed density threshold [6]. Each pixel is labelled with the sequence number of the cardiac cycle in which the pixel intensity level exceeds the threshold, starting from the beginning of the ECG-triggered contrast injection. In addition to the contrast arrival time image, a density image is computed, with each pixel intensity value being representative for the maximal local contrast medium accumulation.

On corresponding basal and hyperemic end-diastolic frame sequences, identical regions of interest (ROI's) are selected. Epicardial coronary arteries, visible on the angiogram, the coronary sinus and the great cardiac vein are excluded from the analyses.

The regional relative flow values are quantitatively determined using the following videodensitometric principle: Q = V/T (Q = regional blood flow, V = regional volume and T = mean appearance time). Since the intensity value in the maximal density image is proportional to the transradiated amount of contrast medium, the regional vascular volume for a user-defined ROI is proportional to the mean radiographic density within the ROI. The mean contrast appearance time is derived from the contrast arrival time image. The myocardial flow reserve for one ROI can thus be calculated as follows:

$$CFR = \frac{Q_h}{Q_b} = \frac{V_h/T_h}{V_b/T_b} = \frac{V_h x T_b}{V_b x T_h} = \frac{D_h x T_b}{D_b x T_h}$$

(D = mean maximum contrast density; h = hyperemic; b = baseline).

On-line

The on-line method as implemented in the Philips Digital Cardiac Imaging System (DCI) uses the same basic principle as the off-line method [17].

However, there are a few relevant differences with the earlier described off-line approach. First of all, the definition of the arrival time is now set at the moment that the contrast density curve exceeds 50% of the maximal density value as calculated for each individual pixel. Secondly, following the mask mode substraction, it is possible to carry out additional corrections for any remaining background intensity values apparent in non cardiac regions. Thirdly, the baseline and hyperemic relative flow images can be matched spatially in an optimal manner on the basis of user-defined landmarks, e.g. coronary bifurcations.

From the sequences of mask mode substraction images, 3 parametric images are constructed:

- A contrast arrival time image (T_{arr}), where each pixel is related to the cardiac cycle in which the density exceeded the 50% of the maximal density achieved.
- A contrast density image (D_{max}), where each pixel intensity value is representative for the maximal value for contrast density in the sequence of subtracted images.
- Finally, a parametric flow image is constructed, in which contrast density is divided by the arrival time.

A fourth image, a MFR image, can be obtained by exactly superimposing both parametric images when these are obtained under baseline and hyperemic conditions. In this last image, each pixel intensity value is representative for the local myocardial flow reserve value. Grey scaling allows quick inspection of the MFR in different areas of the myocardium.

The thoraxcenter experience

At the Thoraxcenter a study has been initiated to compare, in a clinical setting, off-line assessment of MFR, using a cinefilm based analysis system (CAAS, digital matrix 512 × 512) with the corresponding on-line software (DCI, pixel matrix 512 × 512).

Patients

In all cardiac transplant recipients selective coronary angiography is performed as part of their annual follow-up protocol. During this procedure the off-line MFR is also assessed as part of a larger follow-up study. Therefore, this group of patients was suitable to perform this comparative study.

After the DCI system had been installed at the Thoraxcenter, 18 patients (age 46 ± 14, mean ± SD) were included in this study. The mean interval after transplantation was 3.2 ± 1.1 year. All patients were free of acute rejection at the time of the procedure as assessed by right ventricular biopsy. They were investigated without premedication and their vasoactive medication was discontinued the evening before the catheterization.

Methods

Baseline and hyperemic coronary angiography was performed as described. Simultaneous videocamera acquisition and cinefilm exposure was made possible by selecting the CINE-DCI mode on the X-ray generator. A print-out was made of the on-line MFR image with the selected regions of interest, to allow off-line assessment of MFR in identical regions (Figure 11.1).

Statistical methods

Statistical analysis was performed using linear regression analysis and the Wilcoxon Matched-pairs Signed-ranks test for paired analysis. According to the statistical approach proposed by Altman and Bland [18], the individual differences between MFR measured by CAAS and DCI were plotted against individual mean values. Mean value and standard deviation of the signed differences in MFR between both methods were then calculated to assess the agreement between both measurements. Statistical significance was defined as a p value of 0.05 or less.

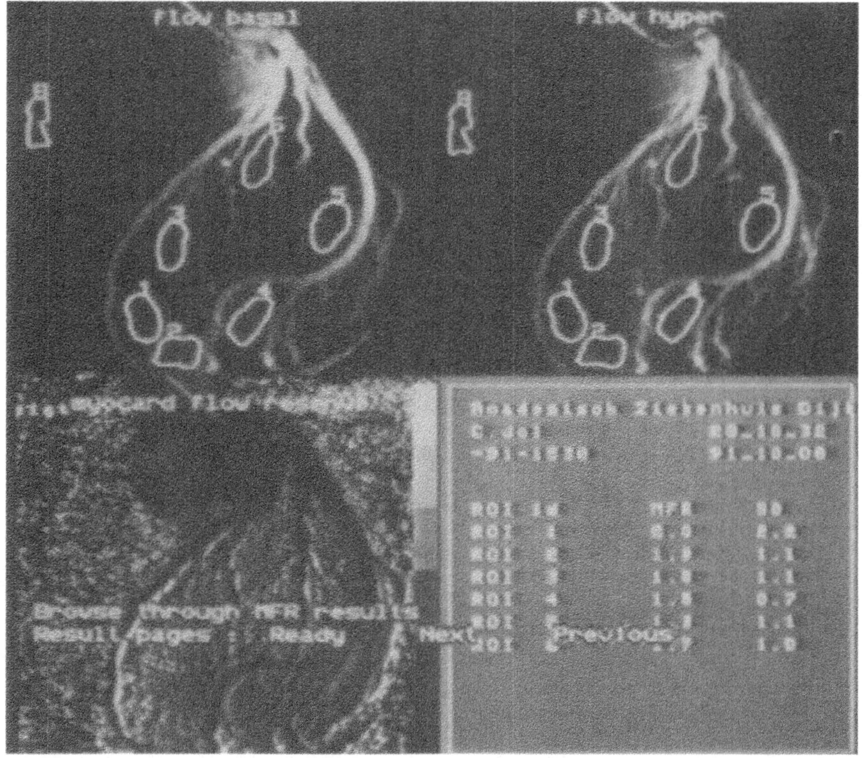

Figure 11.1. Illustration of the image acquisition in this study in a 58 year old male heart transplant recipient. Left: on-line assessment of MFR. Right: off-line assessment of MFR.

Results

A total of 68 ROI's (3.7 per patient, range 3–6) were analyzed with both techniques. Ejection fraction could be assessed in 17 patients and gave a mean value of 69 ± 7%. Mean systolic blood pressure at the time of hyperaemia was 119 ± 15 mmHg and mean diastolic blood pressure was 84 ± 11 mmHg.

Among the patients included in this study, there was no angiographic evidence of collateral circulation or flow limiting stenosis (> 50% diameter reduction) by either visual assessment or quantitative analysis, using automated edge detection.

The linear regression analysis, as shown in Figure 11.2, revealed a reasonable correlation between MFR measurements using the DCI and CAAS system (r = 0.88, = 0.17 + 1.19x, SEE = 0.81). According to the approach of Altman and Bland, as shown in Figure 11.3, the mean difference between

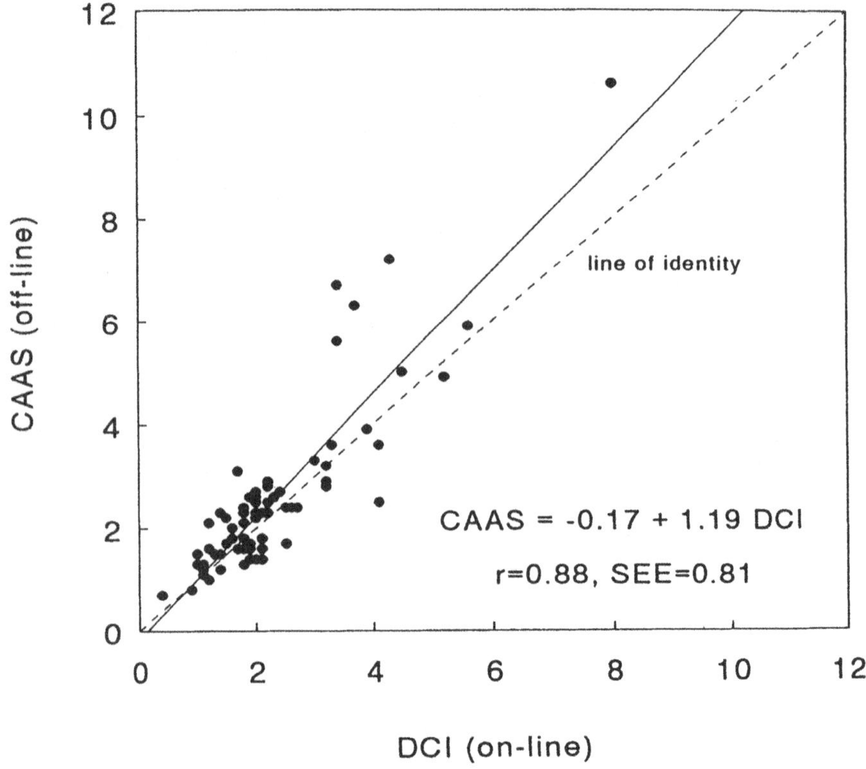

Figure 11.2. Results of comparison of digital and cinefilm measurements: The MFR results of the CAAS are plotted against the results obtained by the DCI system. The results of the linear regression analysis and the line of identity are included in the graph.

both methods was 0.28 ± 0.84 ($p = 0.01$). The DCI system underestimated MFR as compared to CAAS measurements, which was more pronounced for high values of MFR (>5.0 by CAAS; 6 datapoints). For MFR ≤ 5.0, there was no significant difference between MFR measurements by CAAS (mean 2.18 ± 0.87) and DCI (mean 2.10 ± 0.91). The linear regression analysis yielded the following equation: $y = 0.47 + 0.81x$ ($r = 0.85$, $SEE = 0.47$).

Discussion

The functional significance of coronary lesions cannot always completely be evaluated by visual interpretation of stenosis morphology or quantitative measurement of it's geometric dimension [19, 20]. As already stated in this book, the concept of myocardial flow reserve has been developed to provide information concerning the functional significance of a coronary stenosis as

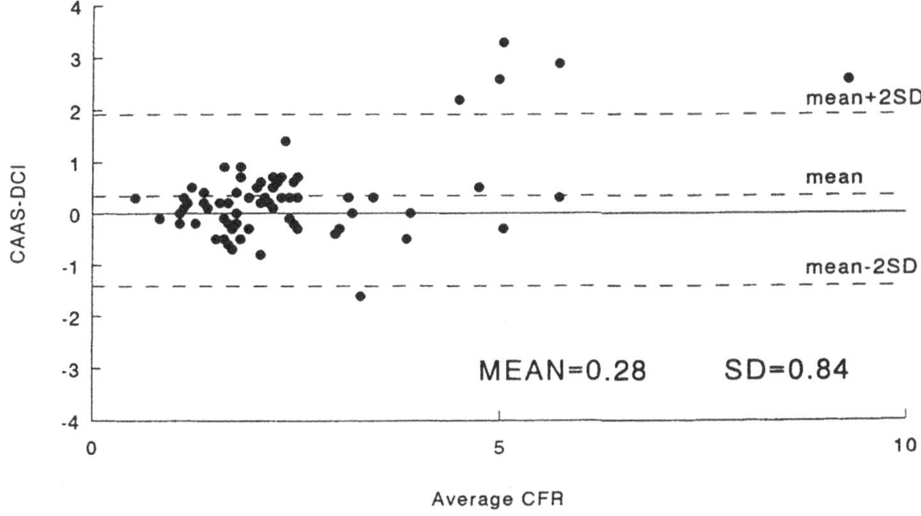

Figure 11.3. Comparison of digital and cinefilm measurements according to the method of Altman and Bland [16]: the differences between CAAS and DCI measurements are plotted against the mean values. The mean difference and 2–fold standard deviation are shown in the figure.

well as concerning the specific characteristics of myocardial flow, which can be relevant in patients with cardiomyopathy, syndrome X or diffuse coronary artery disease. Furthermore, this method can be used to assess the influence of different treatment strategies on myocardial perfusion in multicenter trials.

In vivo validation studies of videodensitometric MFR (VD) have shown excellent results [21, 22]. The validation using intravascular Doppler assessment of blood flow velocity (DOP) is eminently relevant because the methodological approach of both techniques is completely different. In a study of 21 patients undergoing elective PTCA for angina pectoris [21], a good relationship was found between both measurements, irrespective whether the flow was limited by the severity of the stenosis (VD = 0.88 DOP + 0.12, r = 0.85, SEE + 0.38), or whether additional factors were present with potential influence on the outcome of MFR measurements like left ventricular hypertrophy or coronary artery dissection (VD = 0.96 DOP + 0.01, r = 0.87, SEE = 0.34).

Animal experiments, using microspheres, also show a good correlation between videodensitometric measurements of MFR and the application of microspheres (N = 86, r = 0.79, y = 0.58 + 0.81x, SEE = 0.80) (unpublished observations).

Since the analysis of the angiogram includes the selection of ROI's by the observer using a writing tablet interfaced with the computer, this procedure

Table 11.1. Reproducibility of the digital subtraction technique [22].

	Variability (mean ± SD)	
Intra-observer	−0.01 ± 0.07	NS
Inter-observer	0.08 ± 0.52	NS
Short-term	−0.02 ± 0.26	NS
Medium-term	−0.06 ± 0.52	NS
Long-term	0.11 ± 0.63	NS

can introduce some interobserver variability. However, both the inter- and intra-observer variabilities, as well as the short-, medium-, and long-term variabilities of MFR as assessed from CAAS show a reasonable reproducibility of this technique (Table 11.1) [23].

The relation between videodensitometric MFR and the severity of coronary artery disease was assessed in a precision study from the Thoraxcenter by quantitative analysis of coronary artery dimensions. A good relation was found between MFR and the minimal luminal cross-sectional area (r = 0.92, SEE = 0.73) as well as between MFR and the percent area stenosis (r = 0.92, SEE = 0.74) [6]. In visually normal coronary arteries (N = 17) a MFR of 5.0 ± 0.8 was calculated, which differed significantly from the MFR of coronary arteries with obstructive disease (N = 12) providing values between 0.5 and 3.9. Therefore a normal MFR was defined as greater than or equal to 3.4 (2 SD below the mean MFR of angiographically normal coronary arteries) [6, 21, 23]. The measured mean MFR in this study (2.33 ± 1.25 by DCI, and 2.62 ± 1.70 by CAAS), is relatively low, but not an unexpected finding in such a group of patients [24–26].

Where estimated MFR was >5.0 by CAAS, the DCI yielded lower MFR values. One of the reasons for this discrepancy may be the fact that on cine-film the relation between light exposure and it's resulting optical transparency is nonlinear. The nonlinear stages in the transfer function between contrast and videosignal level in the DCI have been corrected for. Moreover, the fixed density threshold, used in the contrast arrival time image to calculate contrast arrival time, is different for both systems. For the off-line system this threshold, expressed in percentage of the brightness scale, was empirically derived by analyzing images in 12 patients with visually normal coronary arteries [6]. A threshold of 12% was defined for the CAAS system to completely exclude the influence of background noise on the calculation of contrast medium appearance times. The DCI system uses a threshold of 50% of maximal pixel intensity for the calculations of contrast arrival time.

Limitations

In the present study, the same imaging system is used for all angiograms. Since the different x-ray and cine film systems may have impact on the image density versus x-ray intensity relationship, this study cannot address the variability in measurements due to equipment characteristics.

The videodensitometric technique itself, also has certain limitations. The use of contrast media, which have substantial vascular effects, may disturb blood flow [12, 27]. Because longterm variability is 0.11 ± 0.63, this approach is only suitable to detect rather large changes in flow reserve (>1.37, mean + 2 SD). Furthermore, a significant learning curve exists for each angiographist to obtain acceptable image quality. Therefore, the feasibility of this technique in multicenter trials remains doubtful.

For all techniques, the MFR is based on the ratio between maximal coronary blood flow and resting flow. The latter is mainly determined by the aortic pressure and heart rate, and therefore slight changes in these 2 parameters can influence MFR measurements. Flow during maximal hyperemia is linearly related to the perfusion pressure. This can result in a scatter of MFR data in a single patient. The recently described hyperemic versus perfusion pressure relationship [28] theoretically overcomes this problem, but is difficult to assess with angiography.

In conclusion, we can state that the digital subtraction technique is a reliable and useful method to assess MFR, both on-line and off-line. The analysis of multiple regions of interest provides flow information from the various subsegments of the coronary artery tree. This method is easily applicable, and less time consuming than other methods to assess MFR. However, since to date only 5% of the European catheterization laboratories (estimation by the industry) are equipped with digital angiographic facilities and the storage capacity for digital images is still limited, there is a need for off-line analysis systems based on conventional cinefilm.

References

1. Klocke FJ. Measurement of coronary flow reserve: defining pathophysiology versus making decisions about patient care. Circulation 1987; 76: 1183–9.
2. Hoffman JIE. Maximal coronary flow and the concept of coronary vascular reserve. Circulation 1984; 70: 153–9.
3. Klocke FJ. Measurements of coronary blood flow and degree of stenosis: current clinical implications and continuing uncertainties. J Am Coll Cardiol 1983; 1: 31–41.
4. Serruys PW, Juillière Y, Zijlstra F *et al*. Coronary blood flow velocity during percutaneous transluminal coronary angioplasty as a guide for assessment of the functional result. Am J Cardiol 1988; 61: 253–9.
5. Zijlstra F, Reiber JC, Juillière Y, Serruys PW. Normalization of coronary flow reserve by percutaneous transluminal coronary angioplasty. Am J Cardiol 1988; 61: 55–60.
6. Zijlstra F, Van Ommeren J, Reiber JHC, Serruys PW. Does the quantitative assessment of coronary artery dimensions predict the physiologic significance of a coronary stenosis? Circulation 1987; 75: 1154–61.
7. Serruys PW, Hermans WRM, Zijlstra F, De Feyter PJ. Coronary Doppler. In Topol EJ (ed): Textbook of interventional cardiology. Philadelphia: WB Saunders 1990: 768–98.
8. Rutishauser W, Simon H, Stucky JP, Schad N, Noseda G, Wellauer J. Evaluation of

roentgen cinedensitometry for flow measurement in models and in the intact circulation. Circulation 1967; 36: 951–63.

9. Rutishauser W, Noseda G, Bussman WD, Preter B. Blood flow measurement through single coronary arteries by roentgen densitometry. Right coronary artery flow in conscious man. Radium Ther Nucl Med 1970; 109: 21–4.
10. Levin DC, Schapiro RM, Boxt LM, Dunham L, Harrington DP, Ergun DL. Digital subtraction angiography: principles and pitfalls of image improvement techniques. Am J Roentgenol 1984; 143: 447–54.
11. Zierler KL. Circulation times and the theory of indicator dilution methods for determining blood flow and volume. In Hamilton WF (Section ed): Circulation: volume 1 (Handbook of physiology; section 2). Washington DC: American Physiological Society 1962: 585–615.
12. Vogel RA. The radiographic assessment of coronary blood flow parameters. Circulation 1985; 72: 460–5.
13. Wilson RF, White CW. Intracoronary papaverine: an ideal coronary vasodilator for studies of the coronary circulation in conscious humans. Circulation 1986; 73: 444–51.
14. Zijlstra F, Serruys PW, Hugenholtz PG. Papaverine: the ideal coronary vasodilator for investigating coronary flow reserve? A study of timing, magnitude, reproducibility and safety of the coronary hyperemic response after intracoronary papaverine. Cathet Cardiovasc Diagn 1986; 12: 298–303.
15. Van der Werf T, Heethaar RM, Stegehuis H, Meyler FL. The concept of apparent cardiac arrest as a prerequisite for coronary digital subtraction angiography. J Am Coll Cardiol 1984; 4: 239–44.
16. Van Ommeren J, Zijlstra F, Serruys PW, Reiber JHC. A rapid angiographic technique to measure relative coronary blood flow. In Young IT, Biemond J, Duin RPW, Gerbrands JJ (eds): Signal processing III: theories and applications. North-Holland, Amsterdam/New York/Oxford/Tokyo, 1986: 1375–8.
17. Reiber JHC, Koning G, Van der Zwet PMJ, Bosch HG, Van Meurs B, Schalij M. Assessment of myocardial flow reserve with the DCI. MedicaMundi 1993; 38: 81–8.
18. Bland JM, Altman DG. Statistical methods assessing agreement between two methods of clinical measurement. Lancet 1986; 1: 307–10.
19. Marcus ML, Armstrong ML, Heistad DD, Eastham CL, Mark AL. Comparison of three methods of evaluating coronary obstructive lesions: postmortem arteriography, pathologic examination and measurement of regional myocardium perfusion during maximal vasodilatation. Am J Cardiol 1982; 49: 1699–706.
20. Schwartz JN, Kong Y, Hackel DB, Bartel AG. Comparison of angiographic and postmortem finds in patients with coronary artery disease. Am J Cardiol 1975; 36: 174–8.
21. Serruys PW, Zijlstra F, Laarman GJ, Reiber JHC, Beatt K, Roelandt JRTC. A comparison of two methods to measure coronary flow reserve in the setting of coronary angioplasty: intracoronary blood flow velocity measurements with a Doppler catheter, and digital subtraction cineangiography. Eur Heart J 1989; 10: 725–36.
22. Storm C, Buis B, Marinus J, Van Benthem A, Van Dijk A, Bruschke A. X-ray videodensitometry vs. intracoronary Doppler flow. Two methods evaluating myocardial perfusion by calculating coronary reserve [abstract]. Eur Heart J 1988; 9 (abstract Suppl 1): 117.
23. Zijlstra F, Den Boer A, Reiber JHC, Van Es GA, Lubsen J, Serruys PW. Assessment of immediate and long-term functional result of percutaneous transluminal coronary angioplasty. Circulation 1988; 78: 15–24.
24. Nitenberg A, Tavolaro O, Benvenuti ?? *et al.* Recovery of a normal coronary vascular reserve after rejection therapy in acute human cardiac allograft rejection. Circulation 1990; 81: 1312–8.
25. McGinn AL, Wilson RF, Olivari MT, Homans DC, White CW. Coronary vasodilator reserve after human orthotopic cardiac transplantation. Circulation 1988; 78: 1200–9.
26. Bortone AS, Hess OM, Eberli FR *et al.* Abnormal coronary vasomotion during exercise in patients with normal coronary arteries and reduced coronary flow reserve. Circulation 1989; 79: 516–27.

27. Hodgson JM, Mancini GBJ, Legrand V, Vogel RA. Characterization of changes in coronary blood flow during the first six seconds after intracoronary contrast injection. Invest Radiol 1985; 20: 246–52.
28. Mancini GBJ, McGillem BS, DeBoe SF, Gallagher KP. The diastolic hyperemic flow versus pressure relation. A new index of coronary stenosis severity and flow reserve. Circulation 1989; 80: 941–50.

12. On-line assessment of myocardial flow reserve

MARTIN J. SCHALIJ, MARIKEN J.A. GELDOF,
PIETER M.J. VAN DER ZWET, ENNO T. VAN DER VELDE,
ELS M. NAGTEGAAL, VOLKERT MANGER CATS,
JOHAN H.C. REIBER & ALBERT V.G. BRUSCHKE

Summary

Myocardial flow reserve (MFR), the ratio between pharmacologically induced hyperaemic flow and baseline flow, is an index of myocardial perfusion. In this study two new techniques were validated by comparing the results with transonic (T) flow measurements. In eight dogs digital (Di) angiographic image processing was used to determine relative flow by maximal contrast density (Dmax) and contrast appearance time (Tarr). In five dogs an 0.46 mm Doppler (Dopp) flow velocity wire was inserted into either the left anterior descending artery (LAD) or the left circumflex branch (LCx) and flow velocity ratios were compared with T flow ratios. T flow and Dopp flow were measured just before injection of non-ionic contrast material (6 ml/s, 7 ml). Hyperaemia was induced by intracoronary administration of 12.5 mg HCl-papaverine. Dmax and Tarr at baseline and hyperaemia were derived from end-diastolic frames after mask-mode background subtraction (Tarr = time from onset of contrast appearance until 50% of Dmax is reached). For each region of interest (ROI), placed over the distal myocardial perfusion bed the average Dmax and Tarr were calculated. From these data DiMFR was obtained. DoppMFR was expressed by the ratio between hyperaemic average peak velocity (APV) and baseline APV. *Results*: LAD TMFR was 3.2 ($\pm$1.5) and LAD DiMFR was 3.6 ($\pm$1.0), $n = 20$, $r = 0.70$. LCx TMFR was 2.8 ($\pm$1.0) and LCx DiMFR was 3.5 ($\pm$1.7), $n = 20$, $r = 0.78$. The difference between TMFR and DiMFR can be explained by the presence of collateral circulation between LAD and LCx which affected DiMFR measurements more than it did TMFR measurements. After insertion of the Dopp wire a stable velocity signal was obtained in all experiments. The introduction of this wire did not result in a measurable flow reduction. DoppMFR was 2.7 ($\pm$0.7) and TMFR was 2.6 ($\pm$0.8), $n = 12$, $r = 0.86$. *Conclusion*: DiMFR is a better index of regional myocardial perfusion than TMFR because DiMFR incorporates the contribution of collateral flow. However, it is a rather complex technique with several theoretical limitations. DoppMFR is a simple technique to assess MFR, but its application is limited to large coronary branches and it does not account for the contribution of collateral circulation.

J.H.C. Reiber and P.W. Serruys (eds): Progress in quantitative coronary arteriography, 173–189.

Introduction

In patients with coronary artery disease selective coronary arteriography plays a pivotal role in clinical decision making. Coronary arteriography is unsurpassed in its ability to show the morphology of coronary arteries, however, it has since long been recognized that no simple relation exists between the visually or quantitatively estimated severity of coronary artery disease and its effects on regional myocardial perfusion [1, 2]. Furthermore, due to inherent limitations of cardiac image acquisition systems, only the larger epicardial coronary vessels with sizes of more than 0.5 mm can be studied [3].

To express in a convenient manner the capacity of the coronary vascular system to increase flow, Gould [4] introduced the concept of myocardial flow reserve (MFR, defined as the ratio between maximal coronary blood flow and basal flow [4]), that has been accepted as a functional index of the severity of disturbances of the coronary circulation [5]. Despite several theoretical limitations, in clinical practice MFR measurements can be used to determine the significance of coronary artery stenosis provided the microcirculation is normal or conversely, to evaluate myocardial microcirculation in the presence of normal epicardial arteries [6].

A number of noninvasive and invasive techniques are available to measure MFR in experimental and clinical settings. Noninvasive imaging techniques such as cine computed tomography, contrast echocardiography and magnetic resonance imaging can be used to study coronary flow and transmural flow distribution. Until now it is not clear to what extent these techniques can be introduced in routine clinical practice. The most promising noninvasive technique presumably is positron emission tomography (PET) which enables repeated measurements of regional myocardial perfusion. A widespread introduction of this method is still hampered by the almost prohibitive financial consequences.

Invasive techniques such as intravascular Doppler ultrasound and digital subtraction angiography have been subject to extensive research for many years [7–13].

Based on the principles of the indicator dilution theory, Rutishauser [8, 9] introduced, more than 20 years ago, a radiographic technique for assessing regional coronary blood flow. The transit time of contrast agent at two sequential locations was determined and after calculation of the volume of the coronary segment absolute flow could be derived. Based on these principles, Vogel [10, 11] developed a digital arteriographic method to measure myocardial flow reserve. Relative flow was represented by the ratio of maximal contrast density and appearance time of contrast. By computing the ratio of hyperaemic flow and basal flow, myocardial flow reserve can be determined. Although, as discussed by Pijls *et al.* [12], several theoretical problems exist, densitometric assessment of relative flow can be used to obtain information about the severity of coronary artery disease. Until recently densitometric assessment of MFR was a time-consuming technique which included several potential sources of errors. A major problem concerned the difficulties in controlling the densitometric aspects which are related to the use of cine-film. The introduction of digital image processing techniques enables the on-line assessment of myocardial flow reserve in routine clinical practice and eliminates the potential photographic source of error.

A more direct method to obtain relative myocardial flow in patients became available with the introduction of the intravascular Doppler guide wire [7], using Doppler flow velocity spectra to assess relative coronary blood flow. The earlier wires had a diameter of at least 0,9 mm (3 F) which affected coronary blood flow significantly, thereby limiting the usefulness of this technique. However, steerable Doppler wires with a diameter of only 0.46 mm have become available. In several studies high correlation coefficients between flow velocity measurements by these Doppler probes and absolute flow measurements were demonstrated [13]. With this technique, myocardial flow reserve can be assessed by comparing the hyperaemic and basal flow values.

In the current study both on-line digital densitometric flow measurements and Doppler flow velocity measurements were used to assess myocardial flow reserve. Both methods were validated by comparing the results with absolute flow measurements.

Methods

Surgical preparation

Mongrel dogs (n = 8) of both sexes weighting between 22 and 46 kg (mean 32 kg) were used in this study. Animal care and euthanasia complied with the guidelines of the Governmental Veterinary Committee of the Netherlands and the Institutional Animal Experimentation Review Committee of the University of Leiden. The dogs were premedicated with ketamine intravenously (10 mg/ml) and anaesthetized with fentanyl and nembutal. Respiration was supported mechanically using a mixture of oxygen and N_2O_2 after placement of an endotracheal tube. During the experiments heart rate and blood pressure were monitored continuously and arterial bloodgas analyses were performed at 10 minute time intervals. Heparine was administered intravenously (1000 U/iv/hr).

A lateral thoracotomy was performed and the pericardium was opened. Both femoral arteries were cannulated to allow simultaneous measurement of the systemic blood pressure and cannulation of the left coronary artery. The femoral veins were cannulated to allow administration of fluids and to insert a temporary pacemaker lead into the right atrial appendage.

Instrumentation

After the pericardium was incised the left anterior descending artery and the left circumflex branch were carefully dissected free and two transonic flow probes (Transonic Systems Inc, USA) were installed.

These ring-mounted Doppler probes enable precise measurement of the coronary blood flow [14, 15]. A stable signal was obtained in all experiments.

A temporary pacemaker lead was inserted via the left femoral vein into the right atrial appendage and connected to a programmable constant current stimulator delivering square pulses of 1.5 ms duration. The hearts were stimulated with a stimulus strength of two times diastolic threshold.

The left coronary artery was selectively cannulated via the left femoral artery using an 8 French Judkins catheter.

Heart rate and systemic blood pressure were monitored continuously.

All data were stored enabling both on-line and off-line analysis using a 16 channel analog-to-digital acquisition and analyzing system based on a 80486 microprocessor.

Angiographic images were obtained using a digital angiographic imaging system (DCI-SX, Philips Medical Systems, The Netherlands), based on a 80486 microprocessor, MFR measurements could be performed on-line.

Doppler flow velocity measurements were made using a flexible and steerable 0.46 mm guide wire with a 12 MHz piezoelectric ultrasound transducer integrated in its tip (Cardiometrics, Inc, USA). Pulse repetition frequency was more than 40Hz with a pulse duration of 0.83 μs and a sampling delay of 6.5 μs. Coupled to the quidewire were a real-time spectrum analyzer, a videocassette recorder and a video page printer.

Acquisition protocols

An optimal X-ray projection separating left anterior descending artery (LAD) and the left circumflex branch (LCx) was chosen. The image intensifier was set into the 7 or 9 inch mode. Flow was measured at baseline and during hyperaemia, induced by the intracoronary administration of 12.5 mg HCl-papaverine. Measurements were made 30 seconds after injection of papaverine. The time interval between each pair of data measurements was at least 10 minutes.

Absolute flow measurements

Absolute coronary flow was obtained using the two transonic flow probes mounted around the LAD and the LCx. For MFR assessment the mean flow was measured just before contrast agent injection and more than two minutes after the last contrast agent injection. During injection of contrast agent absolute flow was recorded continuously to assess the effects on coronary flow.

Angiographic flow measurements

Data acquisition was performed in the 'lock-in' acquisition mode (fixing the kilovoltage of the X-ray system) at 25 frames/s [16]. Acquisition was started two or three cardiac cycles before contrast agent injection to stabilize the imaging system and to allow selection of an appropriate background image at the time of analysis. A non-ionic contrast medium was used (Jopromide 37%). Images were obtained after powered injection of 5 to 7 ml contrast agent in one second (at a flowrate of 5 to 7 ml/s).

During data acquisition the hearts were artificially stimulated just above the intrinsic sinus rhythm synchronized with the DCI X-ray pulses to simulate apparent cardiac arrest [17]. Image acquisition was stopped when venous return became visible.

After image acquisition end-diastolic images were selected for analyzing purposes. The selected consecutive end-diastolic frames in an angiographic run represent one run. The combination of basal and hyperaemic runs are denoted a run-pair. Typically a run consisted of 8 (maximum 11) end-diastolic frames. Next a logarithmic mask mode subtraction was carried out. Finally, the basal and hyperaemic phase-matched logarithmically mask-subtracted images were stored in a temporary file for subsequent analysis.

The data from this temporary file were used to obtain a functional image. Both from the hyperaemic and the basal run two parametric images were generated, a contrast medium arrival picture (CMAP) and a maximal density picture. The contrast medium arrival picture was obtained by determining for each pixel how much time was passed before its density exceeded a threshold level of 50% of the maximal density. In the maximal density image each pixel was assigned the maximal value obtained over all end-diastolic images which were part of the run.

From these CMAP and maximal density pictures a relative flow image was computed by dividing for each pixel the maximal density value by the CMAP value. This was done for both the baseline and the hyperaemic images. Finally the ratio between the maximal relative flow and baseline flow images was expressed as the myocardial flow reserve image.

Before determining the final results in manually drawn regions of interest (ROI's) a background correction was performed. Due to this correction the original mask-mode background subtracted images were corrected as well. ROI's were then drawn over the distal myocardial perfusion bed. The resulting MFR's of each ROI were displayed on a video monitor together with data containing information about the quality of the acquired images. After each experiment time-density curves of each of the ROI's were plotted to judge the quality of the acquired images.

Doppler flow velocity measurements

After cannulation of the left coronary artery the Doppler flow velocity wire (0.46 mm) was inserted into either the LAD or the LCx. Measurements were performed just before contrast agent injection and more than two minutes after contrast agent injection. Doppler signals were analyzed on-line by a Fast Fourier transformation algorithm providing a scrolling grey scale spectral display. Simultaneous display of ECG and DCI pulses enabled synchronization with other measurements. Doppler spectra were recorded on videotape. Only signals obtained with a stable wire position were recorded. The time average of the instantaneous spectral peak velocity (APV) was used for calculations to minimize artifacts caused by wall motion. Myocardial flow reserve was expressed by the ratio between the APV during hyperaemia and the APV at baseline.

Statistical analysis

Statistical analysis was performed using linear regression with calculation of r^2, slope intercept, and SEE. To determine short-term variability of each method and to compare two different methods the average differences and standard deviations were computed.

Results

Effect of contrast agent injection on coronary flow

Contrast agent injection resulted in a reproducible triphasic change of coronary blood flow [2, 20]. Figure 12.1 shows the effects of contrast agent injection (6 ml, flow rate: 6 ml/s) on mean coronary blood flow. Although both basal flow and hyperaemic flow were influenced, the time courses of the effects were different. A short initial increase in flow (coinciding with the passage of contrast material) was followed by a sharp decrease. The nadir was reached after 4.2 s (±0.8) at baseline and after 2.4 s (±0.7) during hyperaemia ($p < 0.005$). Basal flow decreased by 66% (±9.2) and hyperaemic flow by 57% (±0.5, $p < 0.005$). Basal flow returned to normal after 7.9 s (±2.0), whereas hyperaemic flow was restored after 6.2 s (±2.0, $p < 0.005$). After normalization a long lasting (more than 20 seconds) hyperaemic period followed. Even during papaverine induced hyperaemia an additional hyperaemic response was observed in all experiments. These different effects of contrast medium injection on basal flow and hyperaemic flow may hamper a straightforward application of densitometric techniques for the assessment of myocardial flow reserve.

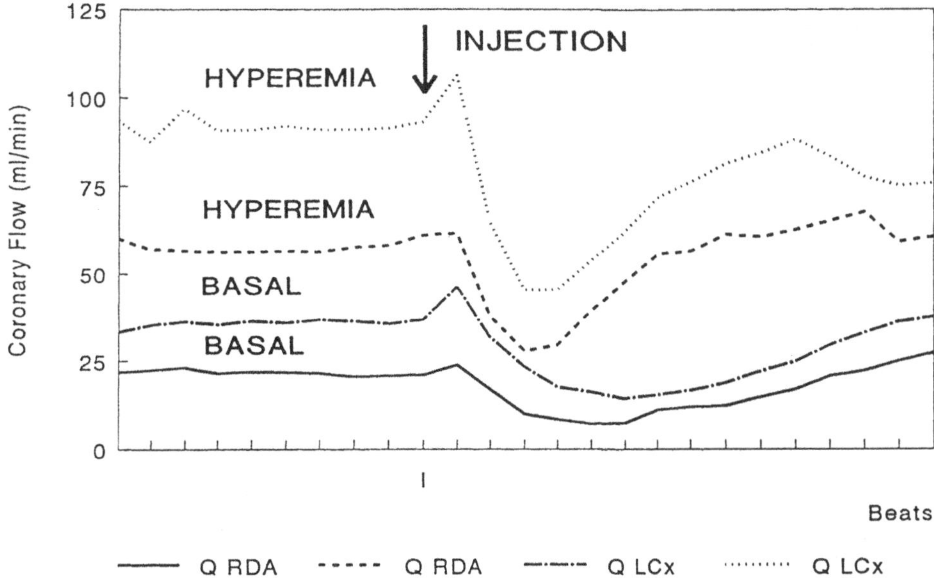

Figure 12.1. Coronary flow changes. The triphasic response caused by contrast agent injection was observed in all experiments. Both basal flow and hyperaemic flow were influenced; however, the time course of the effects was different. A short initial increase of flow (coinciding with the passage of contrast) was followed by a sharp decrease. After normalization a longlasting (more than 20 seconds) hyperaemic period follows. Even during papaverine induced hyperaemia an additional hyperaemic response was observed.

Densitometric myocardial flow reserve

All images were acquired during apnoea and almost motionless images could be obtained in all experiments.

A typical example of such an experiment is given in Figure 12.2. Panels A, C, E, demonstrate the images corresponding to maximal contrast density, the contrast medium arrival time, and the basal flow, respectively. The corresponding hyperaemic pictures are displayed in panels B, D and F. A clear difference in contrast density exists between the basal maximal density image and the hyperaemic maximal density image. In Figure 12.3 the computed myocardial flow reserve image is given. In Figure 12.4 the ultimate results for each of the regions of interest are displayed together with the basal and hyperaemic flow images. Regions of interest were placed over the peripheral myocardial perfusion bed and the corresponding myocardial flow reserves are shown (lower right panel). The corresponding myocardial flow reserve image is also given (lower left panel). The myocardial flow reserve of each ROI, the standard deviation and the number of non-zero pixels are

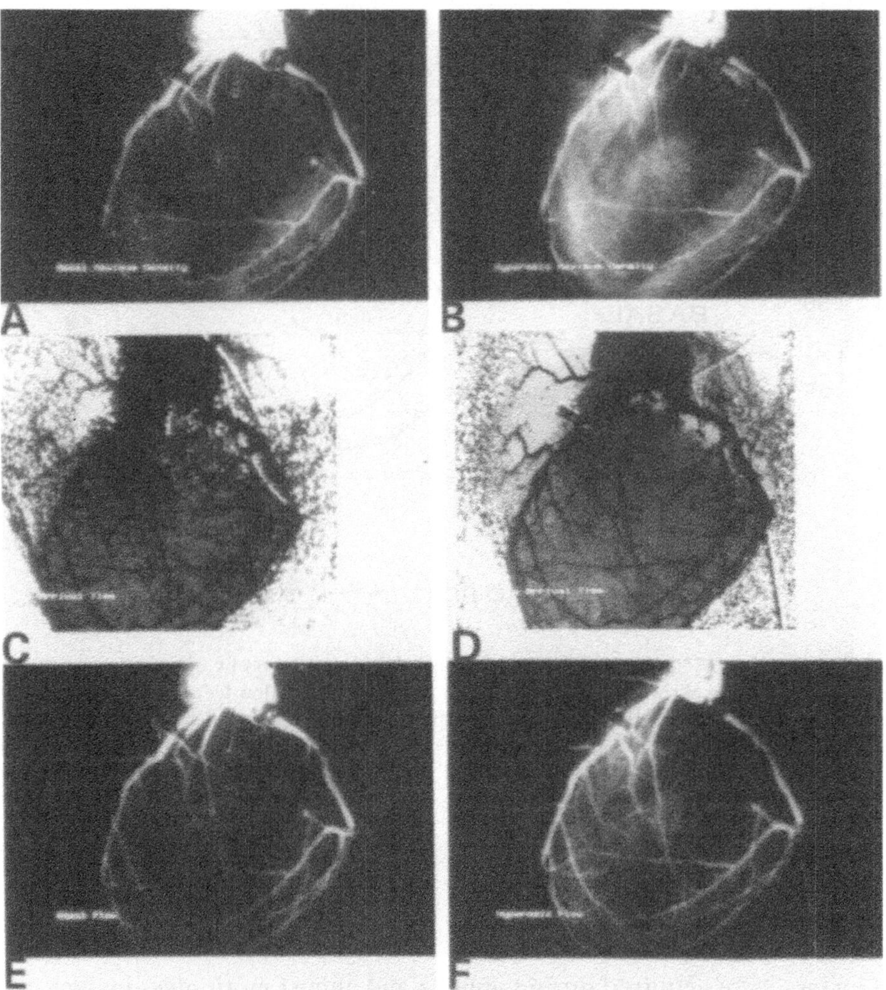

Figure 12.2. Typical example of densitometric assessment of myocardial flow reserve. Panels A, C, E, give the maximal contrast density image, the contrast medium arrival time picture, and the basal flow image, respectively. The corresponding hyperaemic pictures are displayed in panels B, D and F. There is a clear difference in contrast density between the basal maximal density image and the hyperaemic maximal density image.

given as well. The number of non-zero pixels is a reflection of the quality of the image and should be 100.

For each of the ROI's a basal and hyperaemic time versus density curve was reconstructed to reassure the quality of the acquired data.

The corresponding time-density curves of one of the ROI's are given in Figure 12.5. The time-density curve was reconstructed by sampling the aver-

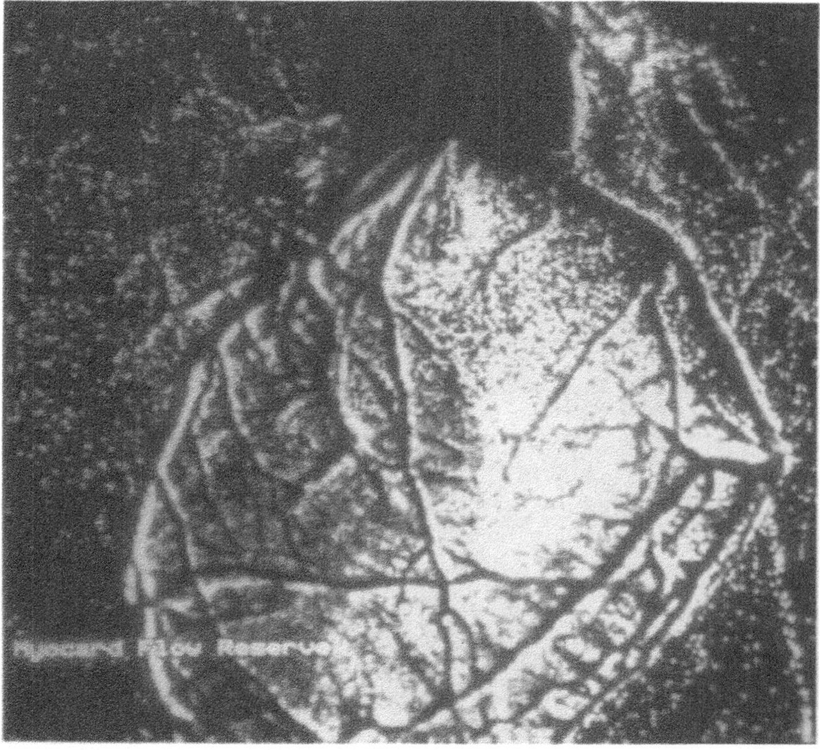

Figure 12.3. Computed myocardial flow reserve image. This image is computed from the data displayed in Figure 12.2.

age pixel density within the ROI's after subtraction of background density. The average density was then plotted against the time. Maximal hyperaemic contrast density was about three times higher than maximal basal contrast density. Basal contrast arrival time was 1.22 beats compared to 0.82 in the hyperaemic situation. This resulted in a MFR of 3.87.

Absolute MFR measured in the LAD was 3.2 (±1.5) compared to a mean densitometric MFR of 3.6 (±1.0, n = 20). The correlation coefficient was 0.70. The mean absolute difference between densitometric MFR and absolute MFR measurements was −0.6 (±1.4). Short-term (10 minutes) variability of the densitometric MFR measurements was good with an average signed difference between the two series of 0.2 (±0.9). The average difference between two consecutive series of absolute MFR measurements was −0.1 (±1.4).

Part of the difference between consecutive MFR measurements was caused by changes in basal flow. The average difference between two basal absolute

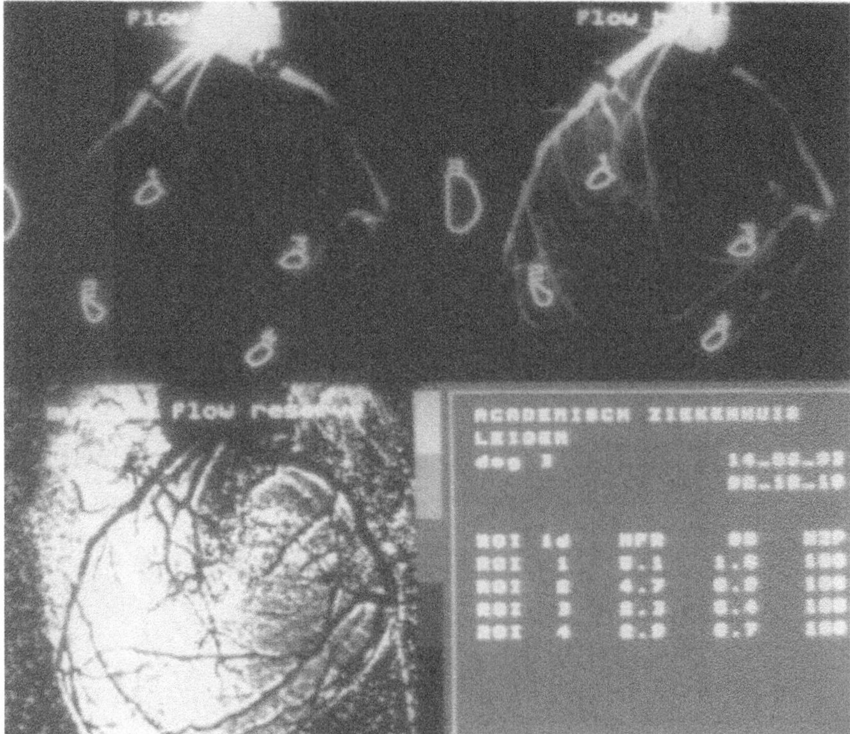

Figure 12.4. The ultimate results for each of the regions of interest are displayed together with the basal and hyperaemic flow images (upper two panels). Regions of interest were placed over the peripheral myocardial perfusion bed and the corresponding myocardial flow reserves are given (lower right panel). The corresponding myocardial flow reserve image is also given (lower left panel). Besides the myocardial flow reserve of each ROI the standard deviation and the number of nonzero pixels are given. The number of nonzero pixels is a reflection of the quality of the image and should be 100 (%).

transonic flow measurements was 6.0, whereas the average difference between two consecutive hyperaemic flow measurements was only 1.0.

Absolute MFR measured in the LCx was 2.8 (±1.0, n = 20) and the corresponding densitometric LCx MFR was 3.5 (±1.7, n = 20). The correlation coefficient was 0.78. The average difference between these two series of measurements was −0.7 with a standard deviation of 1.0. Again, the short-term variability of the densitometric MFR measurements was good with an average difference between the two different series of 1.0 (±0.7). The average difference between two absolute MFR measurements was 1.1 (±0.6). The variability was again caused by changes in basal flow.

The correlation between absolute flow measurements and densitometric relative flow measurements was significant but lower than expected. The

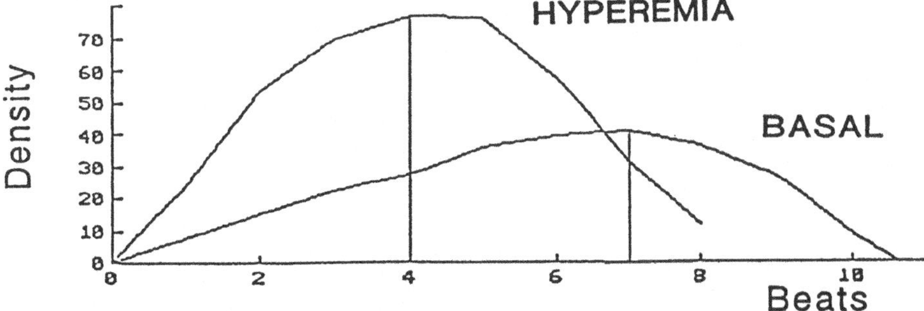

Figure 12.5. Time versus density curve reconstructed to reassure the quality of the acquired data. The time-density curve was reconstructed by sampling the average pixel density within the ROI's after subtraction of background density. The average density was then plotted against the time. Maximal hyperaemic contrast density was about three times larger than maximal basal contrast density. Basal contrast arrival time was 1.22 compared to 0.82 in the hyperaemic situation. This resulted in a MFR of 3.87.

difference may in part be explained by the effects of collateral circulation on regional myocardial blood flow. Figure 12.6 shows an example of collateral coronary circulation. After banding the proximal LAD (arrow), the LAD flow was reduced, and large collaterals between the LAD and LCx became apparent. Flow measured by the transonic flow probe decreased by more than 50%, whereas still a densitometric myocardial flow reserve of 2.5 was still measured over the distal LAD perfusion bed.

Therefore part of the weak correlation between absolute flow measurements and densitometric flow measurements could be explained by taking into account the variable and unknown contribution of collateral coronary circulation. Since densitometric measurements were made over the distal myocardial perfusion bed, these were affected by the collateral circulation to a greater extent than absolute flow measurements, obtained proximal in the large epicardial arteries.

Doppler flow velocity

The introduction of the 0.46 mm Doppler flow velocity wire did not result in a reduction of the coronary blood flow in any of the experiments (n = 5). The wires were placed in the proximal part of either the LAD or the LCx, just distal to the absolute flow probes. Care was taken to avoid side branches between the Doppler element and the transonic flow probes. After insertion of the Doppler wire it was possible to obtain a stable velocity signal for a long period of time in all experiments (Figure 12.7). Normal coronary flow velocity spectra demonstrated a small systolic and a large diastolic velocity component (Figure 12.7). In Figures 12.8A and B an example of the flow velocity spectra obtained in the LAD during respectively basal flow and

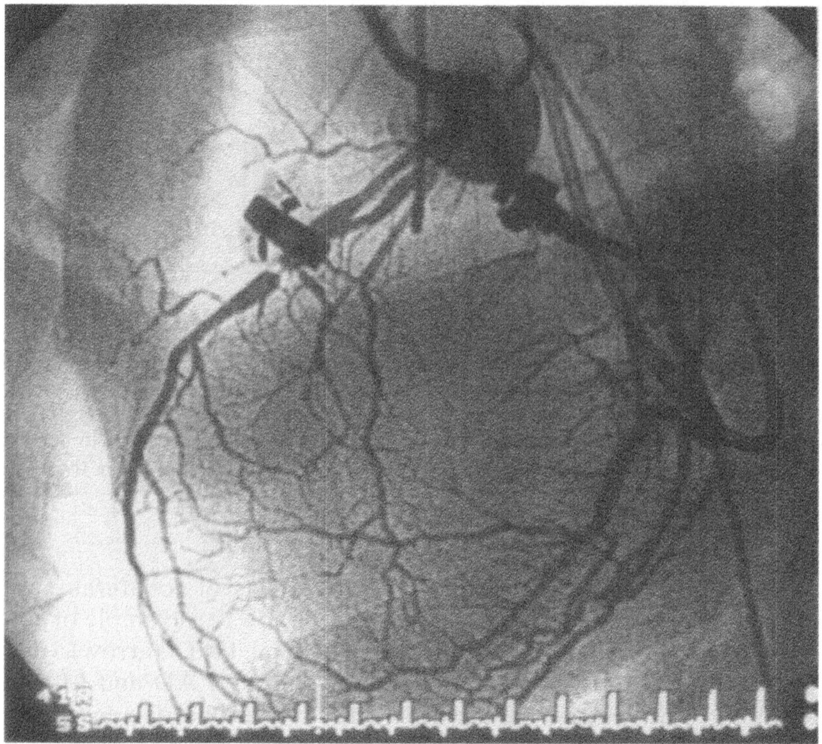

Figure 12.6. After banding of the proximal LAD (arrow), extensive collaterals between LCx and LAD became apparant.

hyperaemic flow is given. Time average peak velocities measured before contrast agent iniection ranged from 14 to 26 m/s (mean 17, SD ± 3.7, n = 18) during basal flow. After papaverine administration the APV increased and ranged from 19 to 55 m/s (mean 39, SD ± 10, n = 18). The average difference between two consecutive series of basal flow velocity measurements was 1.3 (SD ± 2.6), and 0.8 (SD ± 9.4) for two series of hyperaemic flow velocity measurements. The corresponding Doppler myocardial flow reserve was 2.7 (SD ± 0.7) compared with an absolute flow MFR of 2.6 (SD ± 0.8, n = 12). The correlation coefficient between the two methods was 0.86.

Discussion and conclusions

Myocardial blood flow is determined by two variables, namely, the resistance of the myocardial perfusion bed and the perfusion pressure [19]. Maximal

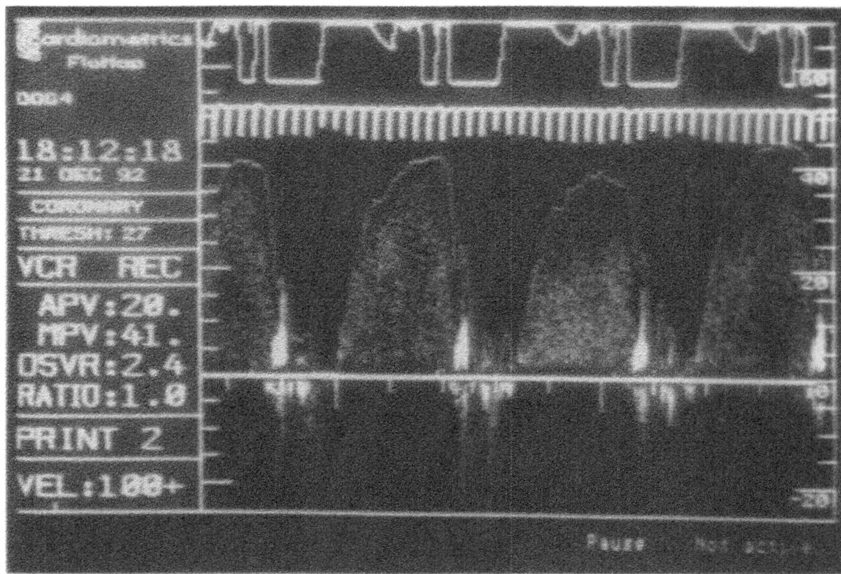

Figure 12.7. It was possible to obtain a stable velocity signal for a long period in all experiments. The coronary flow velocity spectra demonstrated a small systolic and a large diastolic velocity component.

myocardial flow at any given pressure is a function of the total cross-sectional area of the coronary resistance vessels. Myocardial flow reserve at any given pressure is thus a function of the resistance of the myocardial perfusion bed. Because flow reserve depends, among others, on perfusing pressure and basal coronary flow, it is variable and a large range of normal values have been reported. Therefore, MFR measurements in patients must be interpreted cautiously. Despite these limitations, it may be useful to calculate myocardial flow reserve in individual patients to evaluate the severity of coronary artery stenoses in addition to routine selective coronary arteriography, to study microvascular pathology in patients with evidence of small vessel disease and to evaluate the effects of left ventricular hypertrophy on myocardial perfusion. Until now routine clinical application was hampered by time consuming off-line analysis or technical limitations.

In this validation study two different techniques have been discussed enabling on-line assessment of myocardial flow reserve in patients.

Densitometric assessment of myocardial flow reserve

One of the disadvantages of Rutishauser's original technique was that only the flow in proximal epicardial arteries could be measured. Therefore Vogel

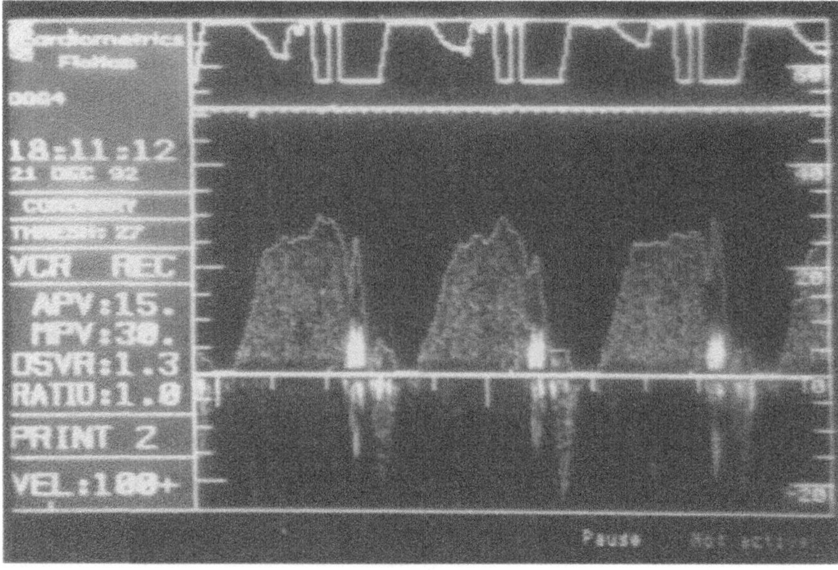

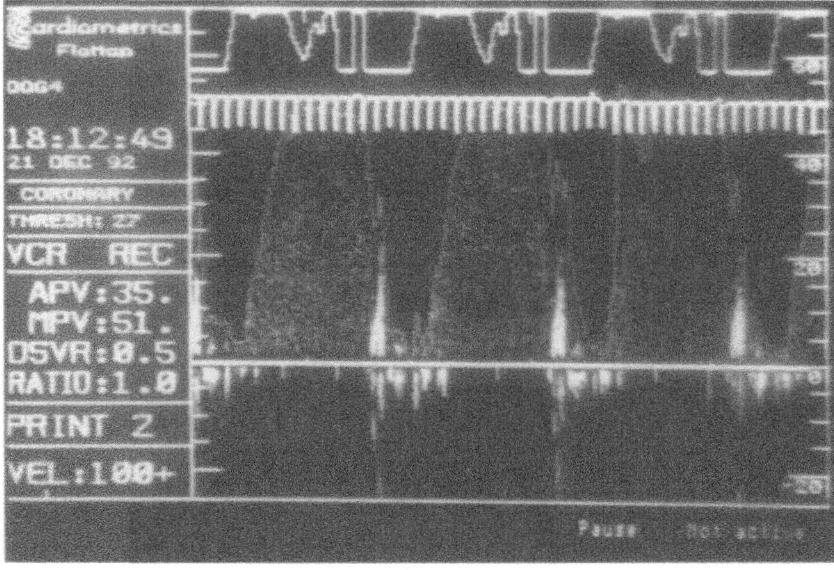

Figure 12.8. An example of the flow velocity spectra obtained in the LAD during respectively basal flow and hyperaemic flow. Time average peak velocities measured during basal flow was 15 (APV, panel A). After papaverine APV increased to 35 (panel B). Corresponding MFR was 2.3.

and co-workers [10, 11] developed a different approach derived from the indicator dilution theory enabling relative flow measurements in the distal myocardial perfusion bed. Arrival time of contrast was used as a flow parameter and by computing the ratio between hyperaemic and basal arrival times myocardial flow reserve could be derived. To improve the results maximal contrast density was used to account for changes in vascular volume.

Theoretical problems limit straightforward application of the indicator dilution theory [12, 18].

One of the premises of the indicator dilution theory is that the dye (contrast agent) does not affect flow. As demonstrated by several investigators and confirmed by the results of this study, contrast agent does affect coronary flow [2, 18]. Flow was reduced by more than 50% after contrast agent injection in all experiments. Furthermore, the time course of the effects was found to be significantly different in the basal and hyperaemic conditions. These different effects on coronary circulation compounds the interpretation of densitometric flow measurements. Another premise of the indicator dilution theory is that the vascular volume remains constant. This is not the case. To overcome this problem Cusma [20] used changes in contrast density to represent changes in vascular volume assuming complete exchange of blood by contrast, but this approach is open to criticism [12]. The use of arrival time of contrast instead of mean transit time is a simplification which may introduce a certain error. Therefore, Pijls *et al.* developed a method using mean transit time of contrast to compare hyperaemic flow before and after interventions. This technique has distinct advantages, however, it does not allow MFR measurements.

In spite of the theoretical limitations inherent to the method, at this time densitometric flow measurement is still one of the most useful techniques to study regional myocardial perfusion.

The results of this validation study corroborate this perception. A significant but rather low correlation was observed between absolute flow measurements and relative flow measurements. Besides the methodological explanations, this may be explained by the different levels at which the measurements were performed. Absolute flow is measured in the proximal portion of large coronary arteries, whereas densitometric flow is measured over the distal myocardial perfusion bed. As demonstrated, the presence of an extensive collateral network affects peripheral flow measurements to a larger extent than it does proximal flow measurements. Therefore, densitometric flow measurements may provide a better index of regional myocardial perfusion than absolute flow measurements. However, it still is a complex technique with several theoretical limitations which warrant further clinical research.

Doppler flow velocity measurements

A number of the limitations of older Doppler flow velocity systems were abolished by the introduction of the new 0.46 mm flow velocity guidewire.

As demonstrated by other investigators Doppler flow velocity correlates well with absolute flow measurements [13]. This was confirmed in this study. Average peak velocities obtained with the Doppler guide wire can be used as relative flow parameters and Doppler flow velocity measurements correlated well with absolute flow measurements. By the introduction of the 0.46 mm guidewire system this technique has come within reach of widespread clinical application. Disadvantages of this method are: a) the need of intracoronary manipulations, thereby introducing a risk of damaging coronary arteries, b) changes in vessel diameter affect flow velocity making it necessary to compute the vessel diameter during basal flow and hyperaemic flow measurements and to correct for changes. Furthermore, the introduction of the wire through a severe coronary artery stenosis may affect coronary blood flow. Because it is still not possible to insert the wire selectively in small coronary arteries without affecting flow, it is difficult to measure differences in regional myocardial perfusion. Despite these limitations the Doppler flow velocity wire can be used to study a number of pathophysiological phenomena in patients.

Conclusion

Digital densitometry enables on-line regional relative flow measurements and despite the theoretical limitations, it may be the most practical technique to study regional myocardial perfusion. Further research is needed to determine its value in clinical decision making. Doppler flow velocity measurements correlated well with absolute flow measurements. It is an easily applicable technique and after the introduction of the 0.46 mm guide wire a number of the existing technical limitations have been solved. However, it is less suitable for the study of local myocardial perfusion and it does not account for the contribution of collateral coronary circulation.

References

1. Harrison DG, White CW, Hiratzka LF *et al.* The value of lesion cross-sectional area determined by quantitative coronary angiography in assessing the physiologic significance of proximal left anterior descending coronary arterial stenoses. Circulation 1984; 69: 1111–9.
2. Klocke FJ. Measurements of coronary blood flow and degree of stenosis: current clinical implications and continuing uncertainties. J Am Coll Cardiol 1983; 1: 31–41.
3. Bruschke AVG, Padmos I, Buis B, Van Benthem A. Arteriographic evaluation of small coronary arteries. J Am Coll Cardiol 1990; 15: 784–9.
4. Gould KL, Libscomb K, Hamilton GW. Physiologic basis for assessing critical coronary stenosis. Instantaneous flow response and regional distribution during coronary hyperaemia as measures of coronary flow reserve. Am J Cardiol 1974; 33: 87–94.
5. Gould KL. Quantification of coronary artery stenosis *in vivo*. Circ Res 1985; 57: 341–53.

6. Hoffman JIE. Maximal coronary flow and the concept of coronary vascular reserve. Circulation 1984; 70: 153–9.
7. Wilson RF, Laughlin DE, Ackell PH *et al.* Transluminal, subselective measurement of coronary artery blood flow velocity and vasodilator reserve in man. Circulation 1985; 72: 82–92.
8. Rutishauser W, Simon H, Stucky JP, Schad N, Noseda G, Wellauer J. Evaluation of roentgen cine densitometry for flow measurement in models and in the intact circulation. Circulation 1967; 36: 951–63.
9. Rutishauser W, Bussman WD, Noseda G, Meier W, Wellauer J. Blood flow measurement through single coronary arteries by roentgen densitometry. I. A comparison of flow measured by a radiologic technique applicable in the intact organism and by electromagnetic flowmeter. Am J Roentgenol 1970; 109: 12–20.
10. Voge' R, LeFree M, Bates E *et al.* Application of digital techniques to selective coronary arteriography: use of myocardial contrast appearance time to measure coronary flow reserve. Am Heart J 1984; 107: 153–64.
11. Vogel RA. The radiographic assessment of coronary blood flow parameters. Circulation 1985; 72: 460–5.
12. Pijls NHJ, Uijen GHJ, Hoevelaken A *et al.* Mean transit time for the assessment of myocardial perfusion by videodensitometry. Circulation 1990; 81: 1331–40.
13. Doucette JW, Corl PD, Payne HM *et al.* Validation of a Doppler guide wire for intravascular measurement of coronary artery flow velocity. Circulation 1992; 85: 1899–911.
14. Drost CJ, Dobson A, Sellers AF, Barnes RJ, Comline RS. An implantable transit time ultrasonic flowmeter for long term measurement of blood volume flow [abstract]. Fed Proc 1984: 538.
15. Vatner SF, Franklin D, Vangitters RL. Simultaneous comparison and calibration of the Doppler and electromagnetic flowmeters. J Appl Physiol 1970; 29: 907–10.
16. Reiber JHC, Koning G, van der Zwet PMJ *et al.* Assessment of myocardial flow reserve with the DCI. Medica Mundi. 1993; 38: 81–8.
17. Van der Werf T, Heethaar RM, Stegehuis H, Meijler FL. The concept of apparent cardiac arrest as a prerequisite for coronary digital subtraction angiography. J Am Coll Cardiol 1984; 4: 239–44.
18. Hodgson J McB, Mancini GBJ, Legrand V, Vogel RA. Characterization of changes in coronary blood flow during the first six seconds after intracoronary contrast injection. Invest Radiol 1985; 20: 246–52.
19. Spaan JAE. Coronary blood flow. Dordrecht: Kluwer Academic Publishers 1991: 333–61.
20. Cusma JT, Toggart EJ, Folts JD *et al.* Digital subtraction angiographic imaging of coronary flow reserve. Circulation 1987; 75: 461–72.

13. Relationship between transstenotic pressure gradients and coronary angiographic parameters

HÅKAN EMANUELSSON, CARL LAMM & MICHAL DOHNAL

Summary

In 20 patients, coronary stenoses were assessed by the combined use of quantitative coronary angiography (QCA) and transstenotic pressure gradient measurements. A fiberoptic pressure sensor mounted on a 0.018" guide wire was used for pressure recordings in 20 patients undergoing percutaneous transluminal coronary angioplasty (PTCA). After intracoronary injection of 125 μg nitroglycerin, multiple angiographic views were taken of the lesion. The pressure sensor was then positioned distal to the stenosis and gradients were recorded before and after intracoronary papaverine injection pre and post PTCA. From pressure and angiographic data, fractional flow reserve (FFR) and stenotic flow reserve (SFR) were calculated. The mean gradient increased from 8 ± 11 mmHg at baseline to 19 ± 12 mmHg after papaverine ($p < 0.001$). There was a curvilinear relationship between angiographic parameters and FFR and SFR, respectively. It may be concluded that the combined information of angiography and pressure gradient recordings facilitates the clinical evaluation of patients undergoing PTCA, in particular if FFR and SFR are calculated from these data.

Introduction

In an early period of coronary angioplasty (PTCA), the recording of transstenotic pressure gradients was routinely performed [1, 2]. It was regarded as an important integral part of the procedure, yielding relevant information about the intervention. The methodology at that time, however, carried several important limitations. Most importantly, since the pressure was measured through the lumen of the balloon catheter lying across the stenosis, there was an intrinsic stenosis gradient created in the system due to the size of the catheter in relation to the minimal luminal diameter. Consequently, there was systematically an overestimation of the pressure gradient. In addition, hydraulic pressure measurement through a long thin catheter is associated with a low frequency response. Mainly due to these drawbacks, most investigators abandoned the routine use of pressure gradient measurement during the PTCA procedure [3]. During recent years, however, new techniques have evolved employing considerably smaller dimensions of the pressure measurement devices [4, 5]. Moreover, other principles, e.g. fiberoptic

J.H.C. Reiber and P.W. Serruys (eds): Progress in quantitative coronary arteriography, 191–206.

tip manometers, have been introduced, yielding a considerably higher frequency response of the pressure signal [6].

The relationship between transstenotic pressure gradient (ΔP), flow (Q) and morphological features of the coronary lesion is described in the equation $\Delta P = fQ + sQ^2$, where the constants s and f contain information regarding the degree of stenosis, reference vessel size, stenosis length and values for blood viscosity and blood density. However, whereas this equation of flow dynamics is valid during experimental conditions where the stenosis parameters can be controlled and exactly measured, it is not yet clarified in detail as to what extent measurement of pressure gradients contribute to the clinical assessment of the stenosis.

Another problem to be addressed is how angiographically equivocal stenoses should be evaluated. In cases of moderate stenosis, the pressure gradient is often low at resting flow. A rise in flow will increase the gradient, and it might therefore be useful to study the pattern of changes in ΔP after inducing a maximal increase in coronary flow.

Consequently, the aim of this investigation was to study the independent value of ΔP in relation to angiographic parameters and to assess the value of derived variables, e.g. coronary flow reserve, to evaluate coronary stenosis severity. In addition, in order to further investigate the sensitivity of the method, pressure gradients were measured at baseline and after intracoronary injection of a vasodilator (papaverine).

Material and methods

Patients

Twenty patients admitted for PTCA were included in this study. There were 8 women and 12 men with a mean age of 58 (48–71 years). All patients had stable angina pectoris, normal left ventricular function and evidence of ischemia on a stress test. Patients with previous acute myocardial infarction, myocardial hypertrophy, valvular heart disease or an open aortocoronary bypass graft on the vessel to be studied were not included for study. The left anterior descending artery (LAD) was studied in 10 patients, the circumflex artery in 5 and the right coronary artery in 5 patients. There were no angiographic signs of collaterals to the affected artery. Patients with stenosis that would be particularly difficult to evaluate by quantitative coronary angiography (QCA), i.e. vessels with diffuse disease, extreme tortuosity or ostial lesions, were not included in the study as well.

Intracoronary pressure measurement

A fiberoptic tip manometer incorporated into a 0.018" guide wire was used for pressure recordings (Pressure Guide™, Radi Medical Systems, Uppsala,

Sweden). This guide wire can be used in regular angioplasty balloons with sufficiently large lumen. The sensor element is situated proximal to a 3 cm soft platinum tip. Light is emitted from a control unit through a beam splitter and is transmitted to the sensor element along an optic fiber integrated in the guide wire. The sensor element consists of a silicone cantilever beam with a mirror integrated into its free end. Deflection of the mirror induced by the elastic movement of the sensor in response to changes in the external pressure modulates the reflected light. The signal is then transmitted back through the same optical fiber and is detected by a photo diode in the control unit. The performance characteristics of the sensor have been described previously in detail [7, 8]. The linear working range of the Pressure Guide™ is −20 mmHg to +300 mmHg and within 0 and 200 Hz. The upper frequency of the interface between the fiberoptic and the electrical system is more than 1 kHz.

Quantitative angiographic measurements

Angiography was performed with the Philips DCI equipment and the quantitative analysis was made using the automated coronary analysis program (ACA-DCI, Philips Medical Systems, Best, the Netherlands) for on-line use. The guiding catheter not filled with contrast medium was used as a scaling device. Contour detection of the stenotic segment, identification of the minimal luminal diameter (MLD) and corresponding reference diameter by interpolation technique is computer-assisted. Mean value of different projections was calculated anticipating a circular coronary lumen.

Using equations of fluid dynamics, the ACA program automatically calculates theoretical transstenotic pressure gradients, assuming a flow velocity of 20 cm/s. By inferring increasing flow rates and combining these with the theoretically calculated pressure drop, a stenotic flow reserve (SFR) value may be calculated for each stenosis [9]. The pressure gradient estimated at maximal flow was used in this study. These calculations are based on the assumption of a standardised aortic pressure of 100 mmHg, resting coronary flow velocity of 20 cm/s and SFR of 5.0 if no stenosis is present. For practical reasons in this study, in order to be able to better correlate with the relative coronary flow reserve (see below), the SFR values were transformed or 'normalized' by division with 5, so that an SFR of 5 corresponds to an SFR_n of 1.

Procedure

After administration of 10.000 I.U. heparin iv. and intracoronary nitroglycerin 100–150 μg, coronary angiograms were performed in at least 2 orthogonal projections. The same projections were used both before and after PTCA. Thereafter, the Pressure Guide™ was positioned with the sensor element distal to the stenosis.

In all patients in which a baseline gradient less than 15 mmHg was found initially or after balloon angioplasty, pressure gradients were also measured during vasodilatation. This was also done in 2 patients with baseline gradients more than 15 mmHg.

Vasodilatation was achieved by intracoronary administration of 125 μg nitroglycerin and 12 mug papaverine into the left coronary artery. If the lesion was located in the right coronary artery, 6 mg papaverine was injected. PTCA was then performed according to clinical practice. Following the procedure, repeat measurements were performed similar to pre-treatment.

Calculations

The proximal pressure was measured through 8 French guiding catheters in the coronary ostium and the mean transstenotic gradient was calculated as the difference of mean proximal and mean distal coronary pressure over 4–8 consecutive beats. The fractional coronary flow reserve (FFR) was calculated according to Gould *et al.* [10]:

$$\mathrm{FFR} = 1 - \frac{\Delta P_{\mathrm{max}}}{P_a}$$

where ΔP_{max} is the maximal pressure gradient and P_a aortic pressure. Pijls *et al.* have further developed this concept by dividing FFR into different components, and by measuring coronary wedge pressure, the contribution of collateral circulation could be calculated [11]. However, since the present study focused on moderately severe stenoses where collaterals have little impact, the original formula proposed by Gould was used. FFR is expressed from 0–1 where the value 1 represents a normal vessel.

Statistical methods

Least squares linear and nonlinear regression analyses were used to define the best fit relations between the pressure gradient and coronary angiographic variables. A p-value of <0.05 was considered statistically significant.

By second order regression functions, FFR and SFR_n were estimated as functions of different variables and 95% tolerance intervals were determined.

Specificity-sensitivity curves were calculated for the prediction of a pressure gradient of more than 15 mmHg for the predictors percent diameter stenosis and SFR.

Table 13.1. Angiographic and hemodynamic data for all patients.

Patient	B/A	D%	A%	MLD (mm)	MLCA (mm2)	Pb (mmHg)	Ppap (mmHg)	FFR	SFR	SFRn	Ppre (mmHg)
1	B	37	60	1.71	2.30	8	19	0.81	4.55	0.91	8
2	B	51	76	1.24	1.31	8	26	0.72	3.38	0.68	28
	A	32	53	1.95	3.01	3	15	0.83	4.62	0.92	7
3	B	39	63	2.21	3.85	5	27	0.70	4.42	0.88	10
	A	18	32	2.68	5.65	1	13	0.85	4.92	0.98	1
4	A	41	65	1.91	2.86	12	21	0.78	4.56	0.91	8
5	B	49	74	1.56	1.91	7	25	0.71	3.82	0.71	21
	A	37	60	1.93	2.95	2	15	0.82	4.61	0.92	7
6	B	71	91	1.18	1.09	46	53	0.42	1.36	0.27	65
	A	43	53	1.87	3.03	9	14	0.84	3.53	0.71	25
7	B	38	52	2.03	3.57	6	19	0.80	4.61	0.92	9
8	B	53	77	1,24	1,21	39	50	0.55	3.22	0.64	31
9	B	54	79	1.32	1.36	1	16	0.79	3.52	0.30	30
10	B	61	85	0.97	0.76	6	35	0.44	2.21	0.44	50
11	B	50	75	1.42	1.58	3	21	0.72	3.72	0.74	23
	A	32	53	1.76	2.46	0	0	1.00	4.60	0.92	7
12	A	32	53	2.68	5.71	3	20	0.80	4.45	0.89	10
13	A	41	65	1.19	1.11	8	18	0.74	3.93	0.79	19
14	A	21	37	2.86	6.49	1	18	0.80	4.85	0.97	3
15	A	30	47	2.60	5.10	5	7	0.92	4.75	0.95	7
16	A	32	53	2.52	5.02	0	15	0.83	4.48	0.90	7
17	A	33	55	1.70	2.29	6	12	0.88	4.51	0.90	9
18	A	22	40	2.62	5.41	1	6	0.93	4.84	0.93	3
19	A	18	34	3.11	7.62	4	8	0.89	4.91	0.99	1
20	A	26	45	2.48	4.88	5	9	0.86	4.79	0.96	4
mean		38	59	1.95	7.13	8	19	0.78	3.02	0.81	15.72
SD		13	16	0.61	1.93	11	12	0.138	0.88	0.88	15.7

B = before PTCA; A: after PTCA; D%: percent diameter stenosis; A%: percent area stenosis; MLD: minimal luminal diameter; MLCA: minimal luminal cross-sectional area; Pb: mean pressure gradient at baseline; Ppap: gradient during papaverine; FFR: fractional flow reserve; SFRn: SFR divided by 5; Ppre: predicted pressure gradient.

Results

Table 13.1 displays baseline and hyperemic angiographic and hemodynamic data as well as calculated values for pressure gradients and flow reserves.

After papaverine injection the aortic pressure decreased by 7 ± 5 mmHg. In 10 patients, measurements were performed before PTCA. In 2 of these, PTCA was not performed due to the combination of an equivocal stenosis angiographically and a low transstenotic gradient. In a third patient, PTCA was performed in spite of a low pressure gradient. In the remaining 7 patients, coronary angioplasty was performed since the stenoses were visually considered significant and the hyperemic gradients were above 20 mmHg. Following PTCA all patients had hyperemic gradients below 21 mmHg.

The individual changes in pressure gradient during papaverine-induced

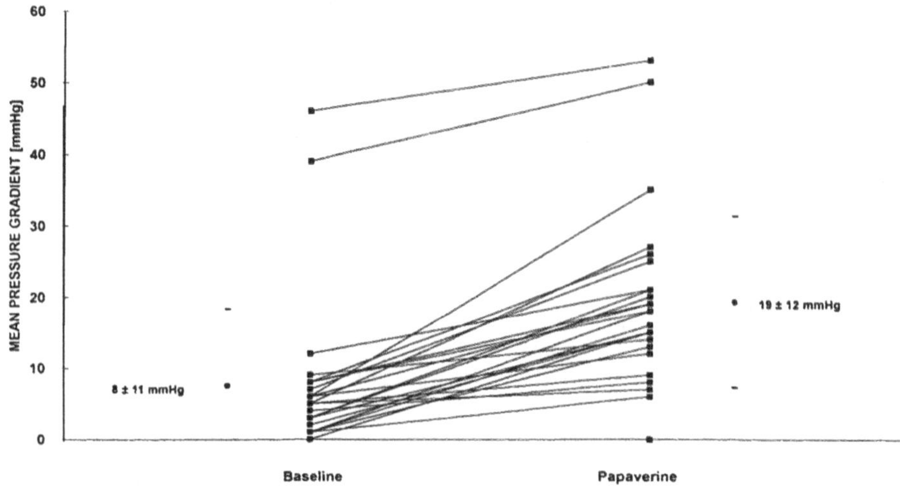

Figure 13.1. Individual pressure gradients at baseline and during papaverine-induced hyperemia.

vasodilatation are shown for all stenoses in Figure 13.1. The mean baseline gradient was 8 ± 11 mmHg and increased during hyperemia to 19 ± 12 mmHg ($p < 0.001$). The relationships between percent area stenosis and pressure gradient at baseline ($r = 0.55$; <0.01) and hyperemia ($r = 0.75$; <0.001), respectively, are visualized in Figure 13.2. Figure 13.3 illustrates the relationship between the maximal measured pressure gradient and the predicted gradient from QCA parameters ($r = 0.79$; $p > 0.001$).

FFR calculated from the pressure measurements and SFR calculated by QCA parameters were compared with angiographic parameters in all patients, see Figures 13.4 and 13.5, respectively. It can be seen that when percent area stenosis exceeds 50–60% flow reserve begins to fall. With both methods, the flow reserve value of 0.70 corresponds to an area stenosis of around 75%. Figure 13.6 shows the correlation between FFR and SFR_n. The correlation coefficient was 0.87 ($p < 0.001$).

Receiver operating characteristic (ROC) curves demonstrating the relationship of sensitivity and specificity with continuously changing values for angiographic parameters to predict a pressure gradient >15 mmHg is displayed in Figure 13.7.

Discussion

For pressure measurement in small vessels like the coronary arteries, the size of the transducer at the site of recording has great impact on the reliability of the pressure value. *In vitro* experimental studies have demon-

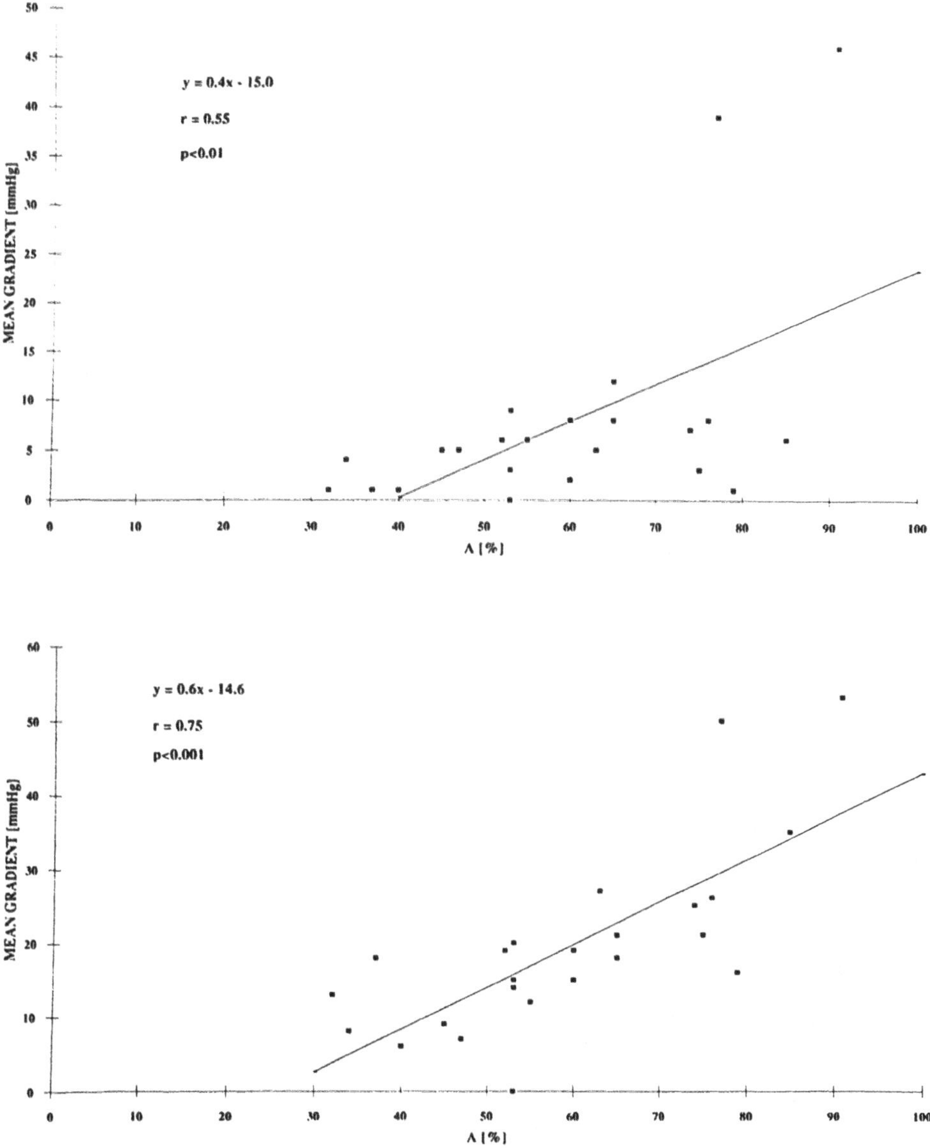

Figure 13.2. Relationships between percent area stenosis (A%) and mean pressure gradient at baseline (Figure A) and during hyperemia (Figure B).

strated that the ratio between the diameter of the pressure device and the MLD of the stenosis is the most important factor contributing to distortion of the recorded pressure gradient [12]. If the ratio is less than 0.4, only a small increase of the gradient will be caused by the pressure transducer itself.

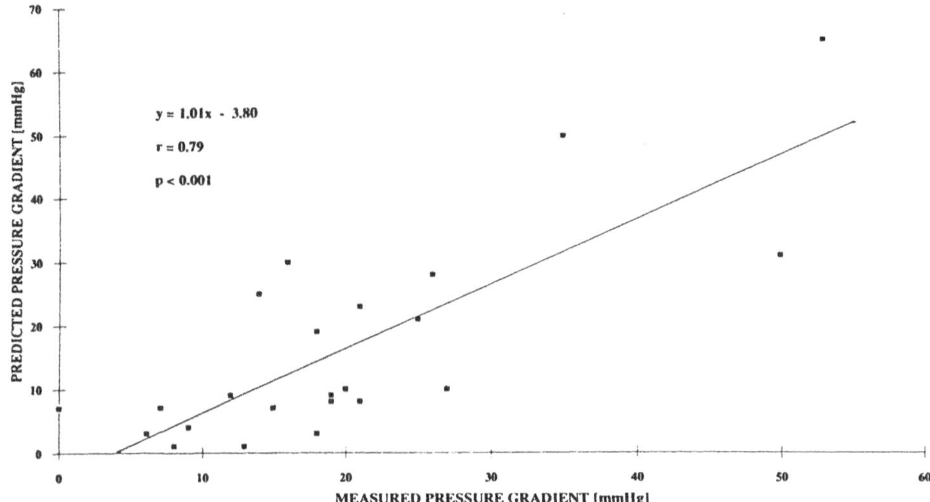

Figure 13.3. Correlation between actually measured pressure gradient and the predicted gradient from angiographic parameters.

In accordance with this, it has been shown in a more recent study that the pressure gradient was only affected to a minor degree by a 0.015'' guidewire in intermediately severe lesions [4]. The extrapolation of these results to the use of Pressure Guide™ in the present study would indicate that in stenoses with an MLD above 1.2 mm, pressure gradients will not be importantly affected by the 0.018'' guidewire.

Administration of papaverine i.c. seems to be of value for assessing intermediately severe coronary stenoses of clinical equivocal significance and with a low or no transstenotic gradient at baseline. In case of appearance of or marked increase of the gradient, implying a reduced coronary flow reserve, the indication for intervention towards the stenosis will be strong. On the other hand, if no gradient is provoked in spite of maximal hyperaemia, this is a case against a coronary intervention. In the presence of clearly significant stenoses with marked pressure gradients at rest, there is no rationale for papaverine provocation, since this would not affect the treatment of the patient.

Another reason for papaverine administration is that it is important to perform measurements under standardized hyperemic conditions if pressure gradients should be correlated with angiographic parameters. This was clearly illustrated in the present study, where the correlation between pressure gradients and stenosis area was considerably improved after papaverine compared to at baseline. An additional contributing factor to explain the relatively close association between pressure gradients and angiographic par-

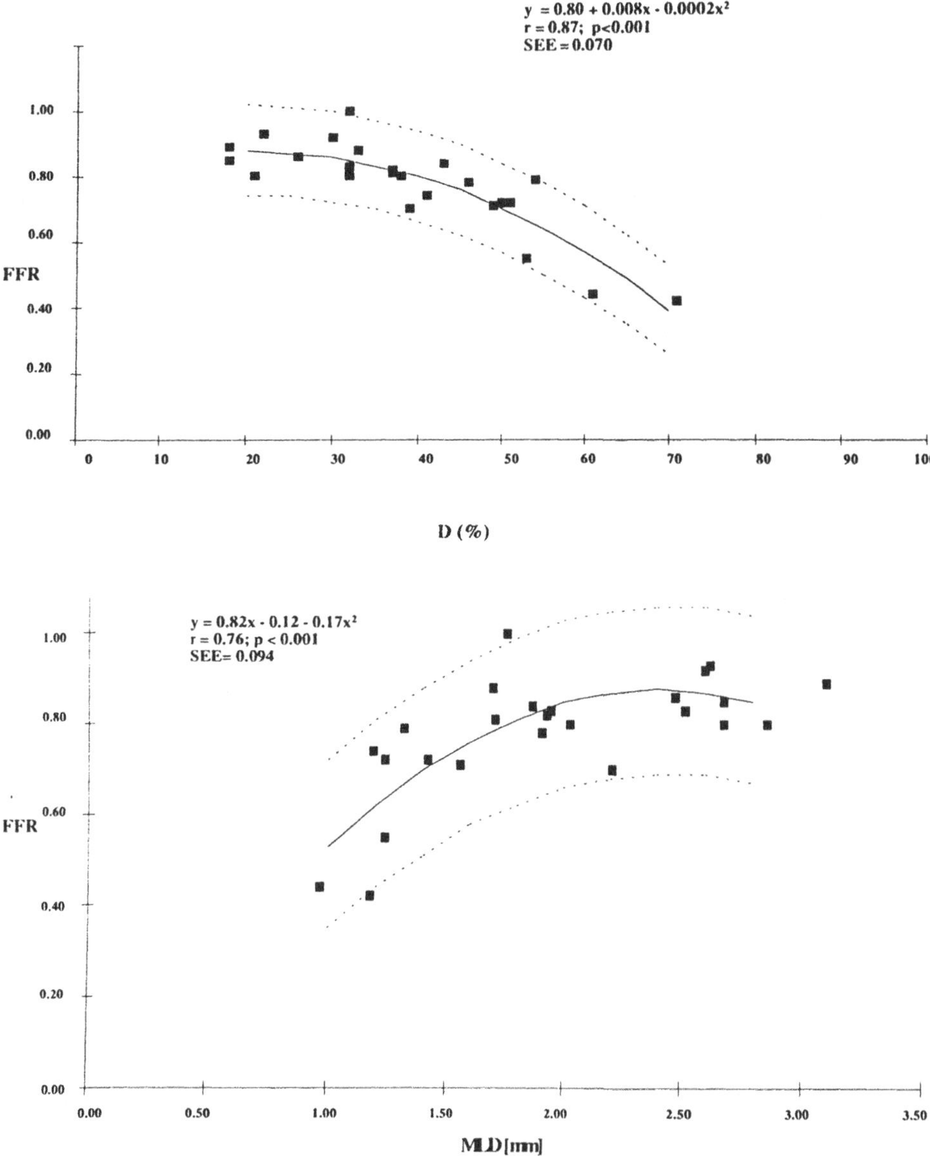

*Figure 13.4*A, B.

ameters is probably the fact that only stenoses optimal for QCA analysis were included in the study.

Coronary flow reserve can be calculated in several ways. In this study, FFR and SFR were used. FFR is defined as the maximal flow in a stenotic artery divided by the maximal flow in the absence of stenosis. It has been

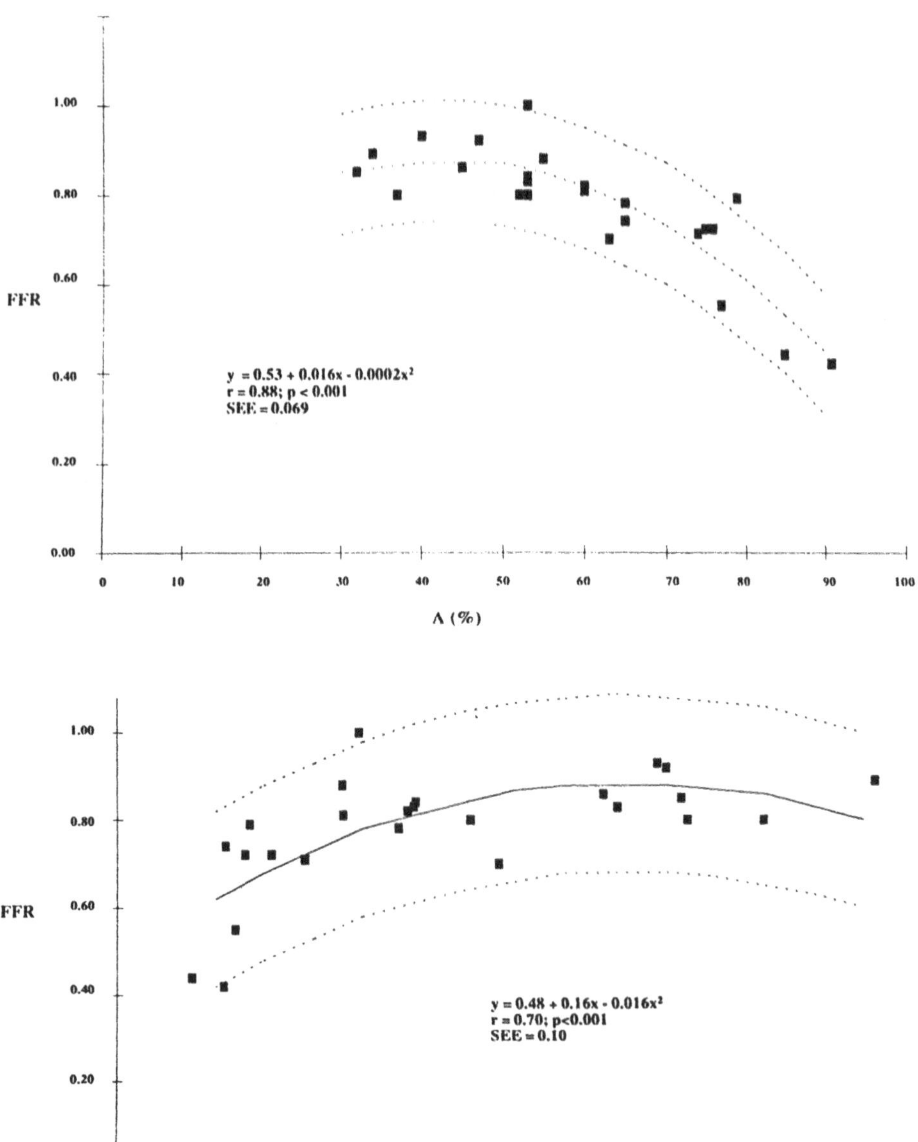

Figure 13.4. Relationships between fractional flow reserve (FFR) and various angiographic parameters: percent diameter stenosis (D%; Figure A), minimal luminal diameter (MLD; Figure B), percent area stenosis (A%; Figure C), minimal luminal cross-sectional area (MLCA; Figure D). 95% tolerance levels are indicated.

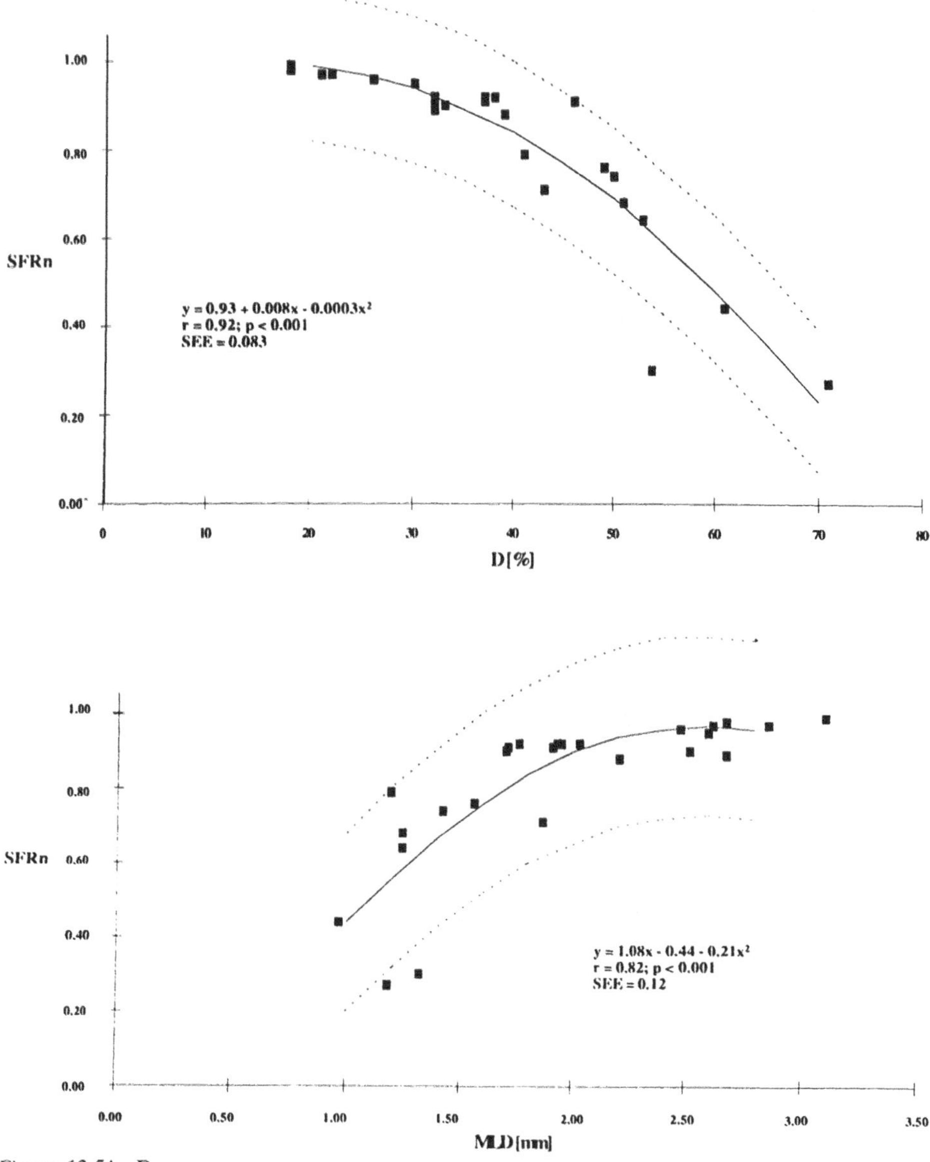

*Figure 13.5*A, B.

demonstrated theoretically and in animal experiments that this quotient can be calculated from intracoronary pressure measurements alone [11]. SFR, on the other hand, is an anatomic-geometric method for determining coronary stenosis severity. It has been derived from integrated angiographic dimensions of length, absolute dimensions and percent narrowing. Calculations have been performed employing theoretical values for aortic pressure and

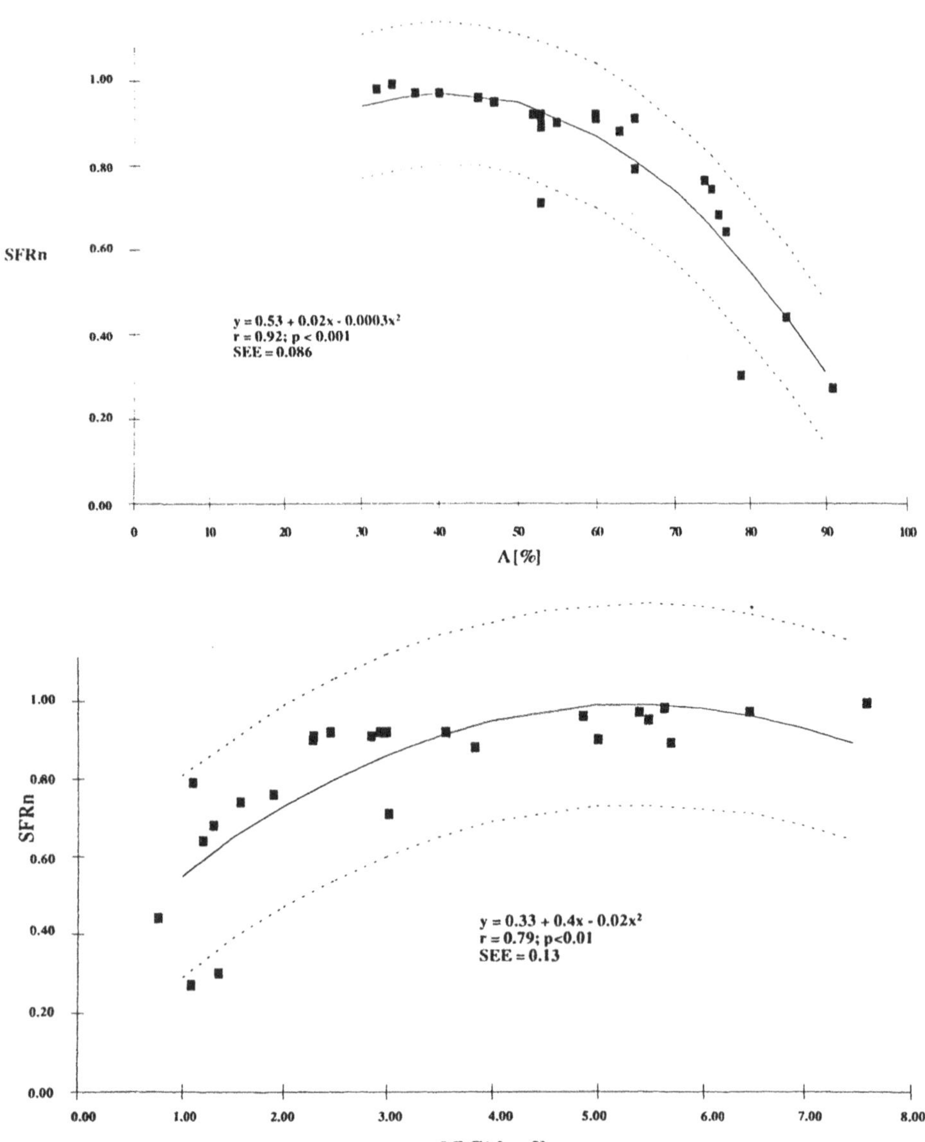

Figure 13.5. Relationships including 95% tolerance levels between normalized stenotic flow reserve (SFR_n in a vessel without stenosis = 1.0) and the same angiographic parameters as in Figure 13.4.

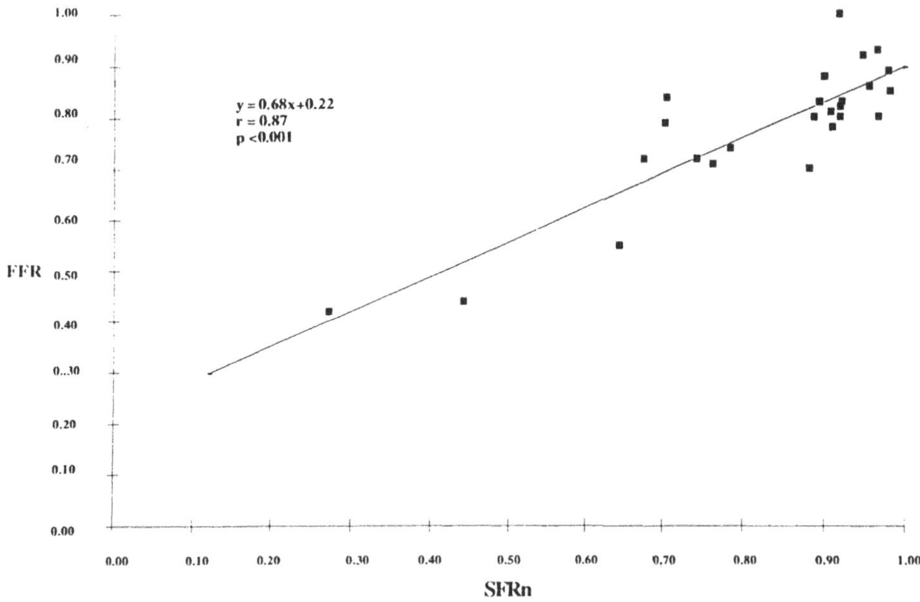

Figure 13.6. Correlation is shown between FFR and SFR_n.

maximal flow in the absence of coronary stenosis [13, 14]. Both FFR and SFR are descriptors of functional stenosis severity independent of all the physiological conditions that may affect absolute coronary flow reserve. In the instrumented dog model, Gould *et al.* found a close correlation between stenotic area and actually measured relative flow reserve by flow meter for progressively severe stenoses [15,16]. In these experiments, normal arterial diameter, stenosis length and physiological conditions were constant and relatively uniform for each stenosis. In contrast, the correlation between angiographic parameters and absolute coronary flow reserve has been poor in humans due to inter-individual variability of these factors [17–20].

In the present study, diameter and area stenosis were curvilinearly related to FFR as well as to SFR and these functions were best described by second degree equations. These relationships were similar to those found under experimental conditions, when progressive narrowings of coronary arteries in dogs resulted in a predictable reduction of the coronary vasodilator response [21, 22].

It was not unexpected that the correlation between SFR and stenotic area should be reasonably good, since SFR is derived from angiographic parameters. Moreover, patients with factors which potentially could affect flow reserve, e.g. previous myocardial infarction, intercoronary collaterals, myocardial hypertrophy, were excluded from the study. On the other hand, it was interesting to find that the correlation between stenotic area and FFR was at least as good as for SFR, in spite of the fact that FFR was calculated

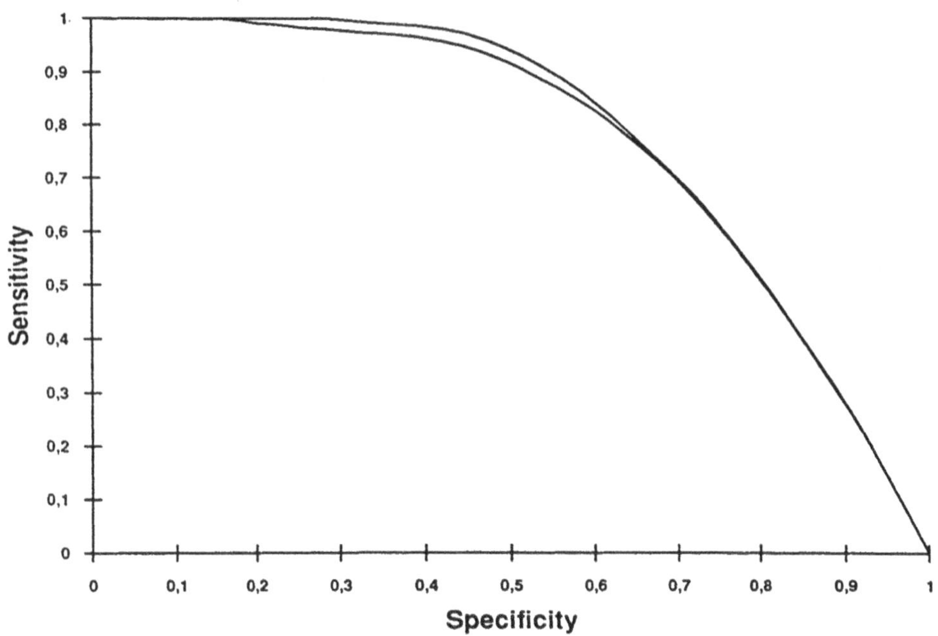

Figure 13.7. Receiver operating characteristic (ROC) curves for percent diameter stenosis (lower curve) and stenotic flow reserve (upper curve) in relation to prediction of a pressure gradient >15 mmHg.

from pressure values only and not from angiographic parameters. There was also a remarkably good correlation between SFR and FFR ($r = 0.87$; $p < 0.001$). It should, however, be pointed out that the 95% tolerance levels were overall 20–30% wider for SFR compared to FFR for the various angiographic parameters. This suggests a somewhat higher reliability for the prediction of FFR as compared to SFR in the individual case.

Another way of exploring the association between pressure gradients and QCA data would be to use receiver operating characteristic (ROC) curves. The ROC curves for prediction of $\Delta P > 15$ mmHg show how sensitivity and specificity vary with changing values of angiographic parameters. A curve with the function of = x would imply that QCA does not contribute to the prediction of a pressure gradient >15 mmHg more than would mere chance. The larger the area under the curve, the higher is the predictive ability of discrimination of the method, i.e. the information obtained from QCA in the present study is helpful in the diagnosis of pathological pressure gradients.

It may be concluded that transstenotic pressure gradients in coronary arteries should be measured during maximal hyperemia in order to obtain optimal sensitivity for evaluating stenosis severity. In addition, during these conditions there is also a closer relationship to coronary angiographic parameters. Expressions of the coronary flow reserve, calculated either from pressure gradient measurement (FFR) or from quantitative angiographic parameters (SFR) also correlated well with the stenotic diameter and area. Thus, calculation of FFR or SFR seems to be of practical value for stenosis assessment in the individual case.

Acknowledgwments

This study was supported by the Swedish Heart and Lung Foundation and Radi Medical Systems AB, Uppsala, Sweden.

We wish to thank Ms Maureen Jehler for preparation of the manuscript and Thomas Lichtneckert, M.D., for invaluable computer support.

References

1. Grüntzig AR, Senning A, Siegenthaler WE. Nonoperative dilatation of coronary-artery stenosis: percutaneous transluminal coronary angioplasty. N Engl J Med 1979; 301: 61–8.
2. Anderson HV, Roubin GS, Leimgruber PP *et al.* Measurements of transstenotic pressure gradient during percutaneous transluminal coronary angioplasty. Circulation 1986; 73: 1223–30.
3. Serruys PW, Wijns W, Reiber JHC *et al.* Values and limitations of transstenotic pressure gradients measured during percutaneous coronary angioplasty. Herz 1985; 10: 337–42.
4. De Bruyne B, Pijls NHJ, Paulus WJ, Vantrimpont PJ, Sys SU, Heyndrickx GR. Transstenotic coronary pressure gradient measurement in humans: *in vitro* and *in vivo* evaluation of a new pressure monitoring angioplasty guide-wire. J Am Coll Cardiol 1993; 22: 119–26.
5. Lamm C, Dohnal M, Serruys PW, Emanuelsson H. High fidelity translesional pressure gradients during percutaneous transluminal coronary angioplasty: correlation with quantitative coronary angiography. Am Heart J 1993; 126: 66–75.
6. Emanuelsson H, Dohnal M, Lamm C, Tenerz L. Initial experiences with a miniaturized pressure transducer during coronary angioplasty. Cathet Cardiovasc Diagn 1991; 24: 137–43.
7. Hök B, Tenerz L, Gustafsson K. Fiberoptic sensors: a micro-mechanical approach. Sensors Actuators 1989; 17: 157–66.
8. Tenerz L, Smith L, Hök B. A fiberoptic silicon pressure microsensor for measurements in coronary arteries. Transducer 1991; 5: 1021–3.
9. Kirkeeide RL, Gould KL, Parsel L. Assessment of coronary stenoses by myocardial perfusion imaging during pharmacologic coronary vasodilation. VII. Validation of coronary flow reserve as a single integrated functional measure of stenosis severity reflecting all its geometric dimensions. J Am Coll Cardiol 1986; 7: 103–13.
10. Gould KL, Kirkeeide RL, Buchi M. Coronary flow reserve as a physiologic measure of stenosis severity. J Am Coll Cardiol 1990; 15: 459–74.
11. Pijls NHJ, De Bruyne B, Kirkeeide RL, Gould KL. Quantitation of relative coronary flow reserve and collateral flow by pressure measurements during maximal hyperaemia: a rapid accurate method for assessing functional stenosis severity at PTCA. Circulation. In press.
12. Leiboff R, Bren G, Katz R, Korkegi R, Ross A. Determinants of transstenotic gradients observed during angioplasty: an experimental model. Am J Cardiol 1983; 52: 1311–7.

13. Gould KL. Identifying and measuring severity of coronary artery stenosis. Quantitative coronary arteriography and positron emission tomography. Circulation 1988; 78: 237–45.
14. Demer L, Gould KL, Kirkeeide R. Assessing stenosis severity: coronary flow reserve, collateral function, quantitative coronary arteriography, positron imaging, and digital subtraction angiography. A review and analysis. Prog Cardiovasc Dis 1988; 30: 307–22.
15. Gould KL, Lipscomb K, Hamilton GW. Physiologic basis for assessing critical coronary stenosis. Instantaneous flow response and regional distribution during coronary hyperemia as measures of coronary flow reserve. Am J Cardiol 1974; 33: 87–94.
16. Gould KL. Pressure-flow characteristics of coronary stenoses in unsedated dogs at rest and during coronary vasodilation. Circ Res 1978; 43: 242–53.
17. Harrison DG, White CW, Hiratzka LF *et al.* The value of lesion cross-sectional area determined by quantitative coronary angiography in assessing the physiologic significance of proximal left anterior descending coronary arterial stenoses. Circulation 1984; 69: 1111–9.
18. White CW, Wright CB, Doty DB *et al.* Does visual interpretation of the coronary arteriogram predict the physiologic importance of a coronary stenosis? N Engl J Med 1984; 310: 819–24.
19. Vogel RA, LeFree M, Bates E *et al.* Application of digital techniques to selective coronary arteriography: use of myocardial contrast appearance time to measure coronary flow reserve. Am Heart J 1984; 107: 153–64.
20. Wilson RF, Laughlin DE, Ackell PH *et al.* Transluminal, subselective measurement of coronary artery blood flow velocity and vasodilator reserve in man. Circulation 1985; 72: 82–92.
21. Gould KL, Lipscomb K. Effects of coronary stenoses on coronary flow reserve and resistance. Am J Cardiol 1974; 34: 48–55.
22. Gould KL, Lipscomb K, Calvert C. Compensatory changes of the distal coronary vascular bed during progressive coronary constriction. Circulation 1975; 51: 1085–94.

14. Intracoronary pressure measurements for calculation of flow reserve

NICO H.J. PIJLS, BERNARD DE BRUYNE, SHERIF EL BILTAGUI, MAMDOUH EL GAMAL, HANS J.R.M. BONNIER, GUY R. HEYNDRICKX, K. LANCE GOULD, RICHARD KIRKEEIDE, G. JAN WILLEM BECH, JACQUES J. KOOLEN, H. ROLF MICHELS, FRANK A.L.E. BRACKE & WILLIAM WIJNS

Summary

Recently, it has been demonstrated how maximum myocardial, coronary, and collateral blood flow can be calculated from arterial, distal coronary, and central venous pressure measurements at PTCA by three pressure-flow equations.

In this chapter, that theory is further elucidated and the concept of fractional flow reserve as an ideal index of functional stenosis significance is explained.

Next, the results of the first human validation studies of these pressure-flow equations are described with encouraging results, and the potentially important clinical implications are discussed. Application in man is demonstrated by some examples and the ease of use of the flow calculations is demonstrated.

Introduction

Since many years it has been widely recognized that the functional significance of coronary artery disease cannot be completely understood from anatomic information obtained by the coronary arteriogram. The shortcomings of the angiogram are most pronounced in the evaluation of PTCA-results, where the edges of the lesion are often hazy and hard to determine, whereas especially in this situation on-line information about the impeding effect of the (dilated) stenosis on blood flow is of paramount importance. Also in diagnostic catheterization, especially in intermediate lesions, determination of the functional significance of the stenosis remains cumbersome. Therefore, many attempts have been made to measure coronary blood flow directly. Most approaches in this field, however, are either crude, inaccurate, laborious, expensive, require complex equipment, or imply certain risks for the patient [1–4]. Of all those methods, only comparison of blood flow velocities by the Doppler wire and ECG-triggered digital subtraction angio-

J.H.C. Reiber and P.W. Serruys (eds): Progress in quantitative coronary arteriography, 207–226.

graphy have gained some clinical application [5, 6]. Both methods, however, only provide information about blood flow through the large epicardial coronary arteries. No information about the contribution of collateral flow to total myocardial perfusion can be obtained. In fact, notwithstanding its importance, quantitative methods to assess collateral flow in conscious man are not available at present. Both in diagnostic catheterization and in PTCA, it would be of great importance if a method would be available that enables measurement of myocardial perfusion by simple means, inexpensively, without extra instruction to the patient, and without prolonging the procedure. It would be of even more importance if the contribution of coronary blood flow (in the stenotic artery) and collateral blood flow to total perfusion of the dependant myocardium could be quantified separately.

Recently, we described the background theory and experimental validation of such a method and introduced three pressure-flow equations for the rapid and accurate calculation of coronary artery flow, myocardial flow and collateral flow by simple measurements of arterial, distal coronary, and central venous pressures [7].

In this chapter, the theoretical background and experimental validation of that method are briefly summarized and the first clinical results will be discussed. Moreover, the concept of fractional flow reserve (FFR) is highlighted as the ideal and most complete index for the functional significance of a coronary artery stenosis. It will be demonstrated how fractional flow reserve can be calculated from pressure measurements and how it can be used in clinical practice.

Theoretical background

Previous attempts to relate transstenotic pressure gradient (ΔP) to the functional significance of a stenosis and its effect on coronary blood flow have been disappointing such that at present only a few centers still routinely perform these measurements [8–14]. In our view, there are three reasons why pressure measurements have not been useful for the assessment of flow.

First, the instrument used for pressure measurement in previous studies (in most cases the balloon catheter) is unsuitable because its size is too large compared with the size of the coronary artery. The crosssectional area of an 80% area stenosis in a vessel with a diameter of 3.0 mm, is almost completely obstructed by a 3F balloon catheter, which is the thinnest catheter available at present (Figure 14.1). Thus, with standard PTCA catheters severe overestimation of ΔP may occur [8, 15].

Second, most previous measurements have been made in the basal state [10–12], in which ΔP is determined primarily by flow as affected by distal coronary autoregulation. Flow and pressure are related to each other by epicardial and myocardial vascular resistances. These resistances are continuously changing under the influence of myocardial oxygen demand, arterial

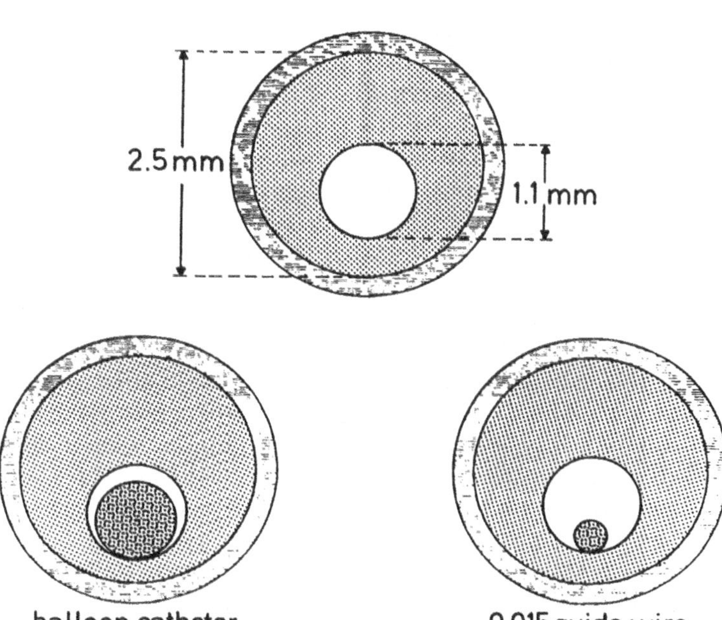

Figure 14.1. Severe overestimation of the transstenotic pressure gradient occurs with a regular 3F balloon catheter across an 80% area stenosis in a 2.5 mm ϕ coronary artery. If, on the contrary, an 0.015" guide wire is used for distal pressure recording, the influence on the gradient is negligible.

pressure, contrast injections, and coronary vasomotion. Therefore, theoretically pressure cannot be related to stenosis severity unless these resistances are known or at least remain constant. This condition can be met by performing pressure measurements during maximum vasodilation of the vascular bed when all resistances in the coronary circulation are close to minimal and presumably constant [2, 6]. As is true for coronary flow reserve, making functional measurements of stenosis severity from pressure measurements after maximum vasodilation is intuitively reasonable since the functional capacity of patients with ischemic heart disease is determined by the maximally achievable blood flow through the stenosis and its dependent myocardium [2, 3, 13, 16, 17]. Although the necessity of maximum vasodilation is generally recognized at present, it has not been applied to measurements of pressure gradient in a number of former studies [9–12, 15].

Third (and this is the most important point), in previous studies for assessing stenosis severity from pressure measurements, coronary flow or improvement of flow has been related to transstenotic pressure gradient or decrease of that gradient, or to transstenotic pressure gradient expressed as a percent of proximal arterial pressure [8–12]. This approach is fundamentally limited because it fails to recognize that the stenosis is only one part of a complex hydrodynamic system, other parts of which may also affect the influence of the stenosis on blood flow.

As explained in Figure 14.2, ΔP is unsuitable as a measure of functional stenosis severity, even if reliably measured with an ultrathin guidewire under maximum vasodilated conditions. From Figure 14.2 it is immediately clear that use of ΔP alone does not make any sense if not the simultaneously measured arterial and central pressure are taken into account.

Therefore, we modeled the coronary circulation in flow-pressure terms after maximum vasodilation, including the contribution of flow through the epicardial coronary artery and the collateral flow to the total myocardial blood flow. In this specific model of maximum vasodilation, measurements of pressures alone enable the calculation of relative maximum flow in the epicardial coronary artery and the myocardium, and the relative contribution of collateral flow. Therefore, this model theoretically provides a good and complete measure of the functional significance of a coronary artery stenosis. Moreover, changes in maximum coronary flow, myocardial flow, and collateral flow as a result of an intervention, can be readily determined in this model by simple pressure measurements under conditions of maximum vasodilation.

Before discussing the model, however, some considerations are necessary about the choice of flow parameters to describe the functional status of the coronary circulation in a clear and optimal way.

Maximum vasodilation and the concept of fractional coronary flow reserve

At this point it is necessary to spend some considerations to the choice of the flow parameter which is the most relevant one to reflect the influence of a coronary artery stenosis on coronary or myocardial blood flow. At a first glance, one should choose absolute blood flow, expressed in ml/min. However, absolute flow is widely varying between different coronary arteries and from one person to another and therefore expressing flow as an absolute volume is meaningless unless the distribution supplied by the artery is known. For this reason other ways to express blood flow in the coronary circulation have been searched for and the concepts of absolute coronary flow reserve (CFR), relative coronary flow reserve (RFR) and fractional coronary flow reserve (FFR) will be discussed shortly (Table 14.1).

Absolute coronary flow reserve was defined by Gould in 1974 as the ratio between hyperemic flow in a coronary artery and resting flow in that same artery. It has been considered as the standard for the functional status of a coronary artery for many years [18]. In clinical practice, however, measuring CFR has limited applications largely due to limited methodology. In addition,

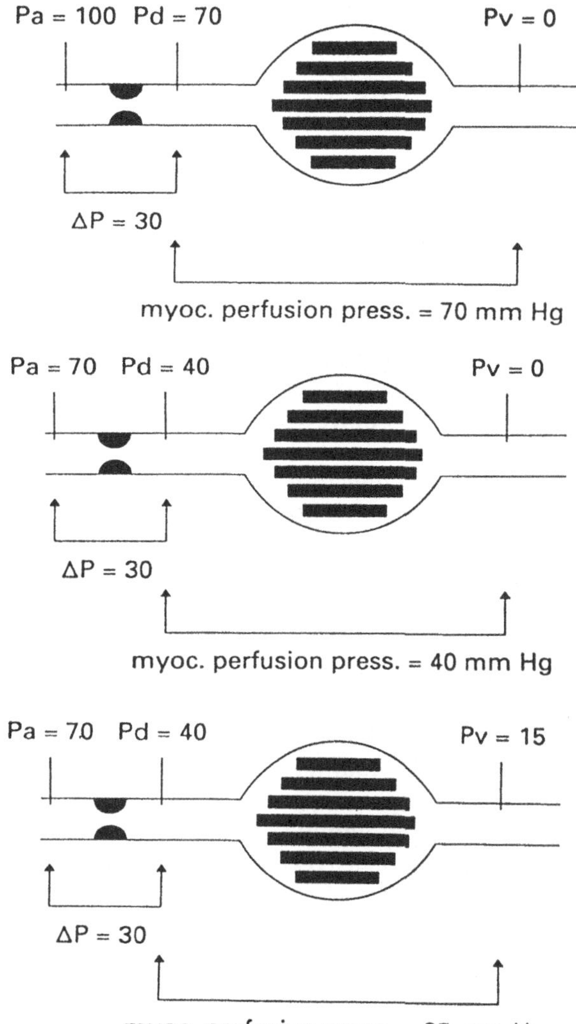

Figure 14.2. Illustration why transstenotic pressure gradient alone cannot be used in any way as a measure of coronary or myocardial blood flow even not if it is measured with an adequately thin pressure-monitoring guide wire under maximum vasodilated circumstances, corresponding with maximum hyperemia and and minimum resistances. In all three examples in this figure trans stenotic pressure gradient at maximum vasodilation equals 30 mmHg. However, the driving pressure over the myocardium (which determines myocardial perfusion at maximum vasodilation) largely varies from 25 to 70 mmHg. Looking at this figure, it is intuitively clear that myocardial flow is not determined by ΔP but by $(P_d - P_v)/(P_a - P_v)$ which is called myocardial fractional flow reserve (FFR_{myo}), and represents that fraction of flow reserve which has still been preserved despite the stenosis. Fractional coronary flow reserve can be defined in a similar way. For further explanation: see text.

Table 14.1. Applications and limitations of absolute, relative, and fractional coronary flow reserve (CRF, RFR, and FFR, respectively).

	Independent of pressure	Easy appl. at PTCA	Applicable to 3–V dis	Assessment of collateral flow
CFR	–	–	+	–
RFR	+	+/–	–	–
FFR	+	+	+	+

because CFR is defined as a ratio, diminished CFR can either reflect decreased maximum flow, increased resting flow, or a combination of both. Because all methods proposed for CFR determination in man, except positron emission tomography, require invasive manipulations or intracoronary contrast injections, true resting conditions in clinical situations are difficult to obtain. Moreover, several physiologic and pathologic conditions unrelated to the stenosis itself, may result in altered CFR for a given fixed stenosis [4, 19–22]. Arterial pressure, heartrate, left ventricular hypertrophy, previous infarction, and a number of other confounding factors all affect absolute coronary flow reserve.

To avoid some of these problems, *relative coronary flow reserve* (*RFR*) was introduced, stimulated by the rapid developments in imaging techniques [19, 23, 24]. RFR is defined as maximum blood flow in a stenotic coronary artery, divided by maximum flow in an adjacent normal coronary artery. In a similar way, relative myocardial flow reserve can be defined. RFR has the clear advantage to be independent of pressure changes because pressure affects the numerator and denominator of the ratio in an identical way. RFR can be reliably assessed non-invasively by positron emission tomography and invasively by videodensitometry [3, 6, 13]. Clinical use of RFR, however, is limited because an adjacent normal distribution is necessary to compare with. Therefore, it can not be used in the presence of three-vessel disease. Even in one- or two-vessel disease one can never be sure that an apparently normal coronary artery in an individual with ischemic heart disease is really normal. Moreover, the imaging methods for reliable assessment of RFR are expensive and only available in a few research laboratories. At last, both absolute and relative coronary flow reserve cannot provide information about the collateral circulation of the heart which, therefore, is mostly neglected.

At this point, *fractional flow reserve* (*FFR*) comes into perspective. Coronary fractional flow reserve (FFR_{cor}) is defined as the ratio of maximum flow in a stenotic coronary artery and normal maximum flow in that same artery, i.e., maximum flow in that artery in the hypothetical case that it would be completely normal. In other words, maximum blood flow in the presence of a stenosis is expressed as a *fraction* (or percentage) of its normal expected value in the absence of a stenosis. This parameter exactly describes to what degree the vessel's function has been affected by disease. If this value is for example 0.44, one knows that this particular coronary artery is stenotic to such a degree that the maximum volume of blood which can stream through that artery, is diminished to 44% of what would be normal. Coronary fractional flow reserve combines the information provided by absolute and relative coronary flow reserve and eliminates their disadvantages: it is independent of pressure changes and other confounding factors affecting absolute flow reserve and is applicable even in three vessel disease when no normal artery is present to compare with (Table 14.1). *Myocardial fractional flow reserve* (FFR_{myo}) is defined in a similar way.

Recently we have developed a set of pressure-flow equations and demonstrated how both FFR_{cor} and FFR_{myo}, as well as the separate contribution of coronary and collateral blood flow to myocardial perfusion, can be easily, rapidly and reliably calculated from simultaneous pressure measurements in the ascending aorta, distal coronary artery and right atrium under the condition of maximum vasodilation of the coronary arteriolar bed and using an ultrathin pressure-monitoring guide wire with a diameter of 0.015" [7].

The experimental validation of these pressure-flow equations has been extensively described elsewhere [7]. Some theoretical explanation, instructions on how to use these equations, as well as some applications in man, will be shortly discussed below.

Pressure-flow equations for calculation of coronary and myocardial fractional flow reserve and quantitative assessment of collateral flow

In Figure 14.3, the coronary circulation is represented. On the left hand side the aorta is depicted and on the right hand side the right atrium. There is one stenotic coronary artery and another coronary artery providing collaterals.

Coronary blood flow, myocardial flow, and collateral flow are indicated by Q_s, Q, and Q_c, respectively. The corresponding resistances are called R_s, R and R_c. Arterial, distal coronary and central venous pressure are indicated by P_a, P_d, and P_v, respectively. If the coronary artery is totally occluded, P_d is called coronary wedge pressure P_w. In case of maximum vasodilation (as can be obtained by intracoronary papaverine or intravenous adenosine administration) R and R_c are presumably minimal and therefore constant, wheras R_s is assumed to be a fixed resistance which can only change by PTCA. Since all blood to the myocardium is provided by the coronary artery and the collateral circulation, this yields $Q = Q_s + Q_c$. If no stenosis is present, R_s equals zero and Q_s equals Q, whereas collateral contribution equals zero. As the stenosis is more severe, Q_s will decrease and Q_c will increase. At total occlusion, $Q_s = 0$ and $Q_c = Q$. The normal values of all flow parameters are denoted by a superfix N. Therefore, $Q^N = Q_s^N$ and $Q_c^N = 0$.

Using this theoretical description of the coronary circulation, we were able to derive the pressure-flow equations presented in Table 14.2. These equa-

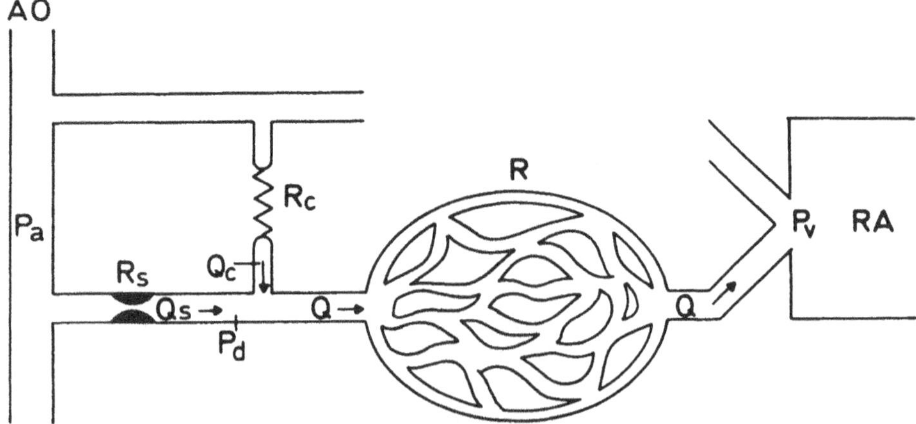

Figure 14.3. Model of the coronary circulation used to derive the pressure-flow equations at maximum arteriolar vasodilation. AO: aorta; RA: right atrium; P_a, P_d, P_v: mean arterial, distal coronary, and central venous pressure, respectively; Q, Q_s, and Q_c: myocardial, coronary arterial and collateral blood flow, respectively; R, R_s, and R_c: resistances of the myocardial vascular bed, the coronary artery stenosis, and the collateral circulation, respectively.

tions express maximally achievable coronary and myocardial blood flow in the presence of a stenosis as a fraction of their normal value, i.e. its value in the case that no stenotic disease is present [7]. Moreover, the collateral flow at maximum vasodilation, also expressed as a fraction of normal maximum myocardial perfusion, can be quantitated. It is important to note that in case of PTCA, if changes in arterial or venous pressure may have occurred during the procedure, the additional equation 4 is to be used for the calculation of P_w at the different values of P_a and P_v as demonstrated in the examples at the end of this chapter. Thereafter, equations 1, 2, and 3 can be used directly and are not dependent anymore on pressure changes.

These pressure-flow equations were validated experimentally in 5 instrumented dogs at different levels of driving pressure over a range of 50 to 150 mmHg and numerous stenoses at each pressure level. This has been described extensively recently [7]. Excellent correlations were found between calculated values of FFR_{cor}, FFR_{myo}, and collateral flow on one hand and maximum coronary blood flow (FFR_{cor}) as directly measured by an epicardial flowmeter on the other hand.

For the application of these equations in man, arterial, distal coronary, and right atrial pressures have to be simultaneously recorded both before and after PTCA after administration of a maximum vasodilatory stimulus (papaverine, adenosine). Together with the values of those pressures, recorded during balloon inflation, the calculations can be made immediately and result in a matrix as demonstrated in the examples at the end of this

Table 14.2. Pressure-flow equations.

1. Myocardial Fractional Flow Reserve (FFR_{myo}):

$$FFR_{myo} = 1 - \frac{\Delta P}{P_a - P_v} = \frac{P_d - P_v}{P_a - P_v}$$

2. Coronary fractional flow reserve (FFR_{cor}):

$$FFR_{cor} = 1 - \frac{\Delta P}{P_a - P_w} = \frac{P_d - P_w}{P_a - P_w}$$

3. Fractional collateral flow (Q_c/Q^N):

$$Q_c/Q_N = (FFR_{myo} - FFR_{cor})$$

4. $$\frac{P_d - P_v}{P_a - P_v} = 1 + R_c/R = \text{constant}$$

Abbreviations: P_a = mean arterial pressure at maximum hyperemia; P_d = mean distal coronary pressure at maximum hyperemia; P_w = mean distal coronary pressure at coronary artery occlusion; P_v = mean central venous pressure at maximum hyperemia; Q^N = normal maximum myocardial blood flow; Q_c = collateral blood flow; R = myocardial resistance at maximum hyperemia; R_c = collateral resistance at maximum hyperemia

From Pijls *et al.*, Circulation 1993; 87: 1354–67

chapter, obtained at one of our clinical experiments. It should be realized what a tremendous amount of information is incorporated in such a matrix, just derived from pressure recordings at maximum vasodilation. The influence of a stenosis on coronary, myocardial and collateral flow can be completely understood from such a matrix and all data are available on-line.

Because pressure is a universal measure and because the equations only use pressures without concern how those pressures are generated, the influence of a number of physiologic phenomenon, such as extravascular compression, coronary capacitance and coronary steal are already accounted for in this model through their influence on measured P_d and P_w. This has been discussed in more detail elsewhere [7]. As far as we know, the only limitation to the use of this model is small vessel disease, distal to the epicardial coronary artery, as may be encountered in diabetes. In that case, the equations (1) and (2) represent maximum flow in the presence of an epicardial stenosis, expressed as a fraction of maximum flow in the absence of that epicardial stenosis but still not normal because of the distal small vessel disease. The value of equation (2) for assessing the increase of maximum coronary flow by PTCA, however, would not be affected by that limitation.

In case of diagnostic catheterization, FFR_{myo} can be determined after introduction of a pressure monitoring guide wire into the coronary artery and administration of a maximum vasodilatory stimulus. In that case, one should consider if this low risk manipulation, is counterbalanced by the extra information provided. Especially in the case of intermediate stenoses on the angiogram, a final decision to dilate or not dilate can be made in this way. To assess maximum coronary flow and collateral contribution separately, use

Table 14.3. Myocardial fractional flow reserve (FFR_{MYO}).

- Based upon firm scientific background
- Well validated in animals and man
- Independent of changes of pressure and heart rate
- Well-defined normal value (1.0), for every artery, every individual, and any hemodynamic state
- Includes collateral circulation
- Applicable in both diagnostic and interventional procedures
- Easily and rapidly obtained by pressure recordings at hyperemia
- If right atrial pressure is not elevated:
- $FFR_{myo} = P_d/P_a$

Therefore: FFR_{myo} is the superior index of functional stenosis severity.

of P_w and therefore balloon inflation is necessary. Therefore, FFR_{cor} and collateral flow cannot be determined at diagnostic catheterization. For the understanding of the significance of a stenosis for the patient, however, FFR_{myo} is the most important parameter which can be easily determined even at diagnostic catheterization (Table 14.3).

If no conditions are present known to be associated with elevated central venous pressure, measurement of P_v may even be neglected without significant influence on FFR_{myo}.

After these theoretical and experimental considerations the first results of some clinical studies to test this theory will be discussed shortly.

Validation of pressure derived myocardial fractional flow reserve by positron emission tomography in man

Hereabove, the theoretical basis and the experimental validation of the concept of fractional flow reserve have been expounded. The following study was designed to validate the concept of fractional flow reserve in man by comparing maximum myocardial blood flow derived from pressure measurements with flow measurement by O^{15} water positron emission tomography. The study population consisted of 18 patients with an isolated proximal or mid left anterior descending stenosis scheduled for PTCA and normal LV function at rest. All patients underwent successively positron emission tomographic determination of maximum myocardial flow, quantitative coronary angiography and transstenotic coronary pressure gradient measurements. Myocardial perfusion images were obtained with an ECAT III (911/01, CTI Inc, Knoxville) one ring device [25].

Regions of interest were placed on the septal and anteroapical segments (stenotic region) and on the lateral segment, supplied by the left circumflex coronary artery and considered as the normal reference region. Myocardial flow measurements were performed at rest and during maximum vasodilation induced by intravenous adenosine (140 μg/kg/min during 5 minutes).

Relative coronary flow reserve was defined as the maximum hyperemic flow in the stenotic region divided by the maximum hyperemic flow in the normal region [25]. Because of the special selection of patients in this study, with a stenotic LAD artery and a normal left circumflex artery, myocardial relative flow reserve as obtained by PET can be assumed to be identical to myocardial fractional flow reserve of the LAD-myocardium in this specific patient population. A high fidelity tip manometer pressure transducer (Camino laboratories San Diego, CA) was advanced through a 7F pigtail catheter into the right atrium. An 8F guiding catheter was advanced into the left main stem. A 0.015" pressure monitoring guide wire as described above was advanced across the lesion enabling the measurement of distal transstenotic pressure during maximal vasodilation induced by intravenous administration of 140 μg/kg/min of adenosine. Right atrial and aortic pressure were recorded throughout the study. As described hereabove, myocardial fractional flow reserve was calculated according to equation (1).

Measurements by PET and pressure recordings were always performed with a time interval of less than 24 hours.

In Figure 14.4, the relationship between pressure-derived FFR_{myo} and FFR_{myo} as determined by positron emission tomography is illustrated. The correlation is excellent over a wide range of flow reserve with a slope close to unity. This excellent correlation is even more impressive because both measurements were performed with up to 24 hours time difference with slightly different arterial and venous pressures. It thereby confirms that fractional flow reserve is independent of pressure changes as predicted by theory [7].

From this study it can be concluded that: transstenotic coronary pressure can be measured easily with the pressure monitoring guide wire, does not carry any additional risk, and can be performed with negligible loss of time. Therefore, FFR_{myo} can readily be calculated during any PTCA procedure since mean aortic pressure is routinely measured through the guiding catheter and mean central venous pressure can be measured by a right atrial catheter or estimated from the neck veins. The determination of FFR_{myo} by pressure measurements during maximal vasodilation is accurate over a wide range of stenosis severities. The calculation takes into account both antegrade flow and collateral flow. A rapid and accurate method to assess maximum myocardial perfusion both before and after PTCA is provided in this way.

Assessment of recruitable collateral blood flow during balloon occlusion in man

As there is no other method available at present to quantitate collateral flow in man, direct validation of the third pressure-flow equation for collateral

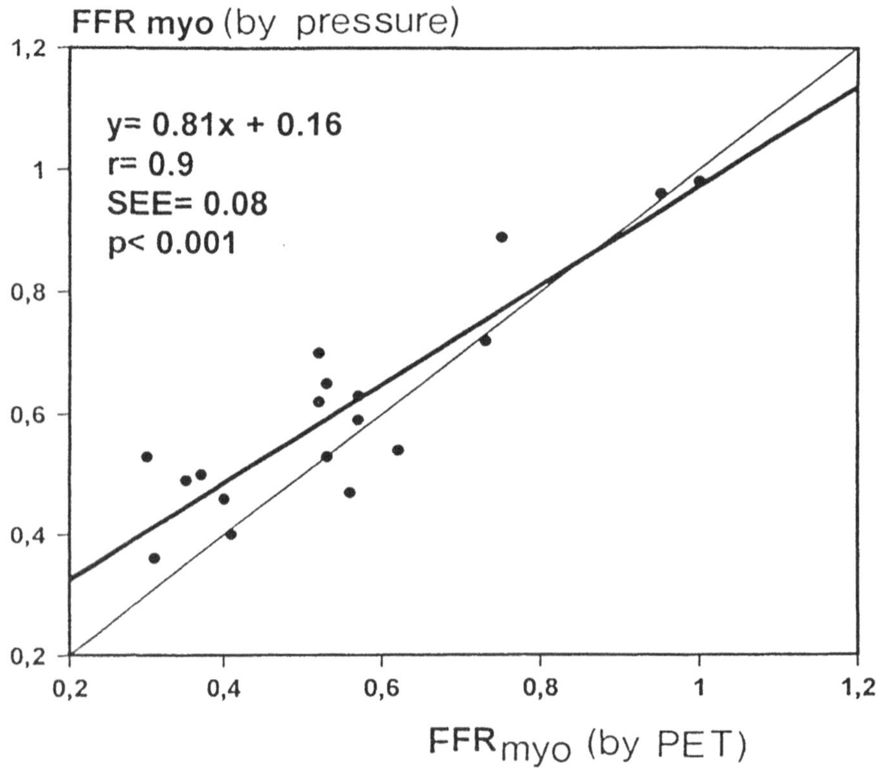

Figure 14.4. Relation between pressure-derived myocardial fractional flow reserve (FFR_{myo}) of the LAD-region and FFR_{myo} obtained by positron emission tomography in 18 patients.

flow assessment is virtually impossible. Indirect evidence, however, can be obtained for the correctness of these calculations in man.

It is well known that the ratio between maximum blood flow and resting blood flow (absolute CFR) is expected to be approximately 5.0 in normal arteries under standard physiologic conditions [18, 20, 26–28] which means that resting flow is approximately 20% of normal maximum flow under standardized conditions. In other words, coronary blood flow should be at least 20% of normal maximum flow to maintain cardiac function at rest. This means that, if recruitable collateral flow to a certain myocardial distribution exceeds 20% of normal maximum flow, no ischemia at rest is expected and that particular part of the myocardium is theoretically protected against acute ischemic events. As will be demonstrated this data provide the possibility to validate the third pressure-flow equations on one hand and may have potentially important clinical implications on the other hand because patients at particular risk for acute ischemic events can be identified.

In a pilot study, 50 patients were selected with stable angina pectoris class

III for at least 3 months and a positive exercise test shortly before the PTCA with clearly distinguishable reversible ECG-abnormalities at exercise. The first inclusion criterium was necessary to assure that collateral circulation had completely developed [29–34] and the second to dispose of a 100% reliable means to indicate or exclude myocardial ischemia at PTCA. As can be easily deduced from equation (3), recruitable collateral blood flow at balloon inflation, expressed as a fraction of normal maximal myocardial flow, can be calculated from arterial, central venous, and coronary wedge pressure during balloon inflation by:

$$Q_c/Q^N = (P_w - P_v)/(P_a - P_v).$$

During balloon occlusion, central venous pressure (P_v) was measured by a 5 F multi purpose catheter in the right atrium and aortic pressure (P_a) by the guiding catheter. Because in this specific study only distal coronary pressure at total occlusion was needed, no special guide wire was necessary and coronary wedge pressure (P_w) could be reliably measured by the central lumen of the inflated balloon catheter after withdrawal of the guide wire. All balloon inflations lasted at least 2 minutes to ensure maximum recruitment of collaterals [29–34]. After a satisfactory result had been obtained or if the operator wished to check the status of the vessel without the balloon in situ, the guide wire was advanced again and the procedure routinely completed. Appropriate calibrations and controls of the different pressure recordings were performed before and after the procedure. During PTCA, the frontal as well as precordial ECG was recorded to check if ischemia was present. Because a positive (ichemic) exercise ECG of every patient was available, comparison of the ECG at balloon occlusion with the exercise ECG could be used as a gold standard for presence or absence of ischemia.

Next, calculated collateral flow was correlated to ischemia, indicated by the ECG. These results are presented in Figure 14.5. The optimal separating value of fractional collateral flow (collateral flow as a fraction of normal maximum myocardial flow) to discriminate between presence or absence of ischemia, is 22%. This value, determined by linear discriminant analysis, is remarkably close to the theoretically expected value of 20% and therefore provides strong evidence for the correctness of collateral flow calculations in man.

The predictive value of the third pressure-flow equation to correctly predict ischemia at coronary artery occlusion, was 95% in this pilot study.

In the past, some other parameters such as visible collaterals on the angiogram, pain, or P_w alone have been used to evaluate ischemia during balloon occlusion. Therefore, also these parameters were compared to our gold standard. The predictive values of these parameters to correctly predict sufficient collateral protection were only 73, 70, and 78% respectively.

During the follow-up of our patients (6 ± 5 months), 3 patients experienced an acute ischemic event. All of them belonged to the group in whom the

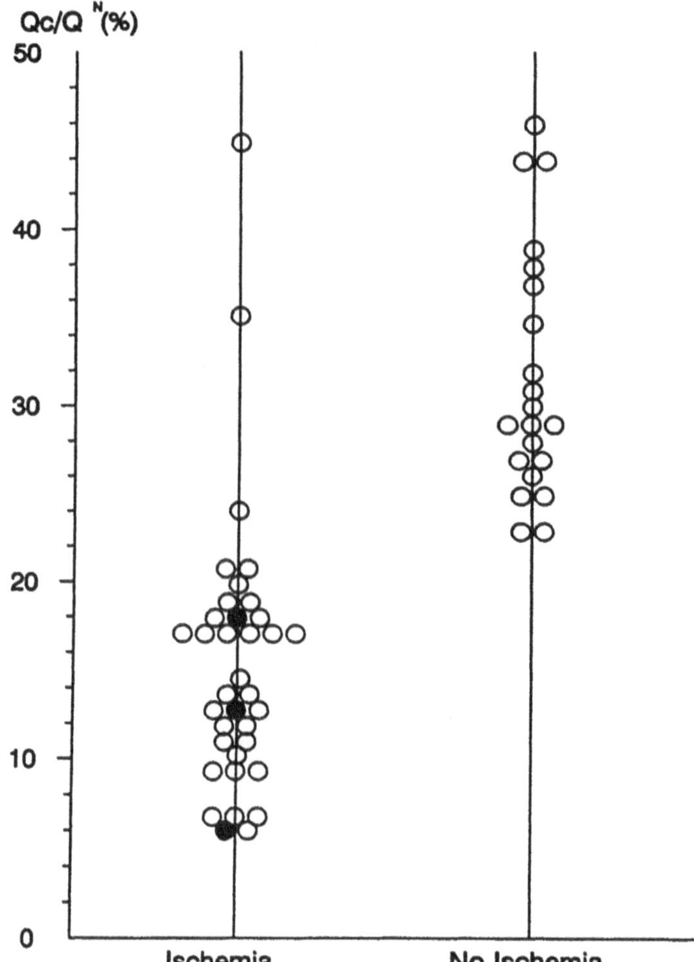

Figure 14.5. Values of recruitable collateral flow during balloon occlusion calculated by equation 3 and expressed as a fraction of normal maximum myocardial flow, and its relation with presence or absence of ischemia during occlusion of the coronary artery. The solid points indicate those patients who experienced an ischemic event during the follow-up.

calculated collateral flow at occlusion was insufficient. These 3 patients had a calculated fractional collateral flow of 6, 13 and 18%, respectively.

It can be concluded that the results of this study provide indirect but strong evidence for the correctness of collateral flow calculation in man according to the third pressure-flow equation. Therefore, for the first time it is possible to quantitatively assess the collateral circulation of the heart in the human cathlab during PTCA in a clinically feasible way. The implications of this study are of direct importance because it helps to predict if a patient is protected by collaterals in case of future acute occlusion of the regarding coronary artery.

Discussion, concluding remarks, and future developments

Patients with ischemic heart disease are limited in their activity as soon as the maximum amount of blood, flowing to their myocardium, is not sufficient anymore to provide an adequate amount of oxygen and substrate to maintain cardiac function. Therefore the best parameter to reflect the functional status of a coronary artery, is the maximum achievable amount of blood which can flow through that artery or to its depending myocardium. In our studies, maximum flow in the presence of a stenosis is related to normal maximal flow, resulting in the concept of fractional flow reserve which has considerable advantages compared to absolute and relative coronary flow reserve (Table 14.1).

From the theory and studies described in this chapter, it may be clear that maximum coronary and myocardial blood flow can be determined by the pressure-flow equations during PTCA by just performing the correct pressure measurements under vasodilated circumstances, using a tiny pressure-monitoring guide wire for distal coronary pressure recording. The measurements can be performed safely, easily and rapidly in conscious man in the catheterization laboratory. According to our first results, the calculations are highly accurate and superior to anatomic data if compared to Positron emission tomography as a gold standard for myocardial flow assessment in man. To calculate flow reserve from pressure measurements, no expensive equipment is needed and the complete procedure is prolonged by only a few minutes. Moreover, the separate contribution of coronary and collateral blood flow to total myocardial flow can be assessed. In fact, this is the first clinical method for quantitative assessment of the collateral circulation in man. Because this method only uses pressures as an endpoint without concern how these pressures are generated, most physiologic phenomenon affecting other methods for flow assessment are already accounted for because these phenomenon are reflected by their influence on pressure.

The definitive value of this method has to be further investigated. Additional confirmation studies in man are warranted. As far as collateral flow is involved, methodology is limited because no gold standard exists for collateral flow assessment in conscious man. Our initial results, however, provide strong indirect evidence for the correctness and applicability of our equation for collateral flow calculation. In case of diagnostic catheterization, FFR_{cor} and collateral blood flow cannot be separately calculated because knowledge of P_w is necessary for calculation of those two parameters. However, FFR_{myo} can be easily determined, even in diagnostic studies by just crossing a stenosis with the pressure-monitoring guide wire and the single administration of a maximum hyperemic stimulus (Table 14.3). Pressure derived functional stenosis assessment can be especially useful in intermediate stenosis and in the post-PTCA setting, where the limitations of the coronary arteriogram are most pronounced. It can also help to better understand data obtained by newer techniques such as angioscopy and intravascular ultrasound imaging. At last, it has been hypothetized that part of the patients with early restenosis, notwithstanding an apparently satisfactory anatomic result, never had adequate functional improvement. Using pressure recordings, further functional improvement at the initial PTCA could be possible in those patients and the restenosis rate accordingly decreased.

Examples

The first example is based on the simple hemodynamic case in which systemic pressures (P_a and P_v) are unchanged during PTCA. Therefore, according to equation (4), wedge pressure P_w is also constant. The superfix $^{(1)}$ indicates values before PTCA and the superfix $^{(2)}$ thereafter.

Before and after a PTCA of one of the coronary arteries, pressure measurements are performed by the pressure monitoring guide wire at maximum coronary hyperemia, induced by intracoronary administration of papaverine or intravenous adenosine.

Mean arterial pressure P_a is 90 mmHg both before and after the procedure, transstenotic pressure gradient ΔP is reduced from 50 mmHg before to 10 mmHg after the procedure, and venous pressure P_v is 0 both before and after the procedure. Coronary wedge pressure, measured during balloon inflation, is 20 mmHg. Therefore;

$$P_a^{(1)} = P_a^{(2)} = 90 \text{ mmHg}, P_d^{(1)} = 40 \text{ mmHg}, P_d^{(2)} = 80 \text{ mmHg},$$
$$P_v^{(1)} = P_v^{(2)} = 0 \text{ mmHg, and } P_w^{(1)} = P_w^{(2)} = 20 \text{ mmHg}.$$

Using equations (2), (1), and (3):

$$FFR_{myo}^{(2)}/FFR_{myo}^{(1)} = (1-10/90): (1-50/90) = 2.0$$
$$FFR_{cor}^{(2)}/FFR_{cor}^{(1)} = (1-10/70): (1-50/70) = 3.0$$
$$Q_c^{(2)}/Q_c^{(1)} = 10/90: 50/90 = 1:5$$

In other words, maximally achievable blood flow through the myocardium increased by a factor 2, maximally achievable blood flow through the dilated artery increased by a factor 3, and collateral blood flow decreased by a factor 5.

By using the equations (1), (2), and (3) (both before and after PTCA), one obtains the values of all flow parameters, expressed as a fraction of normal maximum myocardial blood flow expected in the absence of a stenosis, normalized for pressure changes:

$FFR^{(1)}_{myo} = 4/9 = 28/63 = 0.44$
$FFR^{(2)}_{myo} = 8/9 = 56/63 = 0.89$
$FFR^{(1)}_{cor} = 2/7 = 18/63 = 0.29$
$FFR^{(2)}_{cor} = 6/7 = 54/63 = 0.86$
$Q^{(1)}_{c} = 4/9–2/7 = 10/63 = 0.15$
$Q^{(2)}_{c} = 8/9–6/7 = 2/63 = 0.03$

Moreover, maximum recruitable collateral flow during coronary artery occlusion, expressed as a fraction of normal maximum myocardial perfusion, can be calculated by the equation

$$Q_c/Q^N = (P_w - P_v)/(P_a - P_v) = 20/90 = 0.22.$$

or in summary:

Before PTCA	At balloon inflation	After PTCA	
FFR_{myo}	0.44	0.22	0.89
FFR_{cor}	0.29	0	0.86
Q_c/Q^N	0.15	0.22	0.03

Such a matrix completely describes the distribution of flow in the coronary circulation both before and after PTCA. Moreover, it indicates maximum recruitable collateral blood flow during coronary artery occlusion.

Example 2

The second example demonstrates the calculations when mean arterial and venous pressure do change during PTCA.

A PTCA of one of the coronary arteries is performed. At maximum coronary hyperemia, mean arterial pressure is 96 mmHg before and 80 mmHg after PTCA, ΔP is 45 mmHg before and 15 mmHg after the procedure, and venous pressure is 6 mmHg before and 5 mmHg after the procedure. Coronary wedge pressure is 23 mmHg during balloon inflation. Mean arterial pressure during balloon inflation is 92 mmHg and mean venous pressure during balloon inflation is 6 mmHg.

In this case, with changing P_a and P_v, at first $P^{(1)}_w$ and $P^{(2)}_w$ have to be calculated, using the fact that $(P_a - P_v)/(P_w - P_v)$ is constant according to equation (4). Therefore, $P^{(1)}_w = 24$ mmHg and $P^{(2)}_w = 20$ mmHg. Thereafter, in an identical way as in example 1, equations (2), (1), and (3) are used to calculate that:

$FFR^{(2)}_{myo}/FFR^{(1)}_{myo} = (1–15/75) : (1–45/90) = 1.6$
$FFR^{(2)}_{cor}/FFR^{(1)}_{cor} = (1–15/60) : (1–45/72) = 2.0$
$Q^{(2)}_{c}/Q^{(1)}_{c} = 15/75 : 45/90 = 1 : 2.5$

In other words, maximally achievable blood flow through the myocardium increased by a factor 1.6, maximally achievable blood flow through the dilated artery by a factor 2, whereas collateral flow decreased by a factor 2.5.

By using the equations (1), (2), and (3) (both before and after PTCA) one obtains the values of all flow parameters, expressed as a fraction of normal maximum myocardial blood flow expected in the absence of a stenosis, normalized for pressure changes, whereas maximum recruitable collateral flow at coronary artery occlusion is calculated by $Q_c/Q^N = (P_w - P_v)/(P_a - P_v) = (23–6)/(92–6) = 17/86 = 0.20$.

Before PTCA	At balloon inflation	After PTCA	
FFR_{myo}	0.50	0.20	0.80
FFR_{cor}	0.375	0	0.75
Q^c/Q^N	0.125	0.20	0.05

Such a matrix completely describes the distribution of flow in the coronary circulation both before and after PTCA and at balloon inflation, and is independent of pressure changes.

References

1. Gould KL, Kirkeeide RL, Buchi M. Coronary flow reserve as a physiologic measure of stenosis severity. J Am Coll Cardiol 1990; 15: 459–74.
2. Pijls NHJ. Maximal Myocardial Perfusion as a Measure of the Functional Significance of Coronary Artery Disease. Dordrecht: Kluwer Academic Publishers 1991: 27–37.
3. Gould KL. Identifying and measuring severity of coronary artery stenosis. Quantitative coronary arteriography and positron emission tomography. Circulation 1988; 78: 237–45.
4. Kirkeeide RL, Gould KL, Parsel L. Assessment of coronary stenoses by myocardial perfusion during pharmacologic coronary vasodilation. VIII. Validation of coronary flow reserve as a single integrated functional measure of stenosis severity reflecting all its geometric dimensions. J Am Coll Cardiol 1986; 7: 103–13.
5. Donohue TJ, Kern MJ, Aguirre FV *et al.* Determination of the hemodynamic significance of angiographically intermediate coronary stenoses by intracoronary Doppler flow velocity [abstract]. J Am Coll Cardiol 1992; 19 Suppl. A: 242A.
6. Pijls NHJ. Maximal Myocardial Perfusion as a Measure of the Functional Significance of Coronary Artery Disease. Dordrecht: Kluwer Academic Publishers 1991; 10–39.
7. Pijls NHJ, Van Son JAM, Kirkeeide RL, De Bruyne B, Gould KL. Experimental basis of determining maximum coronary, myocardial, and collateral blood flow by pressure measurements for assessing functional stenosis severity before and after percutaneous transluminal coronary angioplasty. Circulation 1993; 87: 1354–67.
8. De Bruyne B, Pijls NHJ, Paulus WJ, VanTrimpont PJ, Sys SU, Heyndrickx GR. Transstenotic coronary pressure gradient measurement in humans: *in vitro* and *in vivo* evaluation of a new pressure monitoring angioplasty guide wire. J Am Coll Cardiol 1993; 22: 119–26.
9. Meier B, Luethy P, Finci L, Steffenino GD, Rutishauser W. Coronary wedge pressure in relation to spontaneously visible and recruitable collaterals. Circulation 1987; 75: 906–13.
10. Rothman MT, Baim DS, Simpson JB, Harrison DC. Coronary hemodynamics during percutaneous transluminal coronary angioplasty. Am J Cardiol 1982; 49: 1615–22.

11. Chokshi SK, Meyers S, Abi-Mansour P. Percutaneous transluminal coronary angioplasty: ten years' experience. Prog Cardiovasc Dis 1987; 30: 147–210.
12. MacIsaac HC, Knudtson ML, Robinson VJ, Manyari DE. Is the residual translesional pressure gradient useful to predict regional myocardial perfusion after percutaneous transluminal coronary angioplasty? Am Heart J 1989; 117: 783–90.
13. Pijls NHJ, Aengevaeren WRM, Uijen GJH *et al.* Concept of maximal flow ratio for immediate evaluation of percutaneous transluminal coronary angioplasty result by videodensitometry. Circulation 1991; 83: 854–65.
14. De Bruyne B, Meier B, Finci L, Urban P, Rutishauser W. Potential protective effect of high coronary wedge pressure on left ventricular function after coronary occlusion. Circulation 1988; 78: 566–72.
15. Anderson HV, Roubin GS, Leimgruber PP *et al.* Measurement of transstenotic pressure gradient during percutaneous transluminal coronary angioplasty. Circulation 1986; 73: 1223–30.
16. Nissen SE, Gurley JC. Assessment of the functional significance of coronary stenoses. Is digital angiography the answer? Circulation 1990; 81: 1431–5.
17. Pijls NHJ, Uijen GJH, Hoevelaken A *et al.* Mean transit time for the assessment of myocardial perfusion by videodensitometry. Circulation 1990; 81: 1331–40.
18. Gould KL, Lipscomb K, Hamilton GW. Physiologic basis for assessing critical coronary stenosis. Instantaneous flow response and regional distribution during coronary hyperemia as measures of coronary flow reserve. Am J Cardiol 1974; 33: 87–94.
19. Gould KL. Functional measures of coronary stenosis severity at cardiac catheterization. J Am Coll Cardiol 1990; 16: 198–9.
20. Hoffman JIE. Maximal coronary flow and the concept of coronary vascular reserve. Circulation 1984; 70: 153–9.
21. Klein LW, Agarwal JB, Schneider RM, Hermann G, Weintraub WS, Helfant RH. Effects of previous myocardial infarction on measurements of reactive hyperemia and the coronary vascular reserve. J Am Coll Cardiol 1986; 8: 357–63.
22. Klocke FJ. Measurements of coronary flow reserve: defining pathophysiology versus making decisions about patients care. Circulation 1987; 76: 1183–9.
23. Serruys PW, Wijns W, Reiber JHC *et al.* Values and limitations of transstenotic pressure gradients measured during percutaneous transluminal coronary angioplasty. Herz 1985; 10: 337–42.
24. Gould KL. Pressure-flow characteristics of coronary stenoses in unsedated dogs at rest and during coronary vasodilation. Circ Res 1978; 43: 242–53.
25. Bol A, Melin JA, Vanoverschelde JL *et al.* Direct comparison of N^{13}-ammonia and O^{15}-water estimates of perfusion with quantification of regional myocardial blood flow by microspheres. Circulation 1993; 87: 512–25.
26. White CW, Wright CB, Doty DB *et al.* Does visual interpretation of the coronary arteriogram predict the physiologic importance of a coronary stenosis? N Engl J Med 1984; 310: 819–24.
27. Wilson RF, Wyche K, Christensen BV, Zimmer S, Laxson DD. Effects of adenosine on human coronary arterial circulation. Circulation 1990; 82: 1595–606.
28. Marcus M, Wright C, Doty D *et al.* Measurements of coronary velocity and reactive hyperemia in the coronary circulation of humans. Circ Res 1981; 49: 877–91.
29. Rentrop KP, Thornton JC, Feit F, Van Buskirk M. Determinants and protective potential of coronary arterial collaterals as assessed by an angioplasty model. Am J Cardiol 1988; 61: 677–84.
30. Schaper W. Influence of physical exercise on coronary collateral blood flow in chronic experimental two-vessel occlusion. Circulation 1982; 65: 905–12.
31. Pupita G, Maseri A, Kaski JC *et al.* Myocardial ischemia caused by distal coronary-artery constriction in stable angina pectoris. N Engl J Med 1990; 323: 514–20.
32. Fujita M, McKown DP, McKown MD, Hartley JW, Franklin D. Evaluation of coronary

collateral development by regional myocardial function and reactive hyperaemia. Cardiovasc Res 1987; 21: 377–84.
33. Yamanishi K, Fujita M, Ohno A, Sasayama S. Importance of myocardial ischemia for recruitment of coronary collateral circulation in dogs. Cardiovasc Res 1990; 24: 271–7.
34. Sasayama S, Fujita M. Recent insights into coronary collateral circulation. Circulation 1992; 85: 1197–204.

15. Intracoronary Doppler flow velocity in coronary interventions

MORTON J. KERN

Summary

Miniaturization of ultrasound crystals for catheter-based interventions has extended the applications of both intracoronary imaging and Doppler flow physiology to the catheterization laboratory. Intracoronary Doppler-tipped angioplasty guidewires provide important information regarding directly measured blood flow beyond coronary narrowings. These data, acquired at the time of cardiac catheterization, identify the physiologic significance of an observed stenosis, particularly useful for questionable angiographic findings either before or following angioplasty. The Doppler-tipped angioplasty guidewire, by permitting measurement of coronary blood flow velocity not only *proximal*, but also *distal* to coronary obstructions, has provided new insights into the physiologic effects of various mechanical and pharmacologic interventions within the human diseased coronary circulation in regions and under conditions previously unavailable for study. This section reviews the basic principles, technique, validation and the current clinical applications of intracoronary flow velocity during coronary interventions.

Introduction

Miniaturization of ultrasound crystals for catheter-based interventions has extended the applications of both vessel imaging and intracoronary Doppler flow physiology to the catheterization laboratory for the investigation and treatment of coronary artery disease [1–3]. Intracoronary Doppler-tipped angioplasty guidewires provide important information regarding directly measured blood flow beyond coronary narrowings. These data can be acquired at the time of cardiac catheterization to ascertain the physiologic or functional significance of an observed stenosis, particularly useful in the assessment of questionable angiographic findings either before or following angioplasty. The Doppler-tipped angioplasty guidewire, aside from being merely a technical advance over earlier catheter techniques, permits measurement of coronary blood flow velocity not only *proximal*, but also *distal* to coronary obstructions. These data have provided new insights into the physiologic effects of various mechanical and pharmacologic interventions within the human diseased coronary circulation in regions and under conditions previously unavailable for study. The basic principles, technique,

J.H.C. Reiber and P.W. Serruys (eds): Progress in quantitative coronary arteriography, 227–246.

Table 15.1. Applications.

Intermediate (40–70%) Lesion Assessment
Severe lesion management
· Angioplasty
End point
Monitoring complications
Assessing additional lesions
Collateral flow
· Stent
· Atherectomy
Coronary vasodilatory reserve
· Syndrome X
· Transplant coronary arteriopathy
· Saphenous vein graft
· Internal mammary artery
Coronary research
· Pharmacologic studies
· Intra-aortic balloon pumping
· Coronary physiology of valvular disease
· Scintigraphic perfusion imaging correlation

validation and the current clinical applications (Table 15.1) of intracoronary guidewire flow velocity in patients during coronary interventions will be discussed.

Basic principles

Doppler velocity theory

Coronary flow velocity is calculated from the Doppler frequency shift resulting from differences between the transmitted and returning frequency from the moving targets.

$$\text{Velocity} = \frac{(F_1 - F_0)(C)}{(2F_0)(\text{Cos } \phi)}$$

where V = velocity of blood flow, F_0 = transmitting (transducer) frequency, F_1 = returning frequency, C = constant: speed of sound in blood, ϕ = angle of incidence.

There is a direct relationship between velocity and volumetric flow, where volumetric flow = vessel area × flow velocity integral × heart rate [4]. The differences or changes in Doppler coronary flow velocities, thus, can be used to represent changes in absolute coronary flow provided the cross-sectional vessel area remains unchanged. The volumetric flow rate can be calculated with the velocity measurements within 5% of absolute values, assuming a constant vessel diameter and an interrogating angle of <20°. The flow velocity integral can be easily measured by spectral Doppler signal analysis in 3–5 mm vessels which insonifies the parabolic flow profile with the broad beam spread (30° at 5 mm).

The Doppler guidewire

With the advent of a Doppler-tipped angioplasty style guidewire, the major limitations (size and measurements limited to the proximal coronary artery) of Doppler catheters have been overcome making their use nearly obsolete. The Doppler Flowire™ (Cardiometrics, Inc., Mountain View, CA) is a 175 cm long, 0.018" diameter steerable guidewire with a 12 mHz forward-directed transducer at its tip (Figure 15.1). The Doppler guidewire has a cross-sectional area of 0.164 mm^2. The ultrasound beam diverges at 14° from the long axis as measured to the −6 decibel points of the ultrasound beam. A pulse repetition frequency of 40 kHz, pulse duration of 0.83 microseconds and sampling delay of 0.5 microseconds provides satisfactory parameters for spectral signal analysis. The sample volume is 0.65 mm thick by 1.75 mm in diameter and is located an average 5 mm beyond the tip of the guidewire. The spectral velocity analyzer is a real-time Doppler instrument coupled to a video cassette recorder and thermal page printer.

The Doppler guidewire has been validated by Doucette *et al.* [5]. The spectral velocity signals have been found to be highly correlated with absolute volume flow measurements in *in vitro* and *in vivo* studies [5]. Quantitative flow velocity correlations for the two techniques was r = 0.95 in the model cannula and r = 0.85 in the proximal canine coronary artery. The Doppler guidewire accurately measured flow velocity and linearly tracked changes in flow rates in small diameter (3–5 mm) predominantly straight coronary arteries.

Normal coronary flow velocity signal interpretation

Fundamental to using flow velocity as a marker of atherosclerotic flow obstructions is the maintenance of flow velocity, but volume flow, across the epicardial conduit from the proximal to distal part of the artery. Normal coronary flow velocity is maintained over the proximal to distal epicardial regions consistent with both cross-sectional vessel area and absolute volume flow gradually diminishing due to artery branching. To assess normal flow velocity in patients, simultaneous flow velocity measurements in 55 angiographically normal, proximal and distal coronary arteries (right coronary arteries = 12, left circumflex arteries = 19, left anterior descending coronary arteries = 24) were measured [6] (Tables 15.2, 15.3). Coronary hyperemia was produced with intracoronary administration of 8–18 mcg of adenosine. In normal human coronary arteries, distal coronary flow velocity is similar to proximal flow velocity within all 3 major vessels. Proximal and distal mean

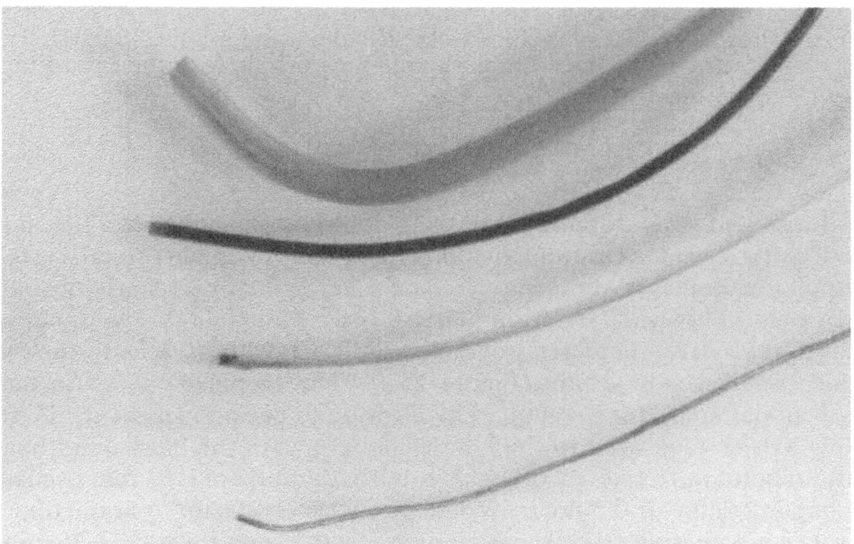

Figure 15.1. Doppler catheters (top 3): 8F Judkins Doppler (Cordis, Corp.); 3F Millar Doppler (Millar Instruments); 3F side-mounted Doppler (NuMed, Inc.) and Doppler angioplasty 0.018" guidewire (bottom). Reprinted with permission from the *American Journal of Cardiology* (See [6]).

velocity in each artery was not different at baseline or hyperemia (Figure 15.2). Among the 3 major coronary arteries, the diastolic velocity integral at baseline was significantly higher for the proximal left anterior descending compared to the proximal right coronary arteries. Hyperemic mean velocity, peak diastolic velocity and diastolic velocity integral were significantly higher in the proximal left anterior descending coronary artery compared to proximal left circumflex and right coronary arteries. The average proximal left anterior descending and circumflex flow velocity values obtained in patients are approximately 30 cm/s (mean diastolic velocity). Peak diastolic velocity ranges from 40–80 cm/s and peak systolic velocity from 10–20 cm/s. Right coronary artery and distal locations may be slightly reduced by ≤15%.

Diastolic-systolic phasic velocity patterns

All 3 coronary arteries show a diastolic predominant pattern in both proximal and distal arterial segments. The normal diastolic/systolic flow velocity ratio >1.5 is maintained in both the proximal and distal segments in patients with normal left ventricles. This pattern is less marked in the right coronary with a significantly lower peak diastolic to systolic flow velocity ratio compared

Table 15.2. Baseline and hyperemia velocity parameters in individual coronary arteries.

	Baseline			Hyperemia[a]		
	LAD (n = 24)	LCX (n = 19)	RCA (n = 12)	LAD	LCX	RCA
Proximal						
Peak D Vel	49 ± 20	40 ± 15	37 ± 12	104 ± 28[b]	79 ± 20	72 ± 13
Mean Vel	31 ± 15	25 ± 8	26 ± 7	66 ± 18[b]	50 ± 14	48 ± 13
D Vel Int	18 ± 11[c]	13 ± 5	11 ± 4	37 ± 55[b]	27 ± ?	22 ± 9
1/3 FF (%)	45 ± 4[c]	44 ± 5	40 ± 5	44 ± 5	43 ± 6	41 ± 4
D/S	2.0 ± 0.5[c]	1.8 ± 0.7	1.5 ± 0.5	2.0 ± 0.5	1.9 ± 0.6	1.9 ± 0.8
Distal						
Peak D Vel	35 ± 16	35 ± 8	28 ± 8	70 ± 17	71 ± 22	67 ± 16
Mean Vel	23 ± 11	21 ± 6	21 ± 9	45 ± 12	45 ± 12	42 ± 9
D Vel Int	13 ± 9	10 ± 3	8 ± 5	9 ± 6	11 ± 8	9 ± 2
1/3 FF (%)	46 ± 2	45 ± 9	39 ± 6	45 ± 3	42 ± 7	40 ± 9
D/S	2.4 ± 0.8[c]	2.1 ± 0.8	1.4 ± 0.3	2.2 ± 1.0	1.9 ± 0.8	1.6 ± 0.3

Notes

[a] All 3 coronary arteries had significantly higher absolute velocity parameters during hyperemia ($p < 0.001$).

[b] LAD vs LCX and RCA.

[c] LAD vs RCA.

Anova: Scheffe F test $p < 0.05$. D = diastolic; D/S = peak diastolic/systolic velocity; D Vel Int = diastolic flow velocity integral (units); Vel = velocity (cm/s); 1/3 FF = one-third flow fraction. Reproduced with permission from Reference #9.

Table 15.3. Baseline and hyperemic velocities in normal and stenotic arteries.

	Baseline			Hyperemia		
	Normal (n = 17)	CAD (n = 27)	p value	Normal (n = 17)	CAD (n = 27)	p value
Proximal						
Mean Vel	28 ± 12	29 ± 17	NS	57 ± 18	45 ± 30	0.06
Peak D Vel	44 ± 17	42 ± 27	NS	88 ± 28	65 ± 44	0.01
D Vel Int	15 ± 9	16 ± 11	NS	30 ± 13	25 ± 20	NS
1/3 FF	43 ± 5	39 ± 7	0.05	43 ± 5	39 ± 5	0.02
Distal						
Mean Vel	21 ± 7	15 ± 7	0.02	45 ± 12	19 ± 12	0.001
Peak D Vel	32 ± 10	21 ± 11	0.01	69 ± 17	27 ± 16	0.001
D Vel Int	10 ± 5	8 ± 6	NS	22 ± 7	9 ± 7	0.001
1/3 FF	42 ± 7	35 ± 6	0.01	42 ± 7	34 ± 9	0.05

D = diastolic; D Vel Int = diastolic flow velocity integral (units); Vel = velocity (cm/s); 1/3 FF = one-third flow fraction. Reproduced with permission from Reference #9.

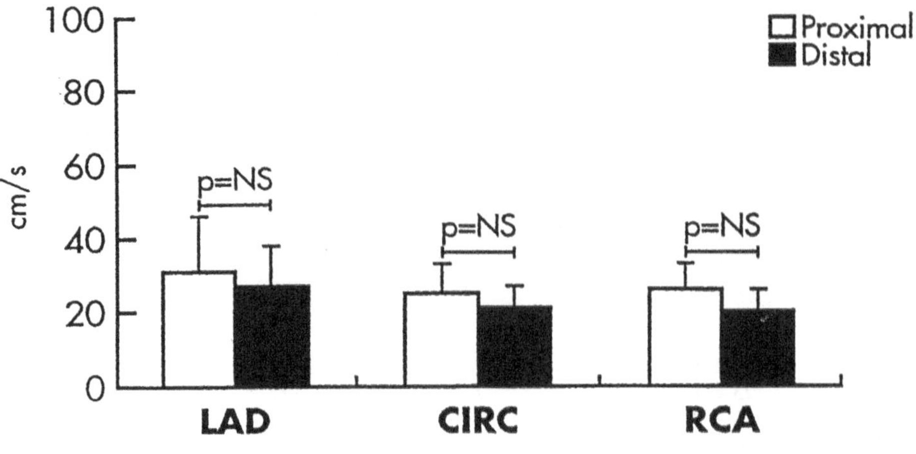

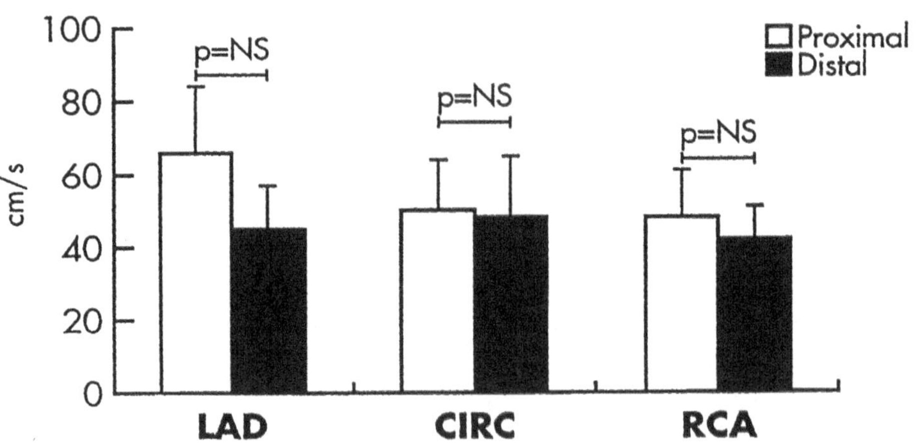

Figure 15.2. Comparison of baseline (top) and hyperemia (bottom) proximal and distal mean coronary blood flow velocity in each angiographically normal artery. Reprinted with permission from the *American Journal of Cardiology* (See [6]).

to left anterior descending coronary artery. The systolic predominant phasic pattern may become diastolic predominant in the posterior descending artery and posterolateral branches over the left ventricle [7].

Lesion management

Limitations and assumptions of doppler velocity for lesion assessment

The measurement of Doppler velocity is a rapid, easy and safe technique to assess the hemodynamically significant lesion with or without associated ischemic stress testing. However, despite the ease of application in daily use, the Doppler guidewire has several limitations. As with all ultrasound-based technology, placement of the transducer as near to parallel to blood flow as possible facilitates accurate peak velocity measurements [4]. The position dependent component of signal acquisition is minimized by utilizing a broad beam spread (27°) which makes most wire positions satisfactory for detecting the highest flow velocities. In tortuous arterial segments, considerable manipulation may be required to achieve satisfactory signals.

Flow velocity distal to severe lesions

The flow velocity findings distal to severe coronary stenoses demonstrate 4 common findings [6–8]: 1) decrease in mean velocity, usually <20 cm/s; 2)

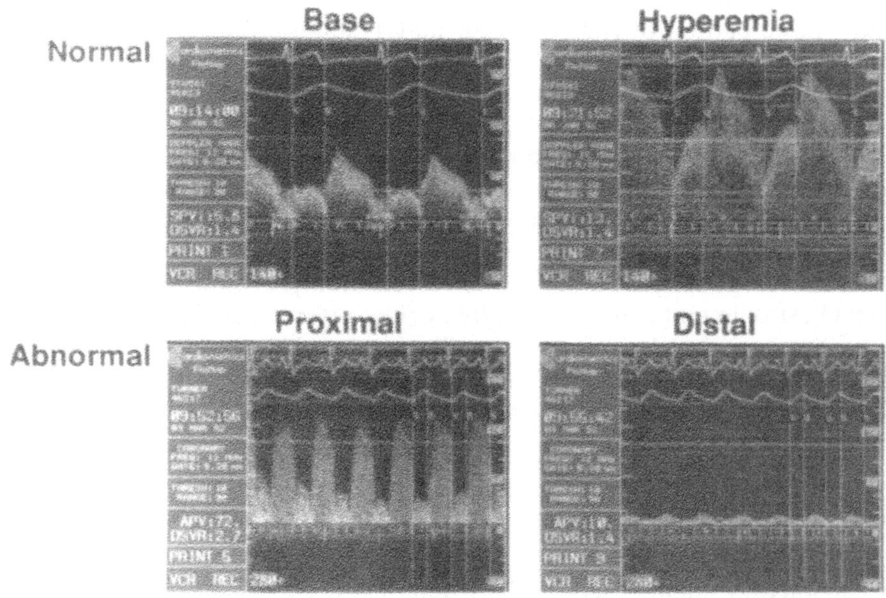

Figure 15.3. Spectral flow velocity at baseline and during hyperemia in a normal coronary artery and in an artery with a significant coronary stenosis. Normal hyperemia exceeds 2.5 fold basal levels and retains its phasic pattern. Abnormal flow velocity distal to a lesion is severely impaired and loses its phasic nature as well as the ability to produce coronary hyperemia.

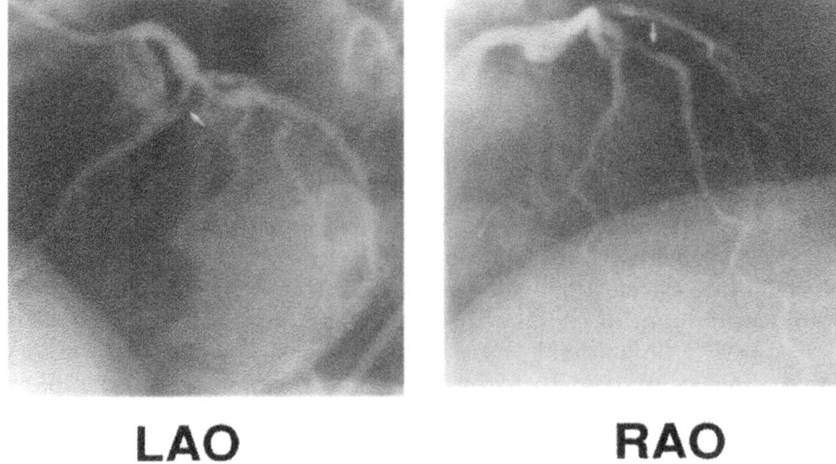

Figure 15.4A. Markedly eccentric lesion (>70% diameter narrowing in left anterior oblique (LAO) projection) in the left anterior descending coronary artery (small arrow). In the right anterior oblique (RAO) view, the lesion is moderate (<50%). Reprinted with permission from the *American Journal of Cardiology* (See [12]).

a mean proximal:distal flow velocity ratio >1.7; 3) an impaired diastolic/systolic phasic pattern of coronary flow and 4) impaired distal coronary hyperemia (<2.0 × basal values).

Normally, the diastolic component of flow velocity is nearly two times the systolic component. A normal diastolic to systolic velocity ratio (DSVR) is usually >1.8 for the left coronary artery. This value may vary normally among vessels, but in severe lesions, a DSVR < 1.4 is common.

Although most studies report a coronary vasodilatory reserve ratio of 3.5–5 in normal patients and experimental animal models, in our and other laboratories, lower values (>2.5) have commonly been observed in patients with chest pain and angiographically normal arteries. It should be noted that in severe coronary lesions, proximally measured flow velocity can produce nearly normal hyperemia (and hence coronary reserve) due to augmentation of branch vessel flow. Flow velocity beyond severe stenoses is universally impaired (Figure 15.3).

Post-angioplasty flow velocity

A satisfactory angioplasty result is demonstrated by near normalization of the 4 features described above. After successful angioplasty, the distal mean velocity is increased (usually >20–30 cm/s). The distal coronary velocity appeared to be more predictive of successful angiographic outcome of balloon angioplasty than did measurements performed proximal to the stenosis [8].

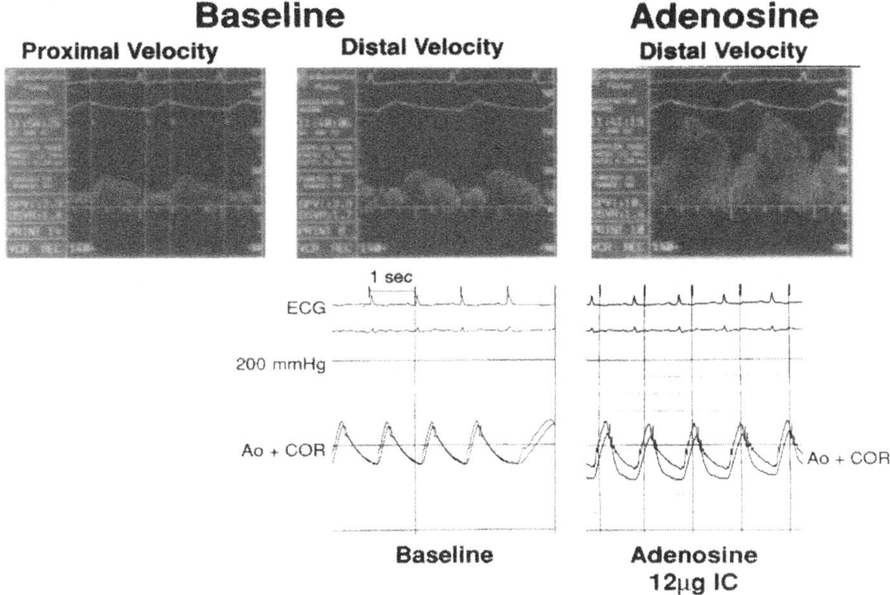

Figure 15.4B. Flow velocity signal (top panels) and translesional gradient (lower panels) at baseline and during maximal hyperemia with adenosine (12 mcg intracoronary). Proximal and distal flow velocity are nearly identical with a ratio of 1.05. The resting gradient is zero. With adenosine, distal flow increases 2.5 × baseline and the hyperemic gradient is 10 mmHg. Despite an equivocal thallium test, angioplasty was not performed. Reprinted with permission from the *American Journal of Cardiology* (See [12]).

Average peak velocity (mean velocity) increased significantly from 19 ± 12 to 35 ± 16 cm/s ($p < 0.01$) in the distal vessel following angioplasty, whereas changes in proximal average peak velocity were increased but to a lesser degree (pre-angioplasty 34 ± 18 cm/s vs post-angioplasty 41 ± 14 cm/s, $p = 0.04$) [9]. Coronary flow reserve was unchanged after angioplasty whether measured in either the distal or proximal coronary artery. In addition, an immediate post-ischemic hyperemic velocity, usually >2 times basal flow which equilibrates over 3–4 minutes to the new post-PTCA basal level is often seen. Failure to observe post-PTCA balloon hyperemia likely indicates continued obstruction to flow at or below the level of the angioplasty site. To assure proper velocity assessment after PTCA, the guidewire tip should be free in the major vessel and the guiding catheter should not obstruct flow into the vessel.

Alterations of phasic coronary flow after PTCA

A multicenter trial has been reported [8], showing coronary balloon angioplasty improved abnormal distal coronary artery flow velocity and normalized

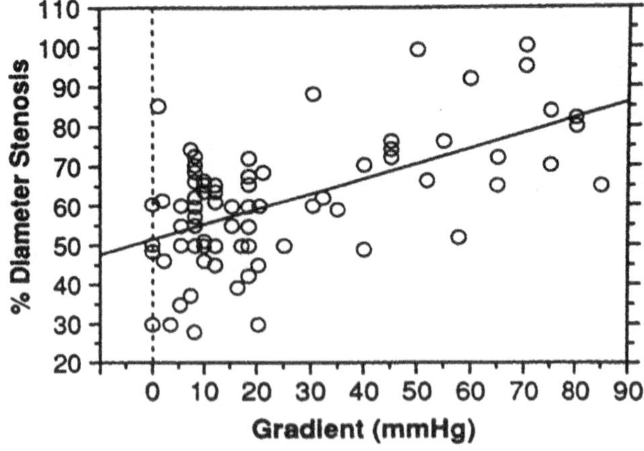

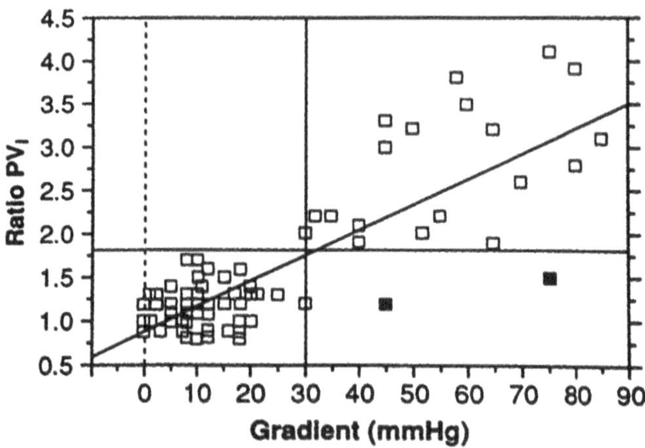

Figure 15.4C. (Top) Correlation between angiography (% diameter stenosis) and translesional pressure gradients (mmHg). (Bottom) Correlation between the ratio of proximal to distal total velocity integral (ratio PVi) and translesional pressure gradients (mmHg). The two black boxes represent the proximal right coronary artery stenosis occurring prior to any branch points. Ratio values >1.7 were nearly always associated with translesional gradients >30 mmHg. Reprinted with permission from the *American Journal of Cardiology* (See [12]).

diastolic/systolic flow velocity patterns. In 38 patients undergoing balloon angioplasty and 12 patients without significant coronary artery disease serving as controls, velocity measurements were performed. Angioplasty increased luminal stenosis diameter from 33 ± 23% to 80 ± 17%. Flow velocity signals demonstrated a marked improvement in the diastolic to systolic average velocity ratio from 1.9 ± 0.6 to 2.8 ± 1.1, a 46% increase from pre-angioplasty values. Significant increases in diastolic to systolic flow ratios occurred

Table 15.4. Clinical data in patients with intermediate lesions.

	Group 1 (<20 mmHg) (n = 56)	Group 2 (≥20 mmHg) (n = 28)	p value
Male (%)	82	74	NS
Age, mean (Range)	57 (28–78)	59 (31–80)	NS
History of MI (%)	26	18	NS
History of prior CABG (%)	5	2	NS
History of prior PTCA (%)	29	37	NS
Diabetes (%)	23	39	NS
Smoking (%)	57	53	NS
Hypertension (%)	79	53	NS
Medications (% of patients receiving)			
Calcium channel blocker	83	91	NS
Nitrates	61	44	NS
Beta blocker	35	35	NS

CABG = coronary artery bypass graft surgery; PTCA = percutaneous transluminal coronary angioplasty: MI = myocardial infraction. Reprinted with permission from the *American Journal of Cardiology* (See [12]).

within 10–15 minutes following successful balloon angioplasty. When measurements were performed in the proximal vessel, phasic diastolic/systolic flow patterns were not significantly different than normal vessel (diastolic to systolic flow ratios = 1.8 ± 0.8 vs 1.8 ± 0.5, p = NS) and diastolic to systolic flow ratios did not increase significantly following angioplasty.

Flow velocity in lesions of intermediate severity

Due to interobserver and intraobserver variability in judging the severity of coronary lesions [10], angiography cannot distinguish the physiologic significance of lesions of severity >40% and <70–80% diameter stenosis. In man, a weak relationship exists between coronary flow reserve, as measured by Doppler techniques, and percent diameter stenosis [11].

In 85 patients with moderate and severe angiographic coronary stenoses, translesional pressure (2.2 tracking catheter) and flow velocity (0.018" Flowire) were measured [12]. There was only a weak correlation with angiography and translesional hemodynamics. However, an excellent correlation was seen, especially for lesions 50–70% narrowed, between translesional flow velocity ratios (proximal/distal velocity integral) and pressure gradients in branched coronary arteries. Ninety-eight percent of coronary narrowings with translesional gradients of ≥30 mmHg are associated with a proximal/distal mean velocity ratio >1.7 [12] (Figure 15.4). The clinical characteristics of the patients with translesional gradients >20 and <20 mmHg are shown in Table 15.4. The flow velocity data for these two groups separated significant differences in distal, but not proximal flow velocity (Table 15.5).

Table 15.5. Flow velocity for patients with intermediate lesions.

	Systolic integral (units)	Peak systolic velocity (cm/s)	Diastolic velocity integral (units)	Peak diastolic velocity (cm/s)	Total flow integral (units)	Mean velocity (cm/s)	S/D ratio
Proximal							
Gradient ≤20 mmHg	8.7 ± 6.0	34 ± 19	22 ± 13	55 ± 25	31 ± 18	35 ± 16	0.7 ± 0.3
Gradient ≥20 mmHg	8.9 ± 5.5	38 ± 21	38 ± 21	65 ± 35	38 ± 20	45 ± 23	0.6 ± 0.2
p value	0.873	0.483	0.0578	0.175	0.121	0.062	0.579
Distal							
Gradient ≤20 mmHg	7.7 ± 5.4	31 ± 18	21 ± 14	49 ± 23	29 ± 18	33 ± 16	0.6 ± 0.2
Gradient ≥20 mmHg	4.6 ± 6.5	17 ± 9	11 ± 8	26 ± 13	14 ± 9	17 ± 9	–
p value	0.038	0.0001	0.0001	0.0001	0.0001	0.0001	0.233
P vs D							
Gradient ≤20 mmHg							
p values	0.0628	0.085	0.449	0.032	0.118	0.075	0.435
Gradient ≥20 mmHg							
p values	0.002	0.001	0.001	0.0001	0.0001	0.0001	0.202
Proximal to distal ratios							
Intermediate vs severe							
Gradient ≤20 mmHg	1.2 ± 0.4	1.1 ± 0.3	1.1 ± 0.2	1.1 ± 0.3	1.1 ± 0.2	1.1 ± 0.3	1.0 ± 2.3
Gradient ≥20 mmHg	2.8 ± 1.9	2.5 ± 1.4	3.6 ± 3.7	2.7 ± 1.3	3.2 ± 1.9	3.9 ± ?	1.0 ± 0.6
t	0.0001	0.0001	0.0001	0.0001	0.0001	0.0297	0.823

The decremental distal flow relative to proximal flow velocity is predicated on a branched tube model, wherein flow is diverted away from the branch with a high resistance (stenosis) to branches with lower resistances. The proximal/distal ratio will not apply in single tubes without branches where the continuity equation mandates equality of flow at any point along the circuit (Figure 15.5). In arteries which are single tube conduits without branches, such as very proximal segments of the right coronary artery or in bypass grafts, the proximal and distal blood flow velocity will be affected equally as determined by the continuity equation. Hence, the transstenotic velocity ratio is not useful for predicting stenosis severity. As described earlier, normal coronary volumetric flow decreases over the proximal to distal course of the epicardial arteries. As the volume is distributed to the branches, the major conduit vessel decreases in cross-sectional area. Since

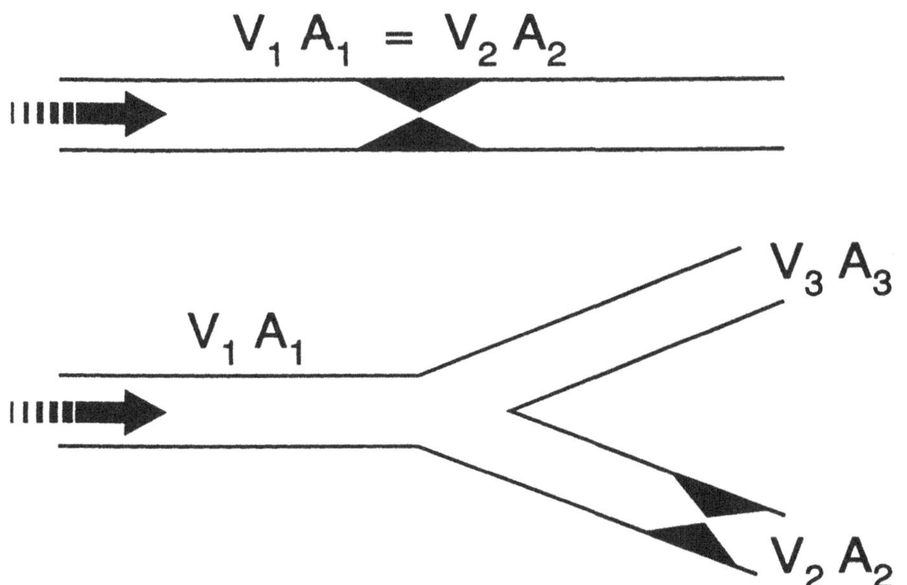

Figure 15.5A. Single and branched tube models. Volume flow equals cross-sectional area × velocity. Single tube model employs continuity equation where as a branched tube model cannot. Flow will be diverted to branch(es) of lowest resistance.

volume flow can be estimated from the product of mean flow velocity and cross-sectional area, velocity is maintained with a proximal to distal flow velocity ratio ≈1. The proximal/distal flow velocity ratio cannot be used in 3 common conditions: 1) non-branching conduits (i.e., saphenous vein grafts, left IMA, proximal right coronary artery); 2) ostial lesions without a proximal velocity and 3) diffuse distal disease with increases in the distal velocity out of proportion to proximal vessel flow.

Angiography alone without objective evidence of ischemia for interventional decision making is common practice in some centers [13]. Coronary flow velocity can assist in important decision making in patients with multiple coronary lesions by confirming translesional flow impairment and facilitate a rational approach to coronary intervention in patients with multiple stenoses of intermediate severity (Figure 15.6) [14].

Continuous flow velocity monitoring during interventions

The use of continuous flow velocity monitoring after angioplasty can identify trend patterns of unstable associated with abrupt vessel closure. Two trend patterns, 1) a constantly declining velocity or 2) cyclic flow variations in the

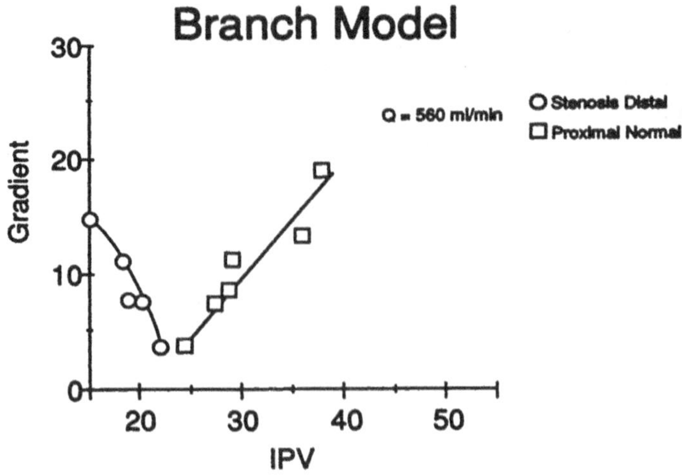

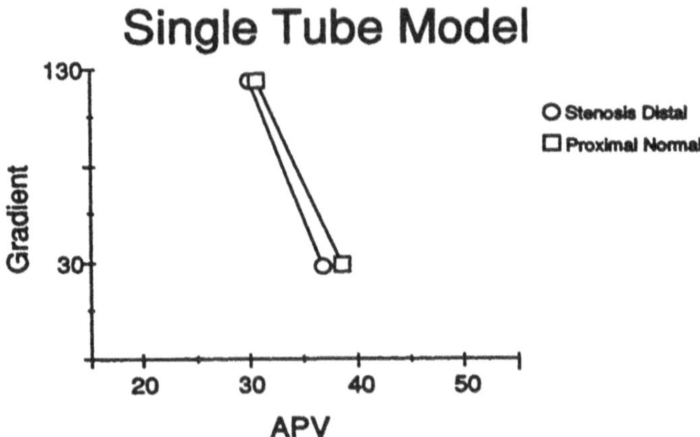

Figure 15.5B. Pump model results of flow velocity of the two arms of branched tube with flow velocity in normal branch (square) and flow velocity distal to lesion with increasing pressure gradient (circles). As pressure gradient across the lesion increases, distal flow falls and flow in normal branch increases.

post-angioplasty period, were associated with abrupt vessel occlusion [15, 16].

A continuously declining post-intervention velocity trend was associated with vessel reocclusion before symptoms, electrocardiographic changes or angiography demonstrated evidence of luminal obstruction [16] (Figure 15.7). This finding was especially relevant in the setting of acute myocardial infarction where recurrent symptoms, or lack thereof, might be unreliable as a

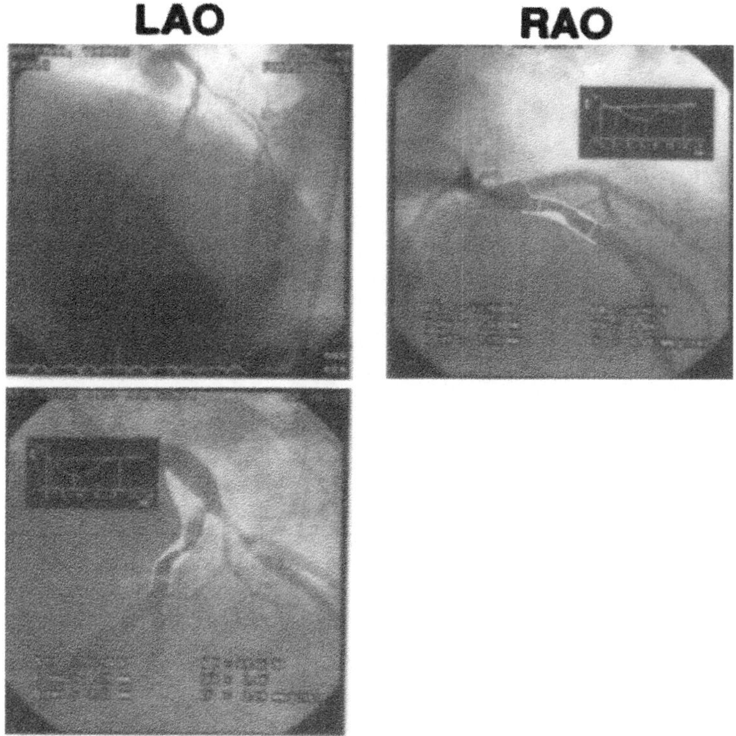

Figure 15.6A. Left anterior descending coronary lesion assessment: LAD lesion 60% narrowing by QCA. Reproduced from [14].

gauge of ischemia. An unchanged and asymptomatic course after immediate mechanical recanalization would likely be attributed to a successful procedure had the operator relied on the symptoms to identify abrupt reocclusion. The velocity trend indicated a pattern of unstable flow preceding silent reocclusion.

Cyclic flow variations associated with intraluminal thrombosis preceding abrupt vessel occlusion [15]. A changing position of the wire tip may cause signal artifact suggesting reduced or lost flow. Should a satisfactory and continuously obtained velocity signal with an intact velocity envelope demonstrate gradually diminishing or rapidly increasing mean velocity trends, an etiology other than wire position is generally responsible.

Continuous velocity trend monitoring is easily incorporated into interventional procedures and demonstrates at least 2 patterns that are associated with abrupt vessel reocclusion. These findings may precede angiographic and

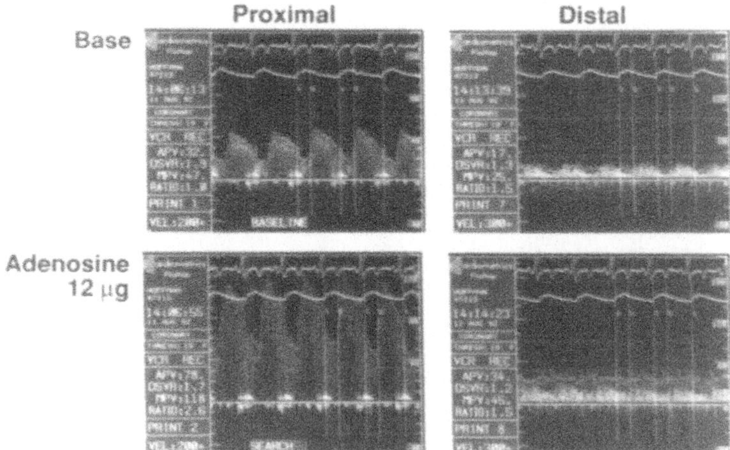

Figure 15.6B. Left anterior descending coronary lesion assessment: Flow velocity distal to the left anterior descending coronary stenosis was impaired (proximal average peak velocity 32 cm/s, distal 17 cm/s, proximal/distal mean flow ratio 32/17 = 1.9). In addition, the distal (not proximal) diastolic/systolic velocity ratio was abnormally low (1.3; normal left coronary diastolic/systolic velocity ratio >1.5). Distal hyperemia was also impaired [distal flow (hyperemic/basal) reserve = 1.42]. Reproduced from [14].

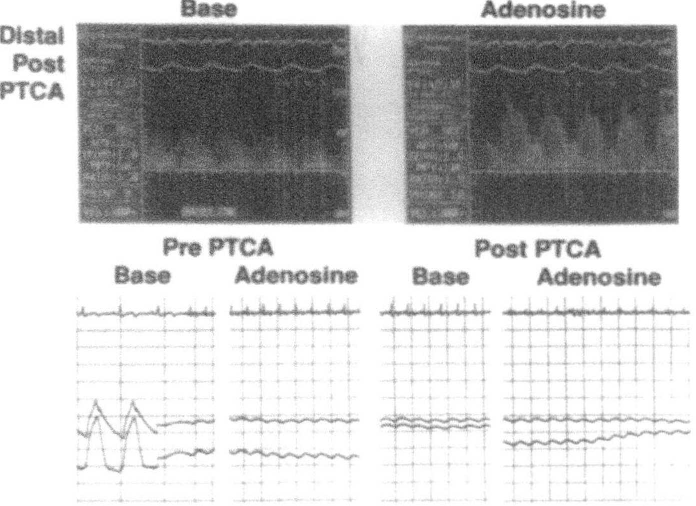

Figure 15.6C. Left anterior descending coronary lesion assessment: (Bottom left) A 40 mmHg gradient at rest increased to 48 mmHg during maximal hyperemia. (Top) After successful coronary angioplasty (stenosis <30% diameter), normal distal phasic flow velocity patterns (diastolic/systolic ratio = 1.6) and improvement of basal flow (mean velocity = 33 cm/s) and distal hyperemia (distal flow reserve = 1.96) can be seen. (Bottom right) The final gradient was 8 mmHg at rest which increased to 20 mmHg during maximal hyperemia. Reproduced from [14].

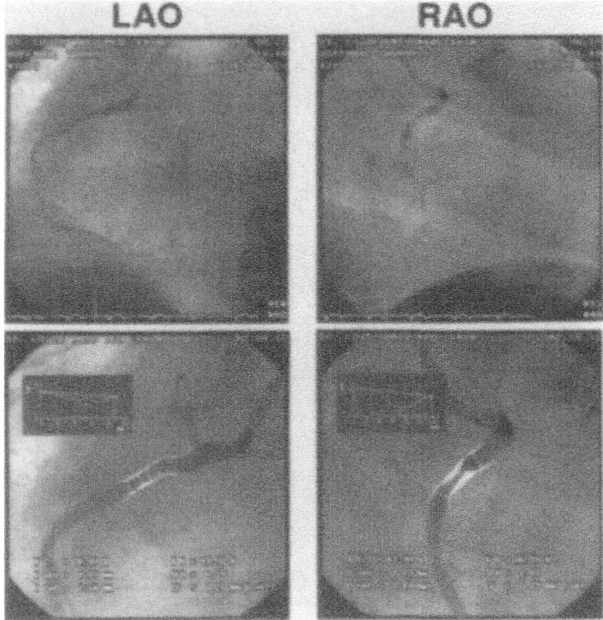

Figure 15.6D. Right coronary lesion assessment: Right coronary artery lesion 63% in 'worst' view. Reproduced from [14].

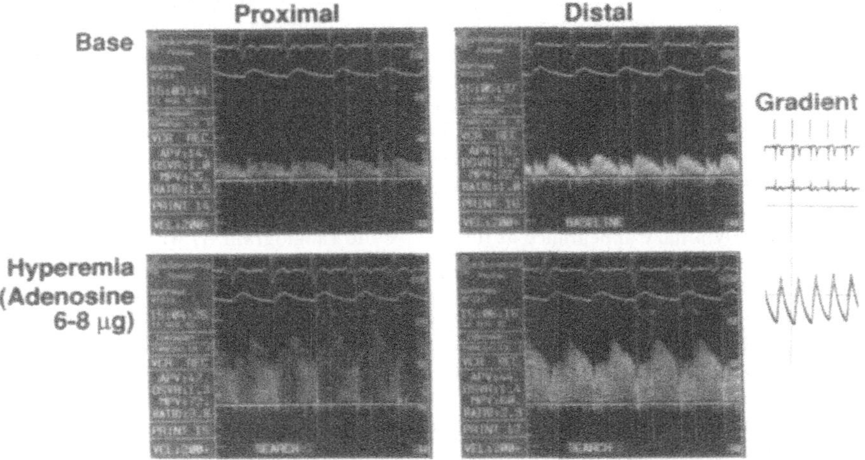

Figure 15.6E. Right coronary lesion assessment: Proximal flow velocity at base and after intracoronary adenosine demonstrated normal hyperemic response. The diastolic/systolic velocity ratio was within normal limits for the right coronary artery. Distal flow velocity was maintained (proximal/distal ratio = 0.9) with the same phasic flow pattern. Distal coronary vasodilatory reserve was normal (hyperemia/basal mean velocity, 44/15 = 2.9). The translesional pressure gradient was zero. Angioplasty was not performed on this artery. With permission from [14].

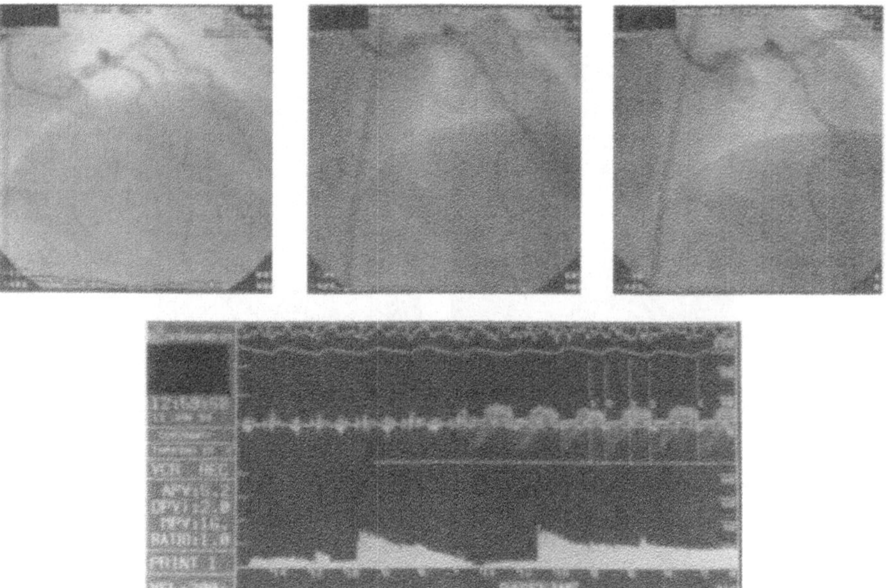

Figure 15.7. Flow velocity trend monitoring during angioplasty in a 41 year old woman with multiple risk factors for ischemic heart disease with an acute anterior myocardial infarction. Emergency angioplasty was performed with an 0.018" Doppler guidewire through a 2.5 mm angioplasty balloon catheter. The initial, mid-point and final angiograms with the corresponding flow velocity trends are shown. The initial flow velocity obtained after crossing the occluded segment with the Doppler guidewire alone was zero (Panel A, velocity trend at A). Positioning the balloon catheter was associated with minimal antegrade flow. After the first dilation (6 ATM × 90 seconds), post-occlusive hyperemia was documented with the elevated flow velocity declining over the next 2–3 minute period (trend pattern B). However, the post-PTCA flow trend after the initial dilations continued to decline. An angiogram taken during the declining trend showed only a hazy appearance at the PTCA site (angiogram B) with satisfactory angiographic flow. Within 3 minutes, the flow velocity fell to zero. Angiography now revealed a subtotally occluded vessel (not shown). The patient had no new ST changes or chest pain. Repeat PTCA was performed with a higher balloon inflation pressure (10 ATM × 120 seconds). The resultant post-occlusive hyperemia was equivalent to inflation #1 (flow trend C), but showed a normal equilibration and stabilization period with the horizontal flow pattern for >10 minutes. Angiography revealed a widely patent left anterior descending coronary artery with a minimally visible PTCA site (angiogram C). Reproduced from [16].

clinical evidence suggesting reocclusion and provide an early warning to suboptimal interventional results.

Conclusion

The measurement of flow velocity using a Doppler guidewire is easily incorporated into the interventional procedures [1] and, in many cases, may be used as the primary guidewire used to cross stenoses. Measurements performed distal to the coronary stenosis appear to be more predictive of lesion significance and outcome than those made proximal to the lesion. Coronary flow reserve measurements appear to be of limited utility immediately following interventions, regardless of whether these measurements are made in the proximal or distal vessel. Measurements of improvement in distal flow velocity parameters appear to reflect angiographic and hemodynamic improvement immediately following interventions [17, 18]. Coronary flow velocity parameters may be routinely used by the interventional cardiologist in decision making, specifically in cases where the angiographic appearance is in question. Studies are currently under way to assess both the usefulness of distal flow velocity measurements in various interventional coronary procedures and to establish the relationship of these various flow parameters to clinical outcome.

Acknowledgements

The author wishes to thank the J.G. Mudd Cardiac Catheterization Team, Dr. Frank Aguirre, Dr. Thomas Donohue, Dr. Richard Bach, Dr. Eugene Caracciolo, Dr. Patrick Serruys of the Thoraxcenter (Rotterdam, The Netherlands) and Donna Sander for manuscript preparation.

References

1. Kern MJ. Intracoronary flow velocity: current techniques and clinical applications of Doppler catheter methods. In Tobis JM, Yock PG (eds): Intravascular ultrasound imaging. New York: Churchill Livingstone 1992: 93–111.
2. Kern MJ, Anderson HV (eds). A symposium: the clinical applications of the intracoronary Doppler guidewire flow velocity in patients: understanding blood flow beyond the coronary stenosis. Am J Cardiol 1993; 71(14): 1D–86D.
3. Wilson RF, Laughlin DE, Ackell PH *et al.* Transluminal, subselective measurement of coronary artery blood flow velocity and vasodilator reserve in man. Circulation 1985; 72: 82–92.
4. Hatle L, Angelsen B. Doppler Ultrasound in Cardiology. Philadelphia: Lea & Febiger 1985: 15.
5. Doucette JW, Corl PD, Payne HM *et al.* Validation of a Doppler guide wire for intravascular measurement of coronary artery flow velocity. Circulation 1992; 85: 1899–911.
6. Ofili EO, Labovitz AJ, Kern MJ. Coronary flow velocity dynamics in normal and diseased arteries. Am J Cardiol 1993; 71(14): 3D–9D.
7. Heller LI, Villegas BJ, Weiner BH. Phasic coronary artery flow following right coronary artery PTCA [abstract]. Cathet Cardiovasc Diagn 1993; 29: 89.

8. Segal J, Kern MJ, Scott NA *et al.* Alterations of phasic coronary artery flow velocity in humans during percutaneous coronary angioplasty. J Am Coll Cardiol 1992; 20: 276–86.
9. Ofili EO, Kern MJ, Labovitz AJ *et al.* Analysis of coronary blood flow velocity dynamics in angiographically normal and stenosed arteries before and after endolumen enlargement by angioplasty. J Am Coll Cardiol 1993; 21: 308–16.
10. White CW, Wright CB, Doty DB *et al.* Does visual interpretation of the coronary arteriogram predict the physiologic importance of a coronary stenosis? N Engl J Med 1984; 310: 819–24.
11. Wilson RF, Marcus ML, White CW. Prediction of the physiologic significance of coronary arterial lesions by quantitative lesion geometry in patients with limited coronary artery disease. Circulation 1987; 75: 723–32.
12. Donohue TJ, Kern MJ, Aguirre FV *et al.* Assessing the hemodynamic significance of coronary artery stenoses: analysis of translesional pressure-flow velocity relationships in patients. J Am Coll Cardiol 1993; 22: 449–58.
13. Topol EJ, Ellis SG, Cosgrove DM *et al.* Analysis of coronary angioplasty practice in the United States with an insurance-claims data base. Circulation 1993; 87: 1489–97.
14. Kern MJ, Flynn MS, Caracciolo EA, Bach RG, Donohue TJ, Aguirre FV. Use of translesional coronary flow velocity for interventional decisions in a patient with multiple intermediately severe coronary stenoses. Cathet Cardiovasc Diagn 1993; 29: 148–53.
15. Anderson HV, Kirkeeide RL, Stuart Y, Smalling RW, Heibig J, Willerson JT. Coronary artery flow monitoring following coronary interventions. Am J Cardiol 1993; 71(14): 62D–69D.
16. Kern MJ, Aguirre FV, Donohue TJ, Bach RG, Caracciolo EA, Flynn MS. Coronary flow velocity monitoring after angioplasty associated with abrupt reocclusion. Am Heart J. 1994; 127: 436–438.
17. Segal J. Applications of coronary flow velocity during angioplasty and other coronary interventional procedures. Am J Cardiol 1993; 71(14): 17D–25D.
18. Younis L, Kern MJ, Bach R *et al.* Post-procedural normalization of coronary flow dynamics following successful atherectomy, PTCA and stenting: analysis by intracoronary spectral Doppler [abstract]. J Am Coll Cardiol 1993; 21(2 suppl A): 79A.

16. The instantaneous hyperemic pressure-flow relationship in conscious humans

CARLO DI MARIO, ROB KRAMS, ROBERT GIL,
NICOLAS MENEVEAU & PATRICK W. SERRUYS

Summary

Background. The limitations and inaccuracies in the measurement of stenosis geometry, especially after coronary interventions, have prompted investigators to use functional indexes of stenosis severity, assessing the reduction of flow induced by the stenosis under study. Coronary flow reserve is greatly affected by the hemodynamic conditions at the time of the measurement and can not be applied for the immediate assessment of the results of coronary interventions.

Aim of the study. In this study the instantaneous relation between coronary flow velocity and pressure in the diastolic phase has been assessed during maximal hyperemia in normal or near-normal coronary arteries (<30% diameter stenosis) in 52 patients and in arteries with ⩾30% diameter stenosis in 24 patients.

Methods. The instantaneous peak coronary flow velocity measured with a Doppler guidewire was plotted against the simultaneously measured proximal coronary pressure, recorded through the guiding catheter. The phase of progressive flow reduction in mid-late diastole was selected in 4 consecutive cardiac cycles at the maximal effect of 8–12.5 mg of papaverine intracoronary. To study the possibility to determine the zero-flow pressure from the intercept of the velocity-pressure relation on the pressure axis, a controlled diastolic cardiac arrest was induced by an intracoronary bolus injection of 3 mg of adenosine in 9 cardiac transplant recipients.

Results. The slope of the instantaneous hyperemic diastolic flow velocity-pressure relation (IHDVPS) could be assessed in 44/52 patients with <30% diameter stenosis (85%) and in 15/24 patients with ⩾30% diameter stenosis (62%). The presence of a flat diastolic flow velocity curve precluded the assessment of the IHDVPS in the patients with the most severe stenoses. The measurement of IHDVPS was highly reproducible (interobserver difference = 2 ± 1%) and showed a moderate beat-to-beat variability (15 ± 7%) The IHDVPS showed no significant correlation with heart rate, mean diastolic aortic pressure, left ventricular +dP/dt, V_{max}, −dP/dt and τ_1, type of vessel studied and cross-sectional area at the site of the velocity recording. The IHDVPS was significantly lower in arteries with ⩾30% diameter stenosis than in normal arteries (0.77 ± 0.52 versus 1.65 ± 0.71 cm s^{-1} $mmHg^{-1}$, $p < 0.0001$).

J.H.C. Reiber and P.W. Serruys (eds): Progress in quantitative coronary arteriography, 247–268.

The study of the velocity-pressure relation during long diastolic pauses showed a curvilinear relation in the lower pressure range between velocity and pressure, with an upwards concavity to the velocity axis and no intercept with the pressure axis in most cases.

Conclusion. The instantaneous flow velocity-pressure relation during maximal hyperemia can be reliably assessed using intracoronary Doppler in the Catheterization Laboratory, has a low inter-observer variability and a moderate beat-to-beat variability, is independent from heart rate, aortic pressure or indexes of left ventricular contractility-relaxation at the time of the assessment. The slope of this relation can distinguish arteries with and without significant coronary stenoses, suggesting that this index is a potential alternative to coronary flow reserve for the assessment of stenosis severity before and after coronary interventions. The curvilinearity of the velocity-pressure relation during long diastolic pauses, possibly due to a significant reduction of luminal cross-sectional area at low pressures, precludes the use of the flow velocity-pressure relation for the assessment of the zero-flow pressure.

Introduction

In the cardiac catheterization laboratory the severity of a coronary stenosis before and after coronary interventions is assessed using morphological techniques to measure absolute and relative dimensions of the stenotic segment. Computer-assisted quantitative angiography has greatly increased the accuracy of these measurements [1] and new techniques, such as intracoronary ultrasound, have the potential to further improve this accuracy in the presence of a lumen of complex geometry such as after coronary interventions [2]. However, multiple geometric characteristics of the stenotic segment (minimal luminal cross-sectional area, length, entrance and exit angles, etc.) must be determined to estimate the stenosis hemodynamics [3, 4]. A complete three-dimensional reconstruction of the stenosis geometry is beyond the possibility of the techniques currently applied to study stenosis morphology, and larger inaccuracies can be expected in the assessment of the results of coronary interventions which induce a severe disruption of the vessel wall [5]. Furthermore, the measurements in the reference segment for the assessment of percent diameter and cross-sectional area reduction are often misleading due to the presence of diffuse atherosclerotic changes or of pre- or post-stenotic ectasia. The use of physiological indexes of stenosis severity, assessing the reduction of flow induced by the stenosis under study, may overcome these limitations. Baseline flow, however, is reduced only in the presence of very severe stenoses, inducing a resistance to flow exceeding the high basal resistance of the distal coronary vasculature. An increase of myocardial metabolic demand or the use of pharmacologic agents inducing a maximal reduction of the distal coronary resistance is required to assess the limitation to the maximal coronary conductance induced by less severe stenoses. The measurement of absolute coronary flow, normalized per unit of viable myocardial mass, is an unequivocal indicator of the adequacy of the maximal myocardial perfusion in the territory of distribution of the artery under study. This measurement, however, can be obtained only with techniques not applicable in humans (radiolabeled microspheres) or not immediately applicable in the interventional laboratory due to their inherent technical complexity (positron emission tomography) [6–8]. The ratio of maximal flow to baseline flow (coronary flow reserve, CFR) is a well-established alternative, well correlated in previous experimental work with the severity of coronary stenoses [9]. As a ratio. however, CFR is influenced by changes in resting myocardial flow and by factors modifying the slope of the flow-pressure relation during maximal hyperemia such as the presence of myocardial hypertrophy and changes in pre-load, heart rate and myocardial contractility [10–12]. Furthermore, the ratio between maximal hyperemic flow, linearly related to changes of driving pressure, and baseline flow, relatively independent from pressure changes in the autoregulatory range, is necessarily variable with the level of aortic pressure at the time of the measurement [10]. Coronary flow reserve, measured in clinical studies using Doppler or videodensitometry, correlated well with the angiographically measured stenosis severity only in very selected subsets of patients [13–15], but this index could not be successfully applied in a large population of patients with coronary artery disease [16]. Furthermore, after coronary interventions the increase in baseline flow and/or the persistence of an impaired vasodilatory response of the distal vasculature, precludes the use of CFR for the immediate assessment of the results of this treatment in the interventional suite [17–23].

To overcome these limitations, Mancini *et al.* [24] proposed the assessment of the instantaneous relation between aortic pressure and coronary flow during maximal hyperemia in the phase of progressive flow decrease in mid- and end-diastole. In their experimental preparation, electromagnetic flowmeters were used to measure coronary flow and left ventricular pressure was used to define the start- and end-points for the measurement, avoiding the phase of rapid cardiac relaxation and the phase of isovolumetric myocardial contraction. In four separate series of experiments [24–27], the slope of the instantaneous hyperemic diastolic flow-pressure relation (IHDFPS) was shown to be independent from changes in heart rate, preload, aortic pressure and cardiac contractility. The IHDFPS was well correlated with the severity of coronary stenoses, showing larger decrements than CFR with increasing stenosis. The measurement of coronary conductance obtained with this index was best correlated with maximal subendocardial conductance measured using radiolabelled microspheres. In humans, selective measurements of instantaneous coronary flow can not easily be obtained in the cardiac catheterization laboratory. Intracoronary Doppler, however, can accurately measure instantaneous flow velocities during the cardiac cycle [28, 29]. Using

Doppler-tipped guidewires, flow velocity can be measured distal to the stenosis, so that the flow changes will certainly reflect the severity of the lesion under study.

Aim of the study: feasibility, reproducibility and independency from the hemodynamic parameters at the time of the assessment of the slope of the instantaneous hyperemic diastolic flow velocity-pressure relation was assessed in 52 arteries with <30% diameter stenosis. Sensitivity and specificity of the IHDVPS for the assessment of a flow-limiting stenosis was established by comparing the measurements of IHDVPS in the control group with the measurements obtained in 24 arteries with ≥30% diameter stenosis. The possibility to estimate the pressure at zero flow ($P_{f=0}$) from the extrapolation of the instantaneous diastolic velocity pressure relation was tested in 9 cardiac transplant recipients after inducing a controlled prolonged diastolic cardiac arrest.

Methods

Patient population

Group I (normal arteries or arteries with <30% diameter stenosis; n = 52) This group included patients undergoing coronary angiography because of suspected coronary artery disease (n = 12), percutaneous coronary interventions in an artery different from the vessel studied (n = 31) and asymptomatic cardiac transplant recipients undergoing control follow-up coronary angiography 1–5 years after transplant (n = 9). Age, sex, clinical characteristics and type of artery studied for the patients undergoing a successful assessment are indicated in Table 16.1. The studied arteries were examined by two experienced angiographers and classified as normal (n = 23) or with minimal lumen irregularities (n = 29). The absence of ≥30% diameter stenosis was confirmed, when necessary, using a subsequently described quantitative angiographic technique. In no cases angiographically visible collaterals originated from the artery studied. None of the cardiac transplant recipients had angiographically visible signs of small coronary vessel disease. In all cases left ventriculography showed a normal left ventricular function in the territory of distribution of the artery studied. Twenty-nine patients (56%) of this group were under antianginal and/or antihypertensive treatment at the time of the study.

Group II (arteries with ≥30% diameter stenosis; n = 24) This group included 21 patients with ≥50% diameter stenosis studied before a coronary intervention and 3 patients with ≥30% but <50% diameter stenosis undergoing a diagnostic coronary angiogram. Patients with acute myocardial infarction, arterial occlusion/subocclusion {Thrombolysis in Myocardial Infarction (TIMI) flow class 0–1} or presence of an open aorto-coronary bypass graft

Table 16.1. Clinical and hemodynamic characteristics of Group I.

Pts	Age	Sex	Hyp.	Vessel	CSA (mm^2)	Aortic pressure range (mmHg)		Flow velocity range (cm/s)		CFR	IHDVPS	IHDVPS variab.	$P_{f=0}$	$P_{f=0}$ variab.	r^2
						max	min	max	min		cm/s /mmHg	%	mmHg	%	
921137	67	M	y	LAD	4.07	96	71	83	39	2.4	1.2	5	32	12	0.85
921335	53	M	n	LCX	9.07	102	85	135	82	2.8	2.5	15	44	16	0.82
921343	67	M	n	RCA	9.38	96	54	63	28	2.5	0.8	13	14	53	0.94
921248	43	M	n	RCA	4.71	108	81	124	65	2.9	1.3	15	22	33	0.81
921238	55	M	n	LCX	4.10	121	91	132	54	2.6	2.4	16	66	13	0.9
920859	45	M	n	LCX	5.85	112	85	176	99	3.0	2.6	9	43	15	0.94
920931	70	M	n	LAD	3.34	100	70	45	14	2.0	0.9	12	52	8	0.90
921117	59	F	n	LAD	5.11	100	69	116	67	2.5	1.6	25	22	41	0.86
921146	45	M	n	LAD	3.43	108	84	119	63	2.7	2.1	10	51	7	0.95
921613	58	M	n	RCA	7.05	88	72	87	60	2.5	1.7	7	34	6	0.84
920613	66	M	n	LCX	5.78	127	97	97	53	3.7	1.4	6	53	8	0.86
921803	42	M	n	LCX	9.49	92	75	107	59	3.1	2.6	6	53	3	0.95
921671	59	M	y	LCX	4.12	139	112	106	76	3.0	1	12	29	35	0.85
921878	45	M	n	LCX	8.59	107	86	131	88	3.0	1.9	8	38	11	0.88
921787	54	F	y	LCX	7.31	111	84	84	59	2.8	1	10	19	36	0.90
921453	71	M	y	RCA	6.27	120	73	67	29	2.2	0.6	19	17	40	0.72
921953	65	F	y	LCX	6.30	80	58	36	24	1.3	0.5	4	5	39	0.91
921645	52	M	y	LCX	1.69	80	63	82	61	1.7	1.1	11	8	55	0.79
921581	53	F	n	LAD	3.88	116	85	64	36	2.1	0.8	7	44	11	0.91
920813	51	M	n	LCX	3.34	75	63	73	60	2.6	3.2	15	55	3	0.85
920705	45	F	y	LAD	14.1	103	87	89	56	4.5	1.6	13	47	8	0.89
922007	58	M	y	RCA		108	88	54	29	3.5	1.5	14	66	7	0.79
922038	56	M	n	LCX		103	84	103	68	3.2	1.5	20	34	33	0.80
921757	42	M	n	LAD	8.82	71	66	78	59	4.5	2.8	33	43	25	0.77
921475	61	M	n	LAD	9.01	102	76	116	58	3.5	2.3	6	48	3	0.93
921097	51	M	y	LAD	10.82	71	58	55	41	2.0	1.1	16	28	26	0.89
921384	50	M	y	RCA	–	75	61	71	40	3.3	2.1	39	31	36	0.75
920966	54	M	y	RCA	–	82	71	82	62	3.5	1.7	16	33	22	0.85
921134	50	M	y	LAD	6.12	105	93	143	99	2.3	3.1	15	59	27	0.78
921922	55	M	y	RCA	–	66	54	51	33	3.0	1.2	21	23	28	0.88
920896	31	F	y	LCX	6.07	94	74	97	50	3.8	1.7	13	36	17	0.81
921961	57	M	y	LCX	7.55	108	79	100	70	3.3	0.9	14	10	49	0.82
920952	67	M	n	SVBG	8.66	121	100	54	25	2.2	1.1	4	73	4	0.72
922002	67	M	n	SVBG	–	86	71	101	53	2.6	2.6	7	44	7	0.78
921548	66	M	y	LAD	17.5	90	73	73	43	1.6	1.6	8	44	6	0.87
930194	53	M	n	LCX	9.89	106	91	37	24	2.0	0.9	11	62	6	0.89
921983	48	M	n	LAD	9.56	90	77	94	71	4.9	1.7	13	34	16	0.92
930053	46	M	n	LAD	3.83	98	83	127	85	2.8	2.8	25	55	13	0.87
930242	68	M	y	LAD	3.84	119	87	85	48	2.7	1.0	7	31	17	0.79
930264	68	M	n	RCA	7.02	98	81	89	52	1.7	2.2	11	56	6	0.85
930131	73	F	n	LCX	7.11	99	77	87	54	3.6	1.4	11	34	17	0.84
930399	47	F	n	LAD	–	118	91	133	80	2.2	1.9	18	44	19	0.84
930090	58	M	y	RCA	5.35	110	79	53	27	2.4	0.8	15	38	36	0.88
921884	57	M	n	LAD	7.26	83	73	98	59	3.8	1.8	16	36	8	0.7
Mean ± SD	55 ± 8					99 ± 18	77 ± 14	93 ± 32	56 ± 21	2.9 ± 0.7	1.7 ± 0.7	14 ± 8	37 ± 16	22 ± 15	0.85 ± 0.07

CSA = cross-sectional area; CFR = coronary flow reserve; IHDVPS = instantaneous hyperemic diastolic velocity pressure slope; $P_{f=0}$ = X-axis intercept; r^2 = squared correlation coefficient.

Table 16.2. Clinical and hemodynamic characteristics of Group II.

Pts	Age yrs	Sex	MI	Hyp	Vessel	DS%	MLCSA	CSA Doppler site	Aortic pressure range (mmHg)	
							mm²	mm²	max	min
1921880	37	F	y	n	LAD	35	1.82	3.30	81	69
1921858	52	M	y	n	LCX	67	1.1	10.2	96	81
1921792	56	M	y	n	LAD	56	1.83	8.76	95	73
1920707	73	M	n	n	RCA	78	0.5	9.5	84	58
1920922	59	M	n	n	RCA	76	1.27	4.64	93	67
920908	63	F	n	n	RCA	55	1.17	6.70	101	78
1921238	55	M	n	n	LAD	68	0.87	2.49	89	70
1920945	69	M	y	y	LAD	55	2.18	4.22	88	75
921504	50	M	n	y	LAD	45	1.46	6.2	96	77
1921834	49	F	y	n	RCA	69	0.59	6.5	125	75
1921118	48	M	y	y	LAD	56	1.06	5.47	95	80
1921774	66	M	n	n	LAD	60	1.02	6.38	67	54
1930228	60	F	y	n	LAD	54	2.49	5.55	112	70
1930201	51	M	y	n	LAD	52	2.07	7.99	111	75
1922038	56	M	y	n	RCA	66	0.79	6.21	62	49
Mean	56					60	1.2	6.20	90	70
± SD	± 10					± 12	± 0.5	± 2.39	± 16	± 10

MI = myocardial infarction; DS% = percent diameter stenosis; MLCSA = minimal lumincal cross-
velocity pressure slope; CFR = coronary 'flow reserve; $P_{R=0}$ = X_{axis} coefficient; r^2 = squared

on the vessel studied were not included in the study. Clinical characteristics and type of vessel studied in the group undergoing a successful assessment are reported in Table 16.2. All patients of this group were under antianginal treatment at the time of the study.

Catheterization procedure

After intravenous administration of 10,000 I.U. of heparin and 250 mg of acetylsalicylic acid, a 7–8 Fr guiding catheter was advanced up to the ostium of the artery studied. The Doppler guidewire was introduced into the proximal or mid-segment of the vessel to be studied (Group I) or distal to the stenosis (Group II). After optimization of the Doppler signal and 3–5 min after intracoronary injection of a bolus of 2–3 mg of isosorbide-dinitrate, baseline flow velocity and proximal coronary pressure were recorded and a cineangiogram was performed in order to measure the cross-sectional area at the site of the Doppler sample volume and the geometric characteristics of the stenosis (when present). The flow velocity measurement was then repeated at the peak effect of an intracoronary bolus injection of papaverine (8 mg: right coronary; 12.5 mg: left coronary and saphenous vein bypass graft) [30]. Care was taken to avoid impairment of flow during maximal hyperemia due to the presence of the guiding catheter in the coronary ostium. If damping occurred, the guiding catheter was withdrawn from the coronary ostium immediately after the injection of papaverine. In 6 cardiac transplant recipients, left ventricular and aortic pressure were measured simultaneously

Flow velocity range (cm/s)		CFR	IHDVPS (cm/s/mmHg)	IHDVPS variab.	$P_{f=0}$ mmHg	$P_{f=0}$ var.	r^2
max	min	%	%				
32	22	2.4	0.7	10	38.6	17	0.83
20	15	2	0.2	13	7.6	27	0.95
47	29	1.8	0.6	7	14.3	24	0.85
50	32	1.5	0.6	19	0	52	0.76
41	18	1.8	1	14	45	5	0.82
33	20	1.5	0.5	24	34	42	0.86
21	12	1.1	0.3	32	26	50	0.70
31	21	1.7	0.6	8	28.7	12	0.72
57	30	1.9	0.7	29	28.9	19	0.60
50	18	1.3	0.5	12	26.6	22	0.92
66	52	1.4	0.7	12	2	70	0.72
38	21	1.7	0.8	10	27.9	9	0.68
202	94	3.3	2.3	11	20	27	0.93
61	37	2.1	0.6	5	9	48	0.94
57	37	1.9	1.5	13	24.7	17	0.92
42	25	1.7	0.7	16	23.4	28	0.79
± 14	± 11	± 0.3	± 0.3	± 8	± 14	± 19	± 0.1

sectional area; CSA = cross-sectional area; IHDVPS = instantaneous hyperemic diastolic correlation coefficient.

using a double sensor high-fidelity pig-tail catheter (Sentron, Roden, the Netherlands). In these cases a previously described automated analysis system [31] was used to measure peak positive and negative first derivative of the left ventricular pressure (+dP/dt and −dP/dt), the maximal velocity of isovolumic left ventricular contraction (V_{max}) and the constant of isovolumic relaxation (τ_1). In all the 9 cardiac transplant recipients, during the phase of maximal hyperemia after papaverine injection, an intracoronary bolus of 3 mg of adenosine was used to induce a prolonged diastolic cardiac arrest. Ventricular pacing was used, when necessary, to restore cardiac contraction.

Quantitative angiographic measurements

The guiding catheter, filmed devoid of contrast medium, was used as a scaling device. A previously validated [32] on-line analysis system operating on digital images (ACA-DCI, Philips Medical Systems, Best, The Netherlands) was used during the catheterization procedure. In this system, after automatic detection of the vessel centerline, a weighted first and second derivative function with predetermined continuity constraints is applied to the brightness profile on each scan line perpendicular to the vessel centerline. In all patients a user-defined diameter was measured at the site of the Doppler sample volume and the corresponding cross-sectional area was calculated assuming a circular cross-section. In Group II, minimal luminal diameter (MLD) was measured and percent luminal diameter stenosis was calculated using an automatic interpolated technique to measure the reference diameter.

Doppler guidewire and flow velocity measurements

The Doppler angioplasty guidewire is a 0.018" (diameter 0.45 mm, cross-sectional area 0.17 mm^2) 175 cm long flexible and steerable guidewire with a very flexible shapable distal end mounting a 12 MHz piezoelectric transducer at the tip (Cardiometrics Inc., Mountain View, CA) [28]. The sample volume is positioned at a distance of 5.2 mm from the transducer and has an approximate width of 2.25 mm due to the divergent ultrasound beam so that a large part of the flow velocity profile is included in the sample volume also in case of eccentric positions of the Doppler guidewire. After real-time processing of the quadrature audio signal, a Fast-Fourier transform algorithm is used to increase the reliability of the analysis [33]. The Doppler system calculates and displays on-line several spectral variables including the instantaneous peak velocity and the time-averaged (mean of 2 beats) peak velocity (Figure 16.1A). The flow velocity measurements obtained with this system have been validated *in vitro* and in an animal model using simultaneous electromagnetic flow measurements for comparison [28]. Mean flow velocity was calculated as time-averaged peak velocity/2, assuming a fully developed parabolic flow velocity profile [29]. Coronary flow reserve was defined as the ratio between maximal flow velocity at the peak effect of the papaverine injection and in baseline conditions.

Instantaneous assessment of the flow velocity-pressure relation

A continuous acquisition of the instantaneous peak Doppler flow velocity, of the pressure measured through the guiding catheter and of the electrocardiogram was performed with a 12 bits analog-to-digital converter (DataQ Instr., Akron, OH) connected to a PC. Electrocardiogram, proximal coronary pressure and instantaneous peak coronary blood flow velocity were sampled at 125 Hz per channel and stored for off-line analysis (Figure 16.1B). Using dedicated software (ACodas, DataQ, Akron, Ohio), the acquired signals were displayed in an X-Y scatterplot, so that the progressive variations of the instantaneous peak flow velocity-pressure loop from baseline to hyperemia could be monitored and 4 consecutive cardiac cycles without recording artifacts could be selected at peak hyperemia. The diastolic interval to be analyzed was selected using as start point the maximal diastolic velocity and as end-point the beginning of the phase of rapid decrease of flow velocity induced by the ventricular contraction (Figure 16.1C). After identification of the interval of analysis for each cycle, linear regression was used to calculate the individual IHDVPS in order to study the variability among different cardiac cycles. Afterwards, the data of the 4 selected diastolic intervals were pooled and the mean IHDVPS was calculated. The reproducibility of the measurements was tested in 10 randomly chosen cases of Group I in which the same 4 cardiac cycles were independently assessed by a second observer. In the 6 patients in whom a left ventricular high-fidelity pressure

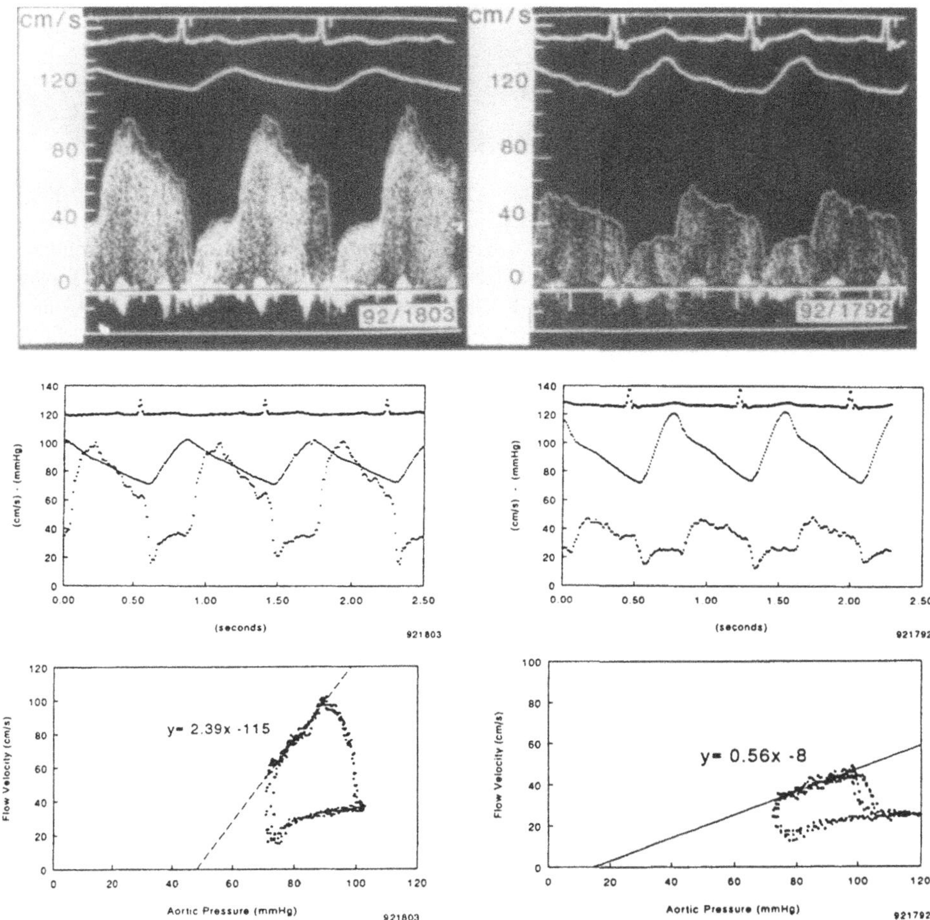

Figure 16.1. (A) Flow velocity measurements during maximal hyperemia in a left circumflex artery with minimal wall irregularities (left side) and in a left anterior descending coronary artery distal to a significant stenosis (56% diameter stenosis). (B) From top to bottom electrocardiogram, aortic pressure and peak velocity of the same beats acquired in a digital format (125 Hz). The maximal velocity and the rapid decrease in velocity due to the beginning of myocardial contraction are used as the start and end point for the analysis of the diastolic hyperemic pressure velocity relation. (C) Pressure flow velocity loop of the same beats. The regression line was calculated from the mid-datapoints of the diastolic interval indicated above. Note the steeper slope of the pressure velocity relation in the normal artery.

was available during the measurements, the slope of the hyperemic diastolic flow velocity-pressure relation was assessed in the same beats using the start- and end-points proposed by Mancini *et al.* (20 ms after peak left ventricular −dP/dt and upstroke of +dP/dt) [24].

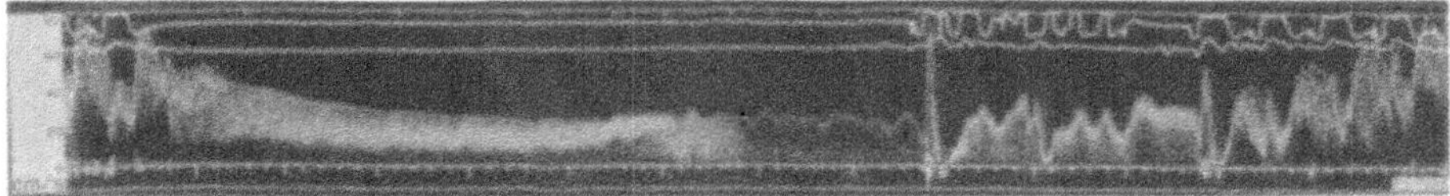

Figure 16.2. Prolonged diastolic pause induced by the intracoronary injection of 3 mg of adenosine during maximal hyperemia induced by papaverine. A progressive decrease of flow velocity and aortic pressure is observed during the 6 seconds of cardiac arrest. In the first beats induced by ventricular pacing, note the presence of a large systolic flow component, indicating refilling of the capacitance of the epicardial coronary artery. The dotted tracing at the top of the Doppler envelope indicates the instantaneous peak velocity (automatically detected on-line and used for the analysis of the pressure-velocity relation).

Velocity-pressure relation during controlled diastolic cardiac arrest

In 9 cardiac transplant recipients a second injection of papaverine intracoronary was performed, followed after 30–45 s by an intracoronary bolus of adenosine 3 mg (Figure 16.2). Using a previously introduced right ventricular pacing catheter, pacing was performed when necessary (4 cases) to restore a normal cardiac contraction. Flushing was reported by 4/9 patients. None of the patients complained of chest discomfort.

Statistical analysis

The results were expressed as mean ±standard deviation (SD). The beat-to-beat variability of the IHDVPS was calculated as the ratio between the standard deviation and the mean of the slopes measured over 4 consecutive cardiac cycles. The mean ±SD of the signed differences of corresponding measurements was used to test the interobserver variability and the variability of the measurements obtained defining the diastolic interval of analysis from the flow velocity signal or from the left ventricular pressure. Covariance analysis was used in Group I to estimate the independency of the IHDVPS from heart rate, mean diastolic aortic pressure, cross-sectional area at the site of the velocity measurements and left ventricular +dP/dt and −dP/dt, Vmax and τ_1. A two-tailed Student's t-test for unpaired data was performed to compare the measurements of IHDVPS in patients with and without >30% diameter stenosis.

To test the linearity of the individual velocity-pressure relations during long diastolic pauses, the data were fit with a linear and a second order polynomial function. A relation was considered non-linear when the coefficient of the second order term of the polynomial fit was significant at $p < 0.01$ and when the F-statistic for the polynomial fit was statistically better at $p < 0.01$ than the linear fit [34].

Results

Feasibility, reproducibility, beat-to-beat variability and dependence on hemodynamic variables of the measurement of IHDVPS

Feasibility A reliable, automatic detection during maximal hyperemia of the progressive decrease in flow velocity in mid-late diastole was obtained in 44/52 patients of Group I (85%) and in 15/24 patients of Group II (62%). A poor quality of the Doppler signal or the presence of multiple artifacts impairing the accuracy of the automatic analysis was the reason for exclusion in all the 8 failed measurements in Group I and in 4 failed measurements in Group II. In the remaining 5 patients excluded in Group II the reason of failure was the presence of a flat diastolic flow velocity curve, without a clear proto-mid diastolic peak usable as start-point for analysis. In all the patients with this pattern a severe coronary obstruction (>75% diameter stenosis) was observed.

Variability The mean difference between measurements of IHDVPS performed independently by two observers (n = 10) was 0.004 ± 0.0001 cm $\cdot$ s^{-1} $\cdot$ $mmHg^{-1}$ (observer 1 minus observer 2), equal to 2 ± 1% of the mean of the two measurements. A beat-to-beat variability of 13 ± 7% was observed in Group I (individual measurements in Table 16.1) and of 15 ± 8% in Group II (Table 16.2). The IHDVPS calculated using start- and end-points for the definition of the diastolic interval derived from the flow velocity tracing or from the left ventricular pressure tracing (n = 6) showed a mean difference of 0.009 ± 0.005 cm $\cdot$ s^{-1} $\cdot$ $mmHg^{-1}$ (measurement with interval selected on the velocity pattern minus measurement with interval selected from the left ventricular tracing, 3 ± 2%).

Dependence on hemodynamic variables In Group I IHDVPS showed no significant correlation with heart rate, mean aortic diastolic pressure, type of vessel studied and luminal cross-sectional area at the site of the Doppler sample volume. In 6 patients of the same group in whom a high-fidelity left ventricular pressure was recorded, no correlation between IHDVPS and +dP/dt, −dP/dt, V_{max} and τ_1 was observed.

IHDVPS in patients with and without coronary stenoses

The patients with and without >30% diameter stenosis in the artery studied showed no significant differences in heart rate (69 ± 12 versus 63 ± 7 beats/min, NS) mean diastolic aortic pressure (88 ± 13 vs 82 ± 7 mmHg, NS) and cross-sectional area at the site of the Doppler measurement (6.9 ± 3.1 vs 6.3 ± 2.2 mm^2, NS). Maximal diastolic velocity was significantly higher in Group I than in Group II (91 ± 31 vs 54 ± 43 cm/s, $p < 0.005$). Coronary flow

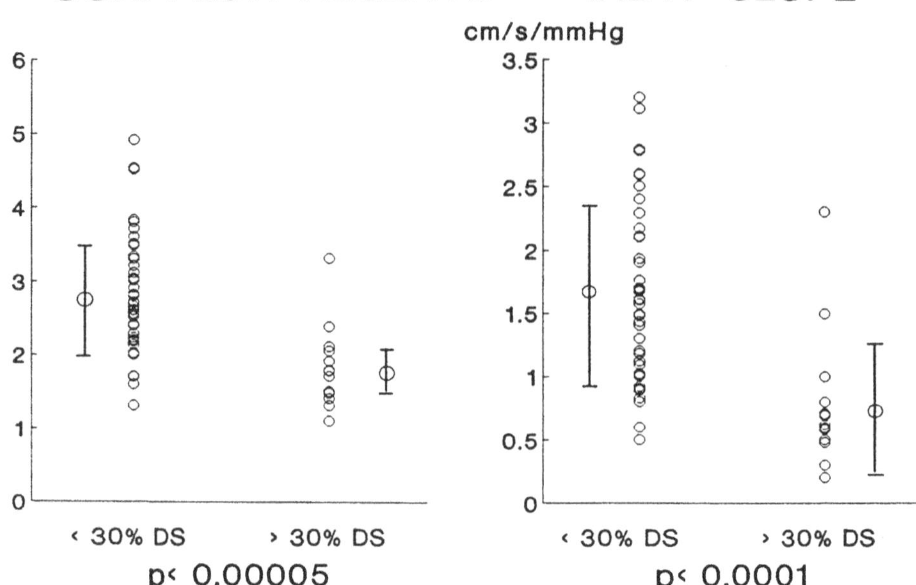

Figure 16.3. Individual measurements of coronary flow reserve and IHDVPS in patients with and without ⩾ 30% diameter stenosis. Both the indices showed a significant difference in the two groups. The measurements of IHDVPS showed a smaller overlap in the two groups and a slightly higher sensitivity in the detection of the absence of ⩾30% diameter stenosis.

reserve was also significantly higher in Group I than in Group II (2.9 ± 0.7 vs 1.7 ± 0.3, $p < 0.00005$). The IHDVPS was significantly higher in the normal or near-normal arteries of Group I than in the arteries with ⩾30% diameter stenosis (1.65 ± 0.71 vs 0.77 ± 0.52 $cm \cdot s^{-1} \cdot mmHg^{-1}$, $p < 0.0001$), (Figure 16.3). A significant correlation was observed between IHDVPS and CFR ($r = 0.51$, $p < 0.0005$). In Group II the IHDVPS showed no correlation with the angiographically measured minimal luminal cross-sectional area and with percent diameter stenosis ($r = 0.39$ and 0.01, respectively, both NS).

IHDVPS during long-diastolic pauses

In 6/9 heart transplant recipients (66%) the injection of 3 mg of adenosine intracoronary was followed by a diastolic pause sufficiently long to induce a reduction of the minimal aortic pressure to ⩽45 mmHg. Two of these patients were excluded because of deterioration of the flow velocity signal in the lower pressure range. Sinus node arrest was observed in 3 patients while a 3rd degree atrio-ventricular block was the cause of the arrest of the left ventricular contraction in the remaining 3 patients.

The individual curves of the 4 longest pauses observed in these patients are plotted in Figure 16.4. The curvilinear relation between velocity and pressure was confirmed by the analysis of the residuals after fitting a linear and a second order polynomial equation (Figure 16.5) and by the F-test, showing that the polynomial fit was better at $p < 0.01$ in 3/4 cases. In order to ascertain whether the curvilinear relation between velocity and pressure was present over the entire range of measurements, an automated calculation of IHDVPS was performed using linear regression over progressively smaller ranges of measurements, starting from the lowest pressure (Figure 16.6) and progressively increasing the lowest pressure by 1 mmHg up to a final smallest range examined including the measurements obtained in the highest 15 mmHg pressure range (Figure 16.6). This series of slopes was then plotted against the corresponding lowest pressure. The results of this analysis showed that a rather constant IHDVPS was present in a pressure range >60 mmHg (Figure 16.6). Similarly, the intercept with the pressure axis showed a progressive increase in the lower pressure range, while stable higher values were observed in the physiologic pressure range.

Discussion

The instantaneous velocity-pressure relation for the assessment of stenosis severity

In this first application in humans of the index proposed by Mancini *et al.* [24–27], special attention was paid to the assessment of the feasibility of the measurement. In the vast majority of the studied arteries the IHDVPS could be assessed. A manual tracing of the peak velocity from the Doppler spectrum could have increased the number of cases with a successful assessment when the presence of artifacts in the automatically detected peak velocity was the reason of failure. This method, however, is cumbersome, requires an-off line analysis so that the results cannot be immediately available at the time of the assessment and is prone to a considerable subjectivity. The presence of a flat diastolic flow velocity curve was the second most important reason of failure in the assessment of the IHDVPS. This pattern was observed only in very severe stenoses for which the assessment of an additional index of functional severity could be considered of limited additional clinical value. Despite a careful selection of the beats analyzed, a relatively large beat-to-beat variability was observed. Respiratory changes can be advocated as a possible explanation but the effect of respiration should be minimal during maximal hyperemia. A technical limitation is the most likely explanation of this variability. The automatic detection of the peak diastolic velocity and, in particular, of the maximal velocity which was used as the start point for analysis and is an essential determinant of the final outcome of the analysis, is very sensitive to the presence of noise. The original method proposed by

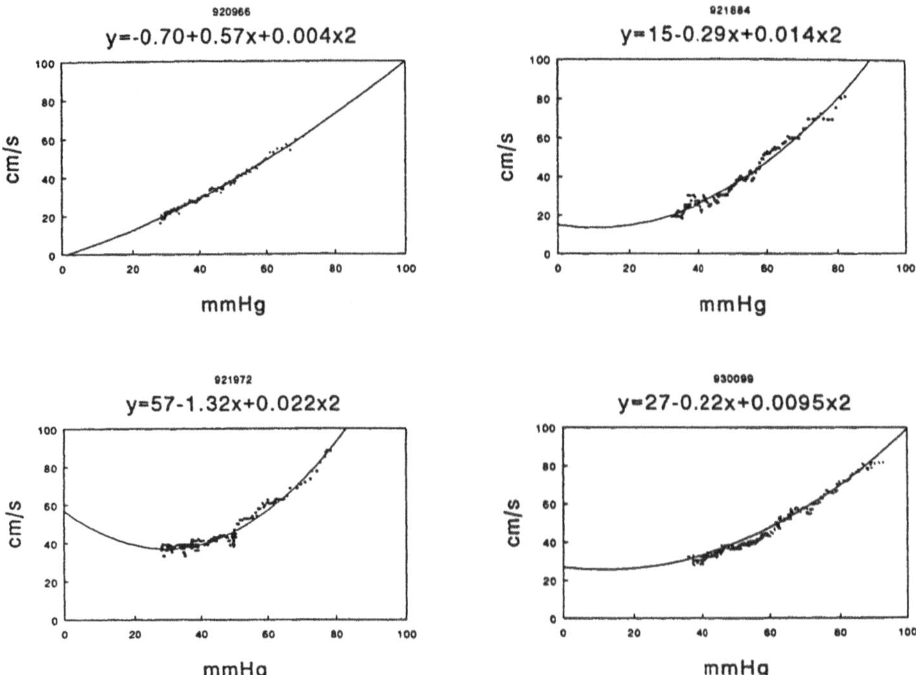

Figure 16.4. The instantaneous hyperemic peak velocity from maximal diastolic velocity to the restoration of cardiac contraction is plotted versus aortic pressure during a prolonged cardiac arrest induced by an intracoronary injection of adenosine 3 mg intracoronary. In all the cases a second order polynomial equation is applied for analysis. In the case in the left upper panel, however, the F-test showed no significant difference between a linear and the displayed second order polynomial function. The curvilinearity in all the other cases is evident and was confirmed by the F-test. Note the absence of the intercept on the pressure axis in these three cases.

Mancini *et al.* [24] required a high fidelity measurement of the left ventricular pressure in order to detect the diastolic interval of interest for analysis. Measurements obtained in a subset of patients demonstrated that the simplified approach used in this study yields results similar to those obtained selecting the interval for analysis from the left ventricular pressure tracing.

Mancini *et al.* [24–27] could independently manipulate the hemodynamic parameters in the animal model used to assess the correlation of CFR and flow-pressure slope with each hemodynamic variable. A similar approach could not be used in a clinical study but the lack of correlation in the population studied between IHDVPS and heart rate, aortic pressure and indices of left ventricular contractility and relaxation at the time of the assessment suggests that also in humans this index is independent from these hemodynamic variables. The IHDVPS measured in arteries with ⩾30% diameter stenosis was less than half the IHDVPS measured in normal or

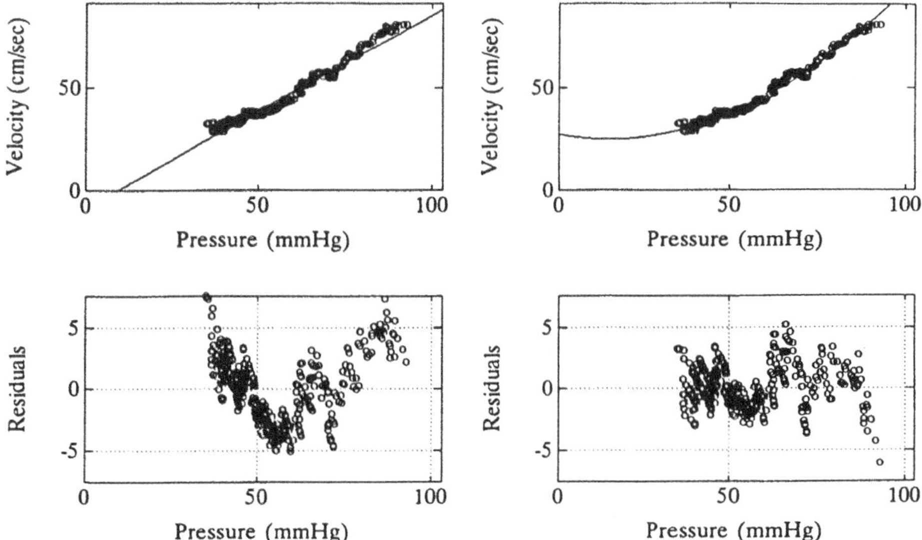

Figure 16.5. Analysis between true measured data points and values estimated applying a linear equation (left panels) and a second order polynomial equation (right panels). When the residuals are plotted against the corresponding pressure an inverted bell-shaped curve is present when a linear model is applied, while the residuals are randomly distributed along the zero line when a second order equation is applied.

near-normal coronary arteries. Due to the small overlap between the two groups, if an arbitrary cut-off of $\geqslant 0.8\,\text{cm} \cdot \text{s}^{-1} \cdot \text{mmHg}^{-1}$ was chosen, the sensitivity and specificity of this index in the detection of the absence of a ≥30% diameter stenosis were 95 and 91%, respectively, with a sensitivity only minimally greater than coronary flow reserve and a similar specificity. The assessment of a larger group of patients with flow limiting stenoses is required to establish the potential advantage of IHDVPS over CFR in the assessment of an impairment of coronary conductance. In particular, these studies should address the usefulness of this index for the assessment of the changes of coronary conductance after coronary interventions. In this setting, the IHDVPS has the great potential advantage over CFR to be independent from changes in baseline velocity and from the hemodynamic conditions at the time of the assessment.

A substantial difference between the approach of Mancini and our approach is the use of flow velocity instead of absolute coronary flow normalized for the myocardial mass. The approach used in this study has the advantage of an easier applicability in the clinical setting but has also the potential disadvantage that the velocity-pressure slope can be influenced by the dimension of the artery under assessment so that slopes measured in arteries of different diameter cannot be compared. The results of this study in normal

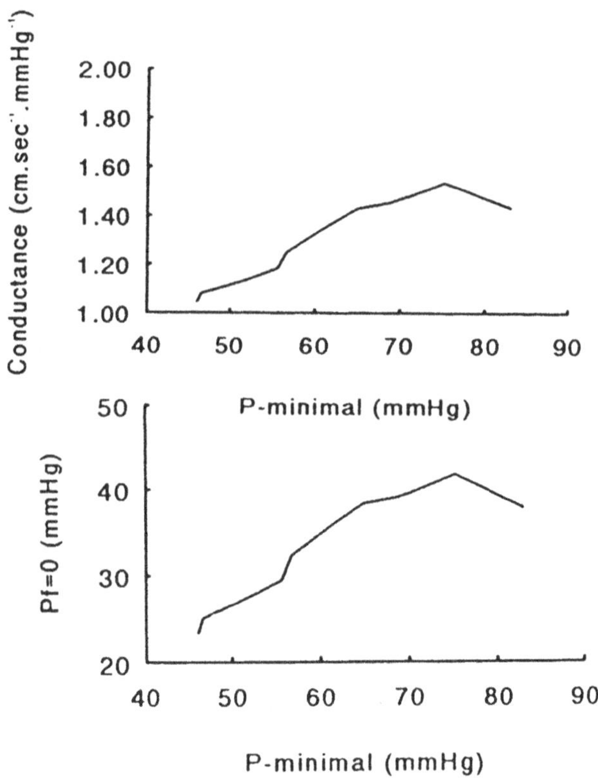

Figure 16.6. The IHDVPS (Conductance) and the X-intercept (P_{zf}) are calculated using linear regression analysis over progressively smaller ranges of measurements, starting in the lowest pressure range and progressively increasing the minimal pressure up to the higher 15 mmHg pressure range. The calculated IHDVPS (Conductance, upper panel) and $P_{f=0}$ (P_{zf}, lower panel) are plotted against the lowest pressure of the sample analyzed. Note the progressive increase in the 30–45 mmHg range and the more stable values at higher pressure.

or near-normal arteries, however, showed that the IHDVPS is independent from the cross-sectional area at the site of the velocity measurement. In the coronary system, the presence of a progressive, moderate increase in total cross-sectional area from proximal to distal has been suggested in accordance with the principles of limited/adaptive vascular shear stress, minimum vascular volume at bifurcations and minimum viscous energy loss [35]. After three-dimensional reconstruction of the arterial tree from orthogonal cineangiograms in humans, Seiler *et al.* [35] calculated a ratio between area of the mother vessel and mean of the areas of the daughter vessels of 1.647, similar to the ratio predicted based on the previously mentioned principles (1.588). These considerations explain why only a moderate decrease of mean velocity, inversely proportional to the moderate increase in total cross-sectional area, occurs from proximal to distal in the epicardial coronary arteries. The maintenance of a relatively constant flow velocity despite the changes in cross-sectional area and in perfused myocardial bed partially limits the inaccuracy consequent to the lack of correction for the perfused myocardial mass which can not be easily determined in humans.

The changes of flow velocity can be considered a reliable indicator of the changes in coronary flow only in the presence of a constant cross-sectional area. The minimal reduction in cross-sectional area occurring during the meso-telediastolic phase of the cardiac cycle is likely to induce a negligible reduction in cross-sectional area and, consequently, a negligible underestimation of the true flow-pressure slope estimated from the flow velocity.

The IHDVPS assesses changes in coronary conductance which can be induced both by the presence of a severe epicardial stenosis and by the presence of an impaired vasodilatation of the coronary microvasculature. A different approach can be used to distinguish these two components of coronary resistance, but this approach requires the additional measurement of the post-stenotic pressure. Gould *et al.* [36] correlated in dogs the severity of experimentally induced coronary stenoses with the changes in the transstenotic pressure gradient-flow velocity relation. Using a high-fidelity pressure transducer mounted on an angioplasty guidewire in combination with a separate Doppler guidewire, this approach was repeated recently in humans [22, 37]. A different analysis of the same recordings can be performed to study the relation between flow velocity and post-stenotic pressure, an indicator of the maximal vasodilatory response of the distal coronary bed. When a high-fidelity pre- and post-stenotic pressure and flow velocity signals are available, two types of relation can be used to separate the functional characteristics of the stenosis and of the distal vascular bed: the instantaneous relation between transstenotic pressure and velocity, assessing the stenosis hemodynamics as in an isolated hydraulic model, independently from the hemodynamic conditions and from the properties of the distal vascular bed, and the relation between flow velocity and post-stenotic pressure, correlated to the conductance of the distal vasculature [22].

The instantaneous velocity-pressure relation for the assessment of the zero-flow pressure

The extrapolation of the pressure-flow relation during a long diastolic pause was used in the original report by Bellamy [38] to assess the pressure at zero flow. His observation that $P_{f=0}$ was higher than the coronary venous pressure has initiated a great deal of experimental work to better define mechanism and physiologic and clinical importance of this phenomenon.

Mechanisms of regulation of the $P_{f=0}$

Bellamy, discussing the importance of a $P_{f=0}$ greater than the coronary venous pressure as a determinant of coronary resistance [39], interpreted this phenomenon as the effect of a vascular waterfall due to active vascular constriction or to the effect of a tissue pressure higher than the intravascular pressure. The lack of a direct demonstration of vascular collapse at the arteriolar level and the persistence of venous outflow after cessation of the arterial flow [40] have suggested alternative mechanisms. The effect of capacitative flow due to the blood stored in the extramural coronary arteries and discharged into the myocardium because of the progressive reduction of epicardial arterial volume at low pressures, suggests that the $P_{f=0}$ at the microvascular level is overestimated by a measurement in a proximal artery. After correction for the capacitative effects, Eng *et al.* [41] calculated a $P_{f=0}$ similar to the right atrial pressure during maximal hyperemia. Canty *et al.* [42], however, confirmed the persistance of a $P_{f=0}$ during maximal hyperemia greater than venous pressure using a capacitance free model. The presence of a large intramyocardial compliance with long time-constants for blood discharge has been proposed as a model alternative to the presence of a vascular waterfall to explain the cessation of flow in the epicardial arteries at a pressure higher than the right atrial pressures [43]. Whatever mechanism is involved in the regulation of the $P_{f=0}$, there is a consensus that the presence of an elevated $P_{f=0}$ (up to 50 mmHg) occurs only in conditions of coronary autoregulation and that much lower pressures are present at the cessation of the arterial flow when the coronary vasculature is maximally vasodilated [44].

Morphology of the diastolic pressure-flow relation

The diastolic flow-pressure relation during maximal hyperemia was found to be concave upwards towards the flow axis in many experimental reports [41, 42, 45]. This curvilinearity may be explained by a discharge of blood from the upstream epicardial vessels and by a progressive increase in vascular resistance due to the pressure-dependent decrease of arterial diameter [45]. If this curvilinearity is ignored or if the pressure-flow relation is not explored in the low pressure range, falsely elevated measurements of $P_{f=0}$ are obtained. In this study the measurements were obtained during a long diastolic pause, with pressures at the end of the period of cardiac arrest <45 mmHg. However, the use of flow velocity instead of flow introduced an additional bias in the estimation of the pressure-flow relation. If the arterial cross-section at the site of the velocity measurement is reduced simultaneously to the reduction in flow velocity, the velocity decrease underestimates the true flow reduction. The phenomenon is relevant for flow velocity measurements obtained in the low pressure range because a curvilinear relation between distending pressure and arterial cross-section is present, with larger changes in cross-section in the low pressure range [46]. Therefore, the marked curvilinearity present in the flow velocity-pressure relation at low pressures, without a positive intercept with the pressure axis, precluded the use of the flow velocity-pressure relation for the assessment of the $P_{f=0}$. The simultaneous use of intracoronary Doppler and two-dimensional ultrasound imaging has the potential to overcome this limitation and allow the estimation of the $P_{f=0}$ in conscious humans in the catheterization laboratory [47]. In the physiologic range of pressures, however, the relation between flow velocity and pressure remained linear so that linear regression could be used to estimate arterial conductance.

Conclusion

The instantaneous velocity-pressure relation during maximal hyperemia can be reliably assessed using intracoronary Doppler in the catheterization laboratory, is highly reproducible, has a moderate beat-to-beat variability and is independent from heart rate, aortic pressure or indexes of left ventricular contractility-relaxation at the time of the assessment. The slope of this relation can distinguish arteries with and without significant coronary stenoses, suggesting that this index is a potential alternative to coronary flow reserve for the assessment of stenosis severity.

The curvilinearity of the velocity-pressure relation during long diastolic pauses precludes the use of the flow velocity-pressure relation for the assessment of the zero-flow pressure.

Acknowledgements

The contribution to the acquisition of the data by the medical, technical and nursing staff of the Catheterization Laboratory is gratefully acknowledged. Dr. C.J. Slager is acknowledged for his contribution and suggestions in the preparation of this manuscript.

References

1. Reiber JHC, Serruys PW, Kooijman CJ *et al.* Assessment of short-, medium-, and long-term variations in arterial dimensions from computer-assisted quantitation of coronary cineangiograms. Circulation 1985; 71: 280–8.
2. Tenaglia AN, Buller CE, Kisslo KB, Stack RS, Davidson CJ. Mechanisms of balloon angioplasty and directional coronary atherectomy as assessed by intravascular ultrasound. J Am Coll Cardiol 1992; 20: 685–91.
3. Young DF, Cholvin NR, Roth AC. Pressure drop across artificially induced stenoses in the femoral arteries of dogs. Circ Res 1975; 36: 735–43.
4. Lipscomb K, Hooten S. Effect of stenotic dimensions and blood flow on the hemodynamic significance of model coronary arterial stenoses. Am J Cardiol 1978; 42: 781–92.
5. Serruys PW, Reiber JHC, Wijns W *et al.* Assessment of percutaneous transluminal coronary angioplasty by quantitative coronary angiography: diameter versus densitometric area measurements. Am J Cardiol 1984; 54: 482–8.

6. Araujo LI, Lammertsma AA, Rhodes CG *et al.* Non-invasive quantification of regional myocardial blood flow in coronary artery disease with oxygen-15-labeled carbon dioxide inhalation and positron emission tomography. Circulation 1991; 83: 875–85.
7. Krivokapich J, Huang SC, Schelbert HR. Assessment of the effects of dobutamine on myocardial blood flow and oxidative metabolism in normal human subjects using nitrogen-13 ammonia and carbon-11 acetate. Am J Cardiol 1993; 71: 1351–6.
8. Gould KL. Identifying and measuring severity of coronary artery stenosis. Quantitative coronary arteriography and positron emission tomography. Circulation 1988; 78: 237–45.
9. Gould KL, Lipscomb K, Hamilton GW. Physiologic basis for assessing critical coronary stenosis. Instantaneous flow response and regional distribution during coronary hyperemia as measures of coronary flow reserve. Am J Cardiol 1974; 33: 87–94.
10. Klocke FJ. Measurements of coronary flow reserve: defining pathophysiology versus making decisions about patient care. Circulation 1987; 76: 1183–9.
11. McGinn AL, White CW, Wilson RF. Interstudy variability of coronary flow reserve. Influence of heart rate, arterial pressure and ventricular preload. Circulation 1990; 81: 1319–30.
12. Rossen JD, Winniford MD. Effect of increases in heart rate and arterial pressure on coronary flow reserve in humans. J Am Coll Cardiol 1993; 21: 343–8.
13. Wilson RF, Marcus ML, White CW. Prediction of the physiologic significance of coronary arterial lesions by quantitative lesion geometry in patients with limited coronary artery disease. Circulation 1987; 75: 723–32.
14. Harrison DG, White CW, Hiratzka LF, Doty DB, Barnes DH *et al.* The value of lesion cross-sectional area determined by quantitative coronary angiography in assessing the physiologic significance of proximal left anterior descending coronary artery stenoses. Circulation 1984; 69: 1111–9.
15. Zijlstra F, van Ommeren J, Reiber JHC, Serruys PW. Does the quantitative assessment of coronary artery dimensions predict the physiologic significance of a coronary stenosis? Circulation 1987; 75: 1154–61.
16. Laarman GJ, Serruys PW, Suryapranata H *et al.* Inability of coronary flow reserve measurements to assess the efficacy of coronary angioplasty in the first 24 hours in unselected patients. Am Heart J 1991; 122: 631–9.
17. Wilson RF, Johnson MR, Marcus ML *et al.* The effect of coronary angioplasty on coronary flow reserve. Circulation 1988; 77: 873–85.
18. Serruys PW, Juilliere Y, Zijlstra F *et al.* Coronary blood flow velocity during percutaneous transluminal coronary angioplasty as a guide for assessment of the functional result. Am J Cardiol 1988; 61: 253–9.
19. Kern MJ, Deligonul U, Vandormael M *et al.* Impaired coronary vasodilator reserve in the immediate postcoronary angioplasty period: analysis of coronary artery flow velocity indexes and regional cardiac venous efflux. J Am Coll Cardiol 1989; 13: 860–72.
20. Segal J, Kern MJ, Scott NA *et al.* Alterations of phasic coronary artery flow velocity in humans during percutaneous coronary angioplasty. J Am Coll Cardiol 1992; 20: 276–86.
21. Ofili EO, Kern MJ, Labovitz AJ *et al.* Analysis of coronary blood flow velocity dynamics in angiographically normal and stenosed arteries before and after endolumen enlargement by angioplasty. J Am Coll Cardiol 1993; 21: 308–16.
22. Serruys PW, Di Mario C, Meneveau N *et al.* Intracoronary pressure and flow velocity from sensor tip guidewires: a new methodological approach for assessment of coronary hemodynamics before and after coronary interventions. Am J Cardiol 1993; 71: 41D–53D.
23. Uren NG, Crake T, Lefroy DC, de Silva R, Davies GJ, Maseri A. Delayed recovery of coronary resistive vessel function after coronary angioplasty. J Am Coll Cardiol 1993; 21: 612–21.
24. Mancini GBJ, McGillem MJ, DeBoe SF, Gallagher KP. The diastolic hyperemic flow versus pressure relation: a new index of coronary stenosis severity and flow reserve. Circulation 1989; 80: 941–50.
25. Mancini GBJ, Cleary RM, DeBoe SF, Moore NB, Gallagher KP. Instantaneous hyperemic

flow-versus-pressure slope index. Microsphere validation of an alternative to measures of coronary reserve. Circulation 1991; 84: 862–70.

26. Cleary RM, Aron D, Moore NB, DeBoe SF, Mancini GBJ. Tachycardia, contractility and volume loading alter conventional indexes of coronary flow reserve, but not the instantenous hyperemic flow versus pressure slope index. J Am Coll Cardiol 1992; 20: 1261–9.
27. Cleary RM, Moore NB, DeBoe SF, Mancini GBJ. Sensitivity and reproducibility of the instantaneous hyperemic flow versus pressure slope index compared to coronary flow reserve for the assessment of stenosis severity. Am Heart J 1993; 126: 57–65.
28. Doucette JW, Corl PD, Payne HM *et al.* Validation of a Doppler guide wire for intravascular measurement of coronary artery flow velocity. Circulation 1992; 85: 1899–911.
29. Serruys PW, Di Mario C, Kern MJ. Intracoronary Doppler. In Topol EJ (ed): Textbook of interventional cardiology, 2nd ed. Philadelphia: Saunders 1993: 1069–1121.
30. Zijlstra F, Serruys PW, Hugenholtz PG. Papaverine: the ideal coronary vasodilator for investigating coronary flow reserve? A study of timing, magnitude, reproducibility and safety of the coronary hyperemic response after intracoronary papaverine. Cathet Cardiovasc Diagn 1986; 12: 298–303.
31. Serruys PW, Wijns W, van den Brand M *et al.* Left ventricular performance, regional blood flow, wall motion, and lactate metabolism during transluminal angioplasty. Circulation 1984; 70: 25–36.
32. Haase J, Di Mario C, Slager CJ, van der Giessen WJ, den Boer A, de Feyter PJ *et al.* *In-vivo* validation of on-line and off-line geometric coronary measurements using insertion of stenosis phantoms in porcine coronary arteries. Cathet Cardiovasc Diagn 1992; 27: 16–27.
33. Di Mario C, Roelandt JRTC, de Jaegere P, Linker DT, Oomen J, Serruys PW. Limitations of the zero-crossing detector in the analysis of intracoronary Doppler: a comparison with fast Fourier transform analysis of basal, hyperemic and transstenotic blood flow velocity measurements in patients with coronary artery disease. Cathet Cardiovasc Diagn 1992; 28: 56–64.
34. Zar JH. Biostatistical Analysis, 2nd ed. Englewood Cliffs: Prentice Hall 1984.
35. Seiler C, Kirkeeide RL, Gould KL. Basic structure-function relations of the epicardial coronary vascular tree. Basis of quantitative coronary angiography for diffuse coronary artery disease. Circulation 1992; 85: 1987–2003.
36. Gould KL. Coronary Artery Stenosis. New York: Elsevier 1991: 41–52.
37. Di Mario C, de Feyter PJ, Slager CJ, de Jaegere P, Roelandt JRTC, Serruys PW. Intracoronary blood flow velocity and transstenotic pressure gradient using sensor-tip pressure and Doppler guidewires: a new technology for the assessment of stenosis severity in the catheterization laboratory. Cathet Cardiovasc Diagn 1993; 28: 311–9.
38. Bellamy RF. Diastolic coronary artery pressure-flow relation in the dog. Circ Res 1978; 43: 92–101.
39. Bellamy RF. Calculation of coronary vascular resistance. Cardiovasc Res 1980; 14: 261–9.
40. Chilian WM, Marcus ML. Coronary venous outflow persists after cessation of coronary arterial inflow. Am J Physiol 1984; 247: H984–90.
41. Eng C, Jentzer JH, Kirk ES. The effects of the coronary capacitance on the interpretation of diastolic pressure-flow relationships. Circ Res 1982; 50: 334–41.
42. Canty JM Jr, Klocke FJ, Mates RE. Characterization of capacitance-free pressure-flow relations during single diastoles in dogs using an RC model with pressure dependent parameters. Circ Res 1987; 60: 273–82.
43. Spaan JAE. Coronary diastolic pressure-flow relation and zero flow pressure explained on the basis of intramyocardial compliance. Circ Res 1985; 56: 293–309.
44. Hoffman JIE, Spaan JAE. Pressure-flow relations in coronary circulation. Physiol Rev 1990; 70: 331–90.
45. Klocke FJ, Weinstein IR, Klocke JF *et al.* Zero-flow pressures and pressure-flow relationships during single long diastoles in the canine coronary bed before and during maximum vasodilatation. Limited influence of capacitative effects. J Clin Invest 1981; 68: 970–80.

46. Nichols WW, O'Rourke MF. In McDonald's blood flow in arteries: theoretic, experimental and clinical principles, 3rd ed. London: Edward Arnold 1990: 77–124.
47. Sudhir K, MacGregor JS, Brzabant SD *et al.* Assessment of coronary conductance and resistance vessel reactivity in response to nitroglycerin, ergonovine and adenosine: *in vivo* studies with simultaneous intravascular two dimensional and Doppler ultrasound. J Am Coll Cardiol 1993; 21: 1261–8.

17. Progress towards improved measurements of coronary vascular dynamics in clinical practice: A comparative summary of new approaches based on measurements during maximal hyperemia

G.B. JOHN MANCINI

Summary

This chapter compares and contrasts three recently proposed methods for measuring coronary vascular reserve. They are all based on measurements obtained during maximal hyperemia. The three methods are instantaneous hyperemic flow versus pressure slope index (*i*-HFVP), the parametric imaging of maximal myocardial perfusion (PIMMP) and a new, pressure derived method (PDM). The advantages and limitations are discussed.

Introduction

Cardiologists have long been trained to make clinical decisions about atherosclerotic coronary disease by making inferences or predictions about the adequacy or inadequacy of coronary blood flow in any given patient. These inferences have been based largely on the patient's symptoms and morphological data, such as provided by the coronary arteriogram. Functional information is available to assist in this process, including the results of exercise or non-exercise (pharmacologic) stress testing. However, many of these methods provide only indirect evidence of the consequences of inadequate blood flow and myocardial perfusion. That is, inadequate perfusion is inferred by detecting new electrocardiographic abnormalities or new wall motion abnormalities. The tests based on radionuclide perfusion imaging, using numerous agents and techniques, come closest to providing a direct assessment of coronary perfusion, at least in a relative sense. Echocardiographic contrast studies, ultra-fast computed tomography and magnetic resonance imaging may also eventually demonstrate a useful role in this area. But clearly, the direct measurement of coronary blood flow and perfusion by practical means remains one of the biggest, unmet, challenges in routine cardiac diagnosis. This continues to spark the many studies designed to get a better and more direct handle on the measurement of coronary blood flow using clinically relevant methods. This is of particular need in the cardiac catheterization laboratory. Positron emission tomography provides both absolute and relative flow data but the technique is not generally available and is not suitable for the catheterization laboratory.

J.H.C. Reiber and P.W. Serruys (eds): Progress in quantitative coronary arteriography, 269–291.

Numerous methods have been proposed to measure various aspects of coronary flow dynamics in the cardiac catheterization laboratory. These include, coronary sinus thermodilution catheters, Doppler velocimeters, diffusible indicators and inert gas clearance techniques, thallium and other perfusion imaging agents, and quantitative digital angiography (predicted and/or measured flow reserves). These methods have been described and discussed in detail over the years and especially in many chapters of this particular series of symposia.

The purpose of this chapter is to summarize some of the most recent information in this field as it relates to the practice of interventional cardiology. The major new developments are related to new technology (the availability of guide-wire mounted pressure and Doppler velocity probes) and a better appreciation of the physiology underlying coronary blood flow and flow reserve.

Significance of maximal hyperemia

The direction of developments in this field can best be appreciated in the context of the physiological phenomena affecting coronary blood flow. The large, major coronary vessels act primarily as conductance vessels whereas the smaller coronary vessels, ranging in size from 10 to 140 microns in diameter, account for most of the resistance to coronary flow. Coronary blood flow is directly dependent on myocardial oxygen consumption and this, in turn, is determined by the heart rate, contractility and wall stress of the heart. The myocardium functions primarily by aerobic metabolism. In the face of an increased demand for work, there are few means available to accommodate an increase in oxygen demand. For example, the myocardium has a limited reserve of glycogen for anaerobic metabolism. And there is only a modest ability to increase oxygen extraction to achieve a venous oxygen saturation much less than the 30% that is already achieved in basal conditions. Accordingly, the major adaptive mechanism for meeting increased myocardial oxygen demand is coronary hyperemia, whereby dilatation of the coronary epicardial, collateral and, most importantly, the arteriolar bed allow for an increased delivery of blood flow and oxygen. Adenosine and other vasoactive substances are felt to be prime mediators of the hyperemic response at the cellular level.

It follows from this that the inadequacy of maximal coronary flow and inadequacy of total, maximal myocardial perfusion are the prime determinants of clinical manifestations of chronic, stable angina. It also follows that the measurement of these parameters would provide the most direct way of diagnosing this illness and the most direct means of determining whether any interventions are warranted. Finally, changes in these parameters would be the most direct indexes upon which to assess the efficacy of any intervention.

The tight coupling between coronary blood flow and myocardial oxygen demand is circumvented in experimental models designed to assess the effects of changes in hemodynamic parameters on coronary blood flow. Thus, in such a perfusion controlled preparation, the myocardial oxygen demand of the heart is not altered despite induction of changes in coronary perfusion pressure. In such experiments it has been well demonstrated that resting coronary blood flow is constant over a rather broad range of coronary perfusion pressures [1]. That is, resting coronary flow is autoregulated over this range of pressures. This autoregulation is achieved by modulations of arteriolar resistance that maintain the constant relation between coronary blood flow and oxygen demand. Resistance decreases when pressure falls and increases when pressure rises, thereby maintaining a constant level of coronary blood flow within a perfusion pressure range of approximately 80 to 140 mmHg. The key point here is that flow remains constant as long as myocardial oxygen demand remains constant. The *level* at which coronary blood flow is autoregulated is dictated by all ambient, prevailing factors affecting myocardial oxygen demand. For example, the level at which regulation occurs will be increased in hypertrophied ventricles, during fever or thyrotoxicosis, in the face of chronic hypertension and so on.

When arteriolar tone is abolished, however, autoregulation is also abolished and flow is no longer coupled to myocardial oxygen demand. In this circumstance, coronary blood flow becomes directly and linearly related to perfusion pressure. Arteriolar tone can be abolished by inducing perfusion pressures that are lower than the pressure range over which autoregulation is in effect or by drugs such as adenosine or papaverine. In the latter circumstance and within the perfusion-controlled experimental framework, the concept of coronary flow reserve, the ratio of maximal to basal hyperemic flow, is both easy to understand and to measure, provided that the coronary perfusion pressure is known and constant. But in the intact preparation, more akin to the situation faced when proposing measurements in patients, variation in the factors affecting coronary flow reserve measurements can lead to confusion if the changing factors are not taken into account (Figure 17.1).

The tight, metabolic autoregulation that occurs in the intact circulation in response to changes in myocardial oxygen demand causes major problems in determining whether any given measure of resting flow is truly 'basal' or not. Moreover, only crude methods are currently available to allow physicians to assess the overall or regional state of myocardial hypertrophy which may lead to high resting flows on a chronic basis even though all other conditions are 'basal'. Accordingly, it is not surprising that coronary reserve measurements, consisting of ratios of hyperemic to basal flows, are rendered quite imprecise and difficult to interpret if basal flow is not fiducial. In contrast, hyperemic flow per gram of myocardium, if truly maximal, is a less ambiguous, less variable parameter. Its prime determinants are perfusion pressure and overall resistance of the vascular bed. To a much lesser extent, heart rate (severe tachycardia) may also affect this measurement.

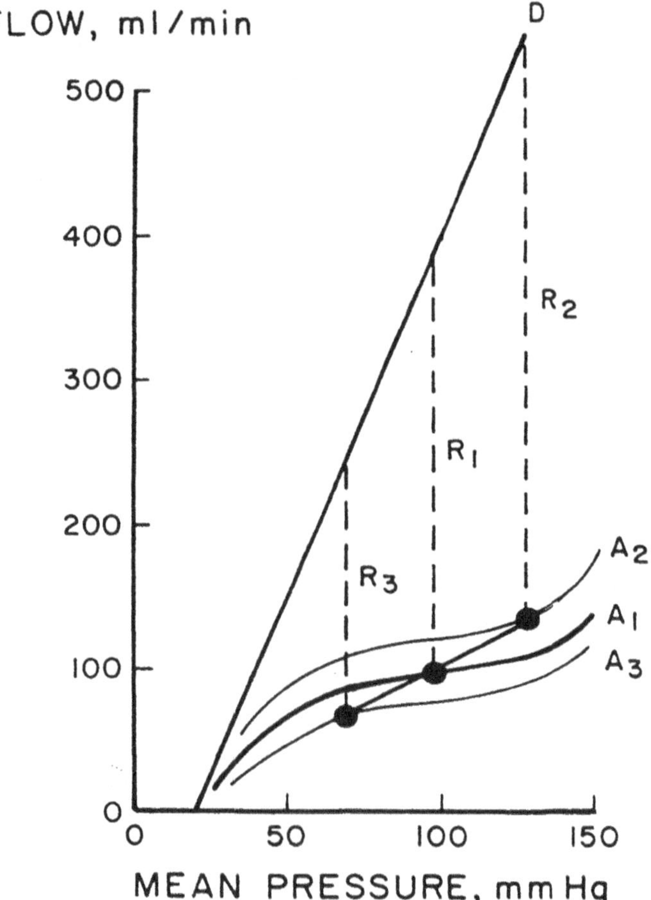

Figure 17.1. This diagram shows the relationship between resting and maximal hyperemic coronary blood flow in a perfusion-controlled animal model (solid line, A1) upon which is superimposed the observed changes in coronary blood flow in the intact preparation (straight line with large dots). The theoretically predicted, new levels of autoregulated, basal flow are shown (A2, A3). Flow reserve, determined by maximal flow divided by basal flow (R1, R2, R3) is clearly pressure dependent in both the perfusion-controlled and intact circumstances although in the latter situation, the increments in basal flow cause the flow reserve ratio to appear less pressure dependent than in the former model. (Reproduced with permission from Reference #1).

Greater cognizance of this simple concept has markedly influenced the direction of research in this field over the past several years. There is now more interest in developing methods of assessing coronary dynamics using indexes that are independent of hemodynamic parameters and, in particular, independent of 'basal' blood flow measurements.

There are three relatively new approaches to the assessment of coronary dynamics in the cardiac catheterization laboratory. All three are independent of basal flow. The first approach to abandon measures of basal flow was the *instantaneous hyperemic flow versus pressure slope index* (*iHFVP*) [2], a concept studied in animal models using traditional technologies. The concept is now being applied in man using angioplasty- and guide-wire mounted pressure and velocity flow probes [3, 4]. The second was *parametric imaging of maximal myocardial flow* (*PIMMP*) [5] based on digital, radiographic coronary imaging. This was also developed in animals and has been applied in several human studies [6, 7]. The third was the *pressure derived method* (*PDM*) [8] of assessing fractional (or relative) maximal coronary, myocardial and collateral blood flow which utilizes ultrathin pressure catheters and may also be measured, perhaps more accurately, with high fidelity micromanometers. There is little published clinical experience with this approach although initial animal validation studies are impressive.

This group of methods is distinct from other methods by virtue of being solely dependent on measurements made during maximal hyperemia, thereby avoiding many of the vagaries induced by variability of basal coronary flow. This chapter will compare and contrast these methods. Other chapters in this book outline the developmental concepts underlying the PIMMP and PDM approaches and will not be repeated extensively here. The background work on the i-HFVP, however, will be reviewed more comprehensively.

The instantaneous hyperemic flow versus pressure slope index

This concept evolved from the above considerations and is based on earlier work performed by Dole and coworkers [9]. In essence, the goal of this approach is to directly measure maximal coronary conductance proximal to a coronary obstruction. This measurement, in its full sense, gives a measure of absolute coronary blood flow (cc per min) per millimeter of mercury, per 100 grams of tissue. This index, therefore, is a measure of maximal coronary conductance, the inverse of minimal coronary resistance.

The concept was developed in four distinct stages. First, studies were undertaken to determine how to best measure maximal coronary conductance in the epicardial arteries of the intact, coronary circulation of animals and to determine whether this approach was truly hemodynamically independent of, or less dependent on, changes in aortic pressure than other available measurements [2]. From these observations, it was determined that the instantaneous hyperemic flow versus pressure slope index (i-HFVP slope index) was the optimal approach to pursue (see below). Secondly, the i-HFVP slope index was validated against microsphere determination of true, maximal conductance in the myocardial perfusion bed [10]. Thirdly, a more detailed investigation of the effects of tachycardia, contractility and volume loading was undertaken [11]. Finally, the relative sensitivity and reprodu-

Table 17.1. Results of stepwise linear regression analysis to determine load dependency of measures of vascular reserve.

	hCBF/AoP	CFR	i-HFVP
Mean hyperemic AoP	0.347	0.465	–
Mean basal AoP	–	−0.288	–
Hyperemic HR	−0.360	−0.162	–
Hyperemic LVEDP	–	–	–
Overall r value	0.486	0.520	–
Results using standardized data			
Mean hyperemic AoP	0.375	0.476	–
Hyperemic HR	−0.353	−0.210	−0.166
Basal LVEDP	–	−0.185	–
Overall r value	0.512	0.540	−0.166

Partial r values are shown. AoP = mean aortic pressure during hyperemia; hCBF = hyperemic coronary blood flow; CFR = coronary flow reserve; LVEDP = left ventricular end – diastolic pressure; HFVP = hyperemic flow versus pressure slope index; HR = heart rate. (Adapted with permission from Reference 2.)

cibility of the i-HFVP slope index was compared to other measures of flow reserve [12].

The initial study looked at several parameters of vascular reserve including: traditional coronary flow reserve. All of the traditional parameters exhibited hemodynamic dependency, especially the coronary flow reserve parameter (see Table 17.1). In contrast, the i-HFVP exhibited only minimal heart rate dependency (a lowered value with severe tachycardia) and appeared to be a more sensitive index of stenosis severity than the traditional coronary flow reserve index.

Figure 17.2 shows the derivation of the i-HFVP slope index (see legend). Figure 17.3 shows the effects of increasing mean aortic pressure on the measurement of CFR. The curves representing control levels, mild stenosis and severe stenosis all increase as pressure increases. Figure 17.4 shows the actual hyperemic and basal coronary blood flow values from which the traditional CFR is derived. One can see that *both* basal and hyperemic flow increase with increasing pressures. This relatively parallel change in the intact coronary circulation tends to minimize the pressure dependency of CFR that is predicted from the perfusion controlled model wherein perfusion pressure and myocardial oxygen demand are divorced from one another and resting flow remains constant. The changes in basal and hyperemic flow that were noted in the intact animal model, however, were not perfectly proportional and, therefore, CFR still demonstrated dependency on ambient aortic perfusion pressure. In contrast, Figure 17.5 shows that the i-HFVP was stable and independent of increasing pressure levels.

The next phase of development was to determine whether the i-HFVP actually bore some relation to maximal *myocardial* conductance [10]. This

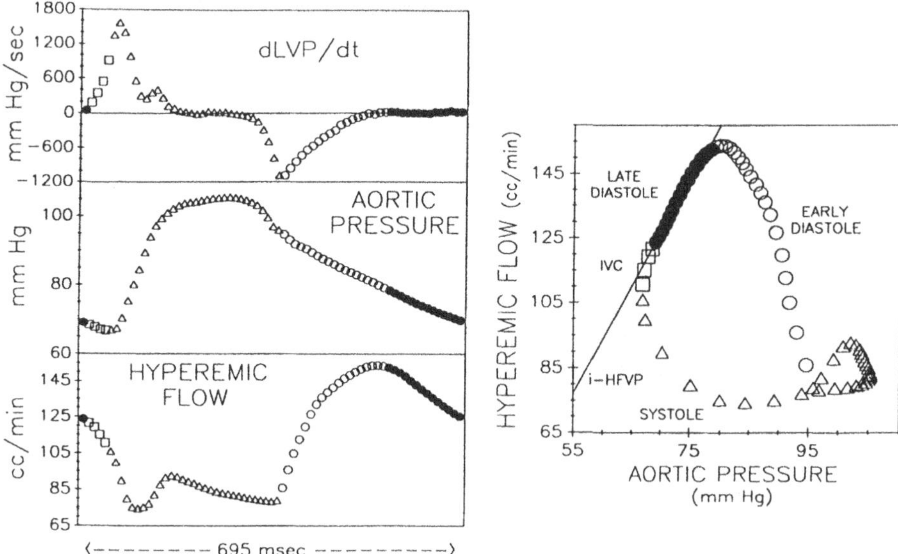

Figure 17.2. Left panel: plots of computer outputs of an average of eight heart cycles acquired during maximal hyperemia in a dog. Shown is differentiated left ventricular pressure (dP/dt); this is provided to help clarify phases of the cardiac cycle. Also shown are average aortic pressure and hyperemic flow tracings. Note that maximal coronary flow occurs preferentially in diastole. These two tracings were combined to form the flow-pressure loop in the right panel. Phases of the cardiac cycle are shown by different symbols: squares = isovolumic contraction (IVC); triangles = systole; open circles = early diastole (including isovolumic relaxation); solid circles = late diastole. The i-HFVP slope index is measured during late diastole. Each symbol represents the average data originally acquired at 200 Hz but displayed at 100 Hz. Right panel: graphic representation of hyperemic coronary flow vs. aortic pressure data from the left panel is shown. The data inscribe a flow-pressure loop that proceeds in a counterclockwise direction through phases of the cardiac cycle. The portion of the curve during late diastole (solid circles) is relatively linear. i-HFVP slope index is calculated by performing least-squares linear regression on these points. The slope of this regression divided by perfusion bed weight equals the i-HFVP slope index (ml/min/mmHg/100g), which is a measure of maximal coronary conductance. (Reproduced from Reference 10, with permission.)

study showed that the i-HFVP slope index measurement in normal and stenotic arteries was not significantly different from the transmural and subendocardial maximal myocardial conductances measured by microsphere methods. The best correlations were obtained between the i-HFVP and these subendocardial maximal conductances.

The relation between the i-HFVP slope index and radiolabelled microsphere measurements was strongest with the subendocardial and weakest with the subepicardial coronary perfusion data. This is probably because subendocardial blood flow is largely dependent on diastolic coronary perfusion and this is the time period during which the i-HFVP slope index is

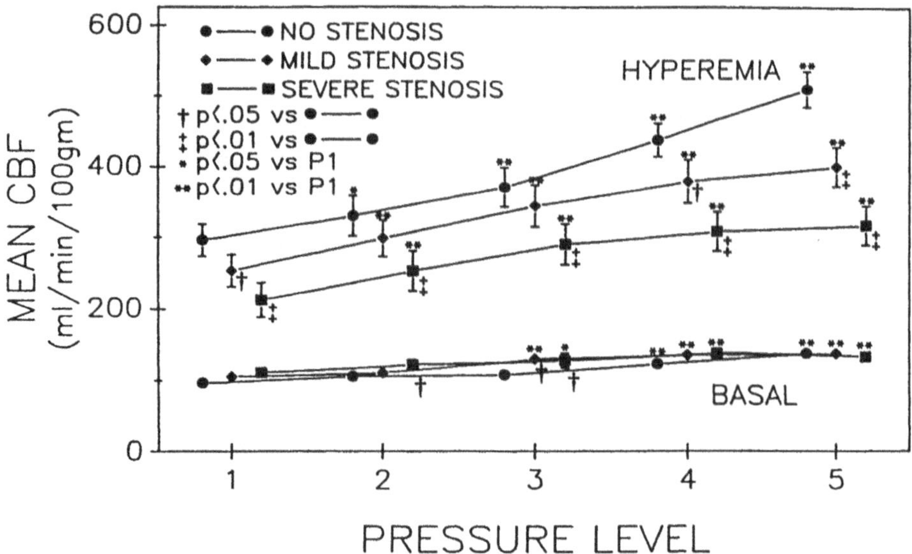

Figure 17.3. CFR is plotted vs. incremental levels of aortic pressure (1 to 5) for the conditions of no stenosis, mild stenosis and severe stenosis. (Reproduced with permission from Reference 2.)

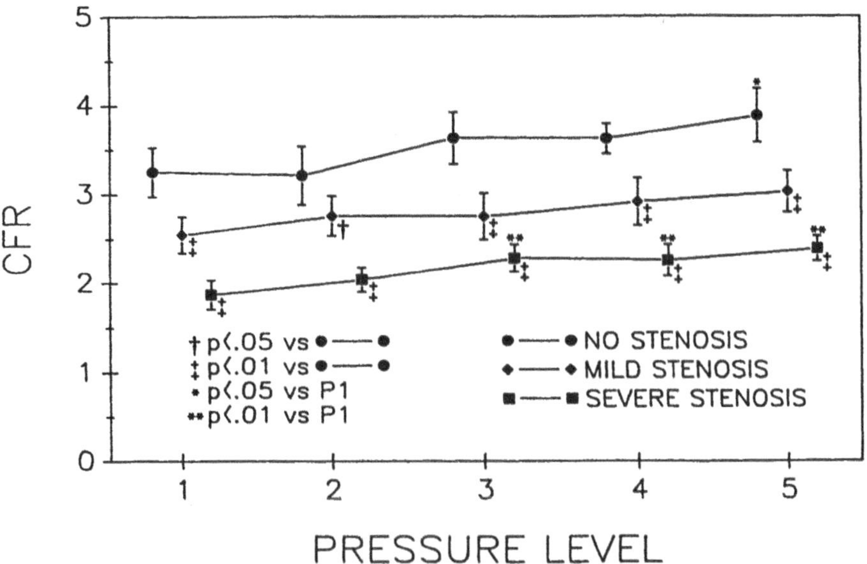

Figure 17.4. Mean coronary blood flow (CBF) is plotted in the same format as Figure 17.3. Note that both hyperemic and basal flow increase with increasing pressure. (Reproduced with permission from Reference 2.)

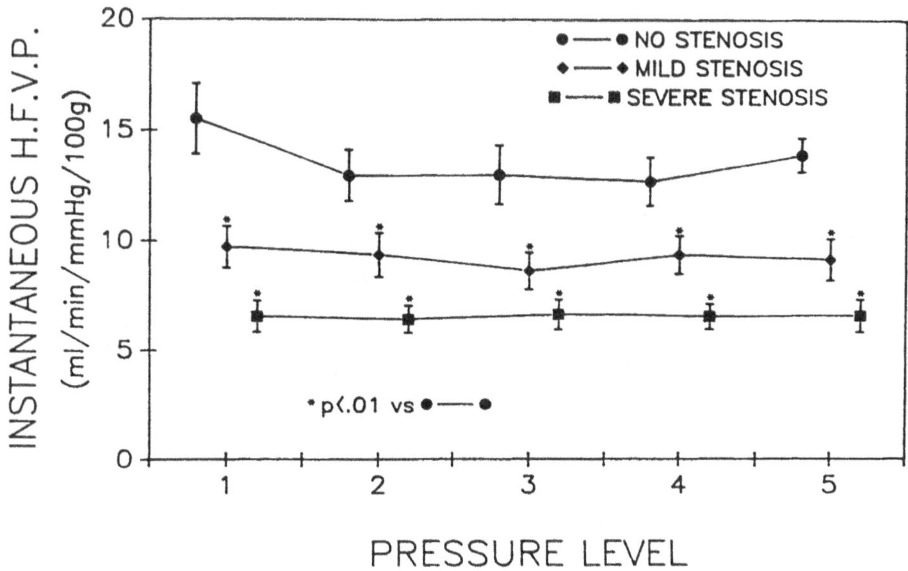

Figure 17.5. The i-HFVP slope index is shown in the same format as Figures 17.3 and 17.4. No pressure dependency is evident. (Reproduced with permission from Reference 2.)

derived. Subepicardial and midmyocardial blood flows are not as restricted to the diastolic interval as is subendocardial flow. Consequently, they would not be as likely to parallel changes in the i-HFVP slope index.

A systematic difference was noted in the frequency with which the individual i-HFVP slope index determinations actually fell within the 95% confidence intervals for maximal coronary conductance derived from the microsphere data (Figure 17.6). We proposed two major factors to account for these findings. The first is the fact that microsphere measures of flow represent a mean flow over a rather prolonged period of time (minutes), whereas the i-HFVP slope index is derived from instantaneous diastolic hyperemic flow data. Accordingly, we expected that the absolute coronary conductance value, derived from the microsphere perfusion measurements, would be less than that derived from the flowmeter values. We also predicted that this disparity would be minimized in the presence of a coronary stenosis.

Indeed, Figure 17.7 shows a superimposition of the diastolic relation between hyperemic coronary flow and aortic pressure used to determine the i-HFVP slope index and the microsphere-derived flow versus pressure data with the associated 95% confidence intervals (C.I.). In the nonstenotic state (upper panel), the data used to derive the i-HFP slope index inscribe a slope that is steeper than the slope of the m-HFVP slope index and, as well, is steeper than the slope of the uppermost C.I. In contrast, in the presence of a stenosis (lower panel), the data used to derive the i-HFVP slope index

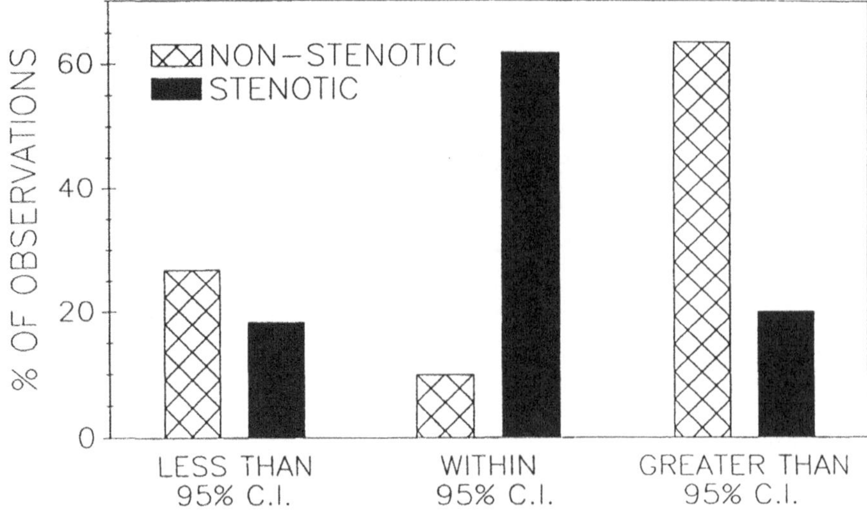

Figure 17.6. Bar graph showing frequency with which individual i-HFVP slope index values fell within the 95% confidence intervals (C.I.) derived from the subendocardial microsphere data of individual dogs. Although the strongest relations were between the i-HFVP slope index and either transmural or subendocardial microsphere-derived hyperemic flow versus pressure (m-HFVP) slope index, this illustration points out systematic differences in the relation depending on the presence or absence of a stenosis. Subendocardial m-HFVP slope index was overestimated by the i-HFVP slope index in normal beds, whereas subendocardial m-HFVP slope index values in stenotic beds were more accurately reflected. (Reproduced with permission from Reference 10.)

inscribe a slope that is nearly identical to the m-HFVP slope index and falls well within the slope range inscribed by the C.I.

A second important factor is the distinct difference in flows measured by the epicardial coronary flow probes and by the radiolabeled microspheres. The latter measures flow from all sources including collateral flow, whereas the former measures only flow through the epicardial coronary artery. Disparities between such measurements would be exaggerated in the presence of a stenosis if collateral flow during hyperemia to the compromised bed is substantial. Accordingly, one would expect relative preservation of myocardial perfusion even in the face of impaired epicardial coronary blood flow if collateral flow is recruited from other sources not measured with the flow probe. This could account for the proportion of i-HFVP slope index values in stenotic beds that were below the 95% confidence intervals established from the perfusion data (i.e., the epicardial measurements tended to overestimate the actual severity of the subendocardial perfusion deficit). Indeed, there was one study, which was excluded from analysis, in which collateral flow was extensive enough to maintain totally normal transmural myocardial perfusion in the presence of a stenosis that induced frank impairment of

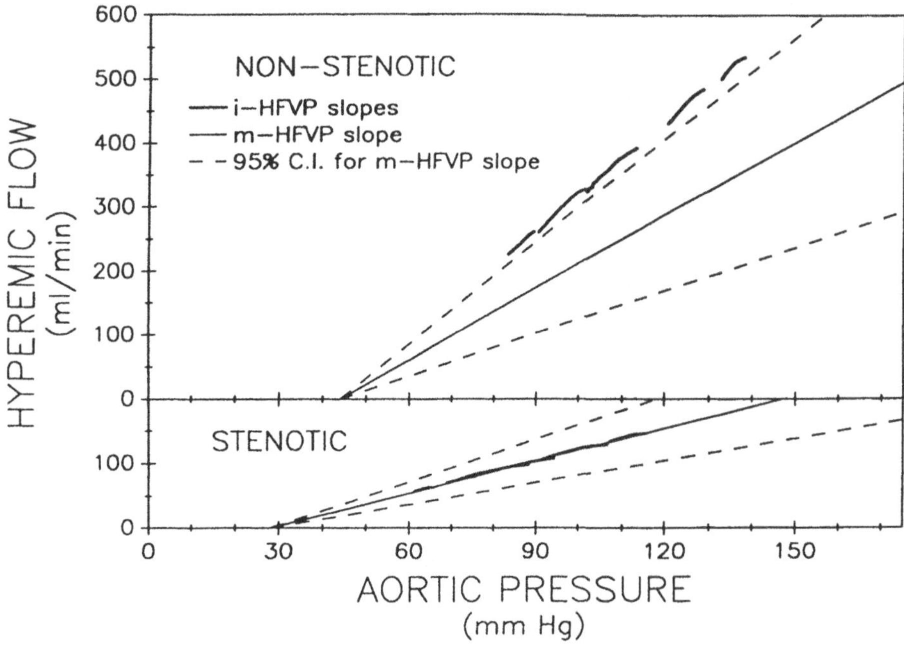

Figure 17.7. See text for details. (Reproduced with permission from Reference 10.)

epicardial flow. In the remaining studies, it is impossible to know whether collateral flow was recruited or, if it was, to what degree.

A subsequent study showed that the i-HFVP slope index was unaltered by changes in heart rate, saline volume loading and dobutamine induced changes in contractility. In contrast, traditional coronary flow reserve measurements showed the expected changes of a decrease with increasing heart rate and acute, volume loading (Figures 17.8 and 17.9). In addition, with altered contractile state, traditional coronary flow reserve changed but the i-HFVP did not (Figure 17.10).

Finally, a direct comparison between the relative sensitivity of the i-HFVP and CFR was undertaken in an animal model. Figure 17.11 shows that the i-HFVP showed a proportionately greater fall with increasing degrees of stenosis than did the CFR. This is especially evident in those settings where CFR might be falsely elevated due to an increase in perfusion pressure during the observation period. Subanalysis of this circumstance demonstrates a markedly increased sensitivity of the i-HFVP compared to CFR (Figure 17.12). Moreover, this study also demonstated that the i-HFVP was far more reproducible than the CFR and this was largely due to alterations in basal flow throughout the observation period that affected the CFR dramatically but were irrelevant to the measurement of i-HFVP.

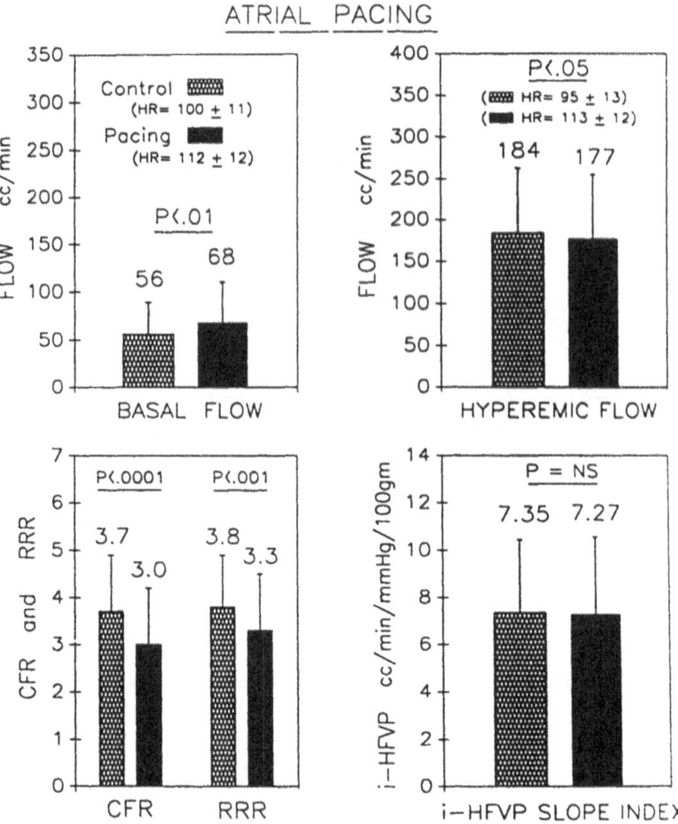

Figure 17.8. Effects of atrial pacing. The bars and numbers above each column represent, respectively, 1 SD and the mean values for each variable. p values compare control values and values during pacing. RRR = resistance reserve ratio defined as basal coronary resistance divided by hyperemic coronary resistance. Resistance is defined as the mean aortic perfusion pressure divided by mean coronary blood flow. (Reproduced with permission from Reference 11.)

Parametric imaging of maximal myocardial perfusion

This method, proposed by Pijls *et al.* [5], is based on the theory that at maximal vasodilation of the myocardial vascular bed, the maximally achievable blood flow through the myocardium is inversely proportional to mean transit time (T_{mn}) of contrast material. The T_{mn} is determined from ECG-triggered, digital coronary angiograms obtained during papaverine-induced, maximal coronary vasodilation. Contrast material is used as a perfusion agent and videodensitometry is used to construct time-density curves that resemble dye-dilution curves. Pijls *et al.* argued that prior attempts to use this concept were limited by lack of a specific focus on T_{mn}, the only reliable and physio-

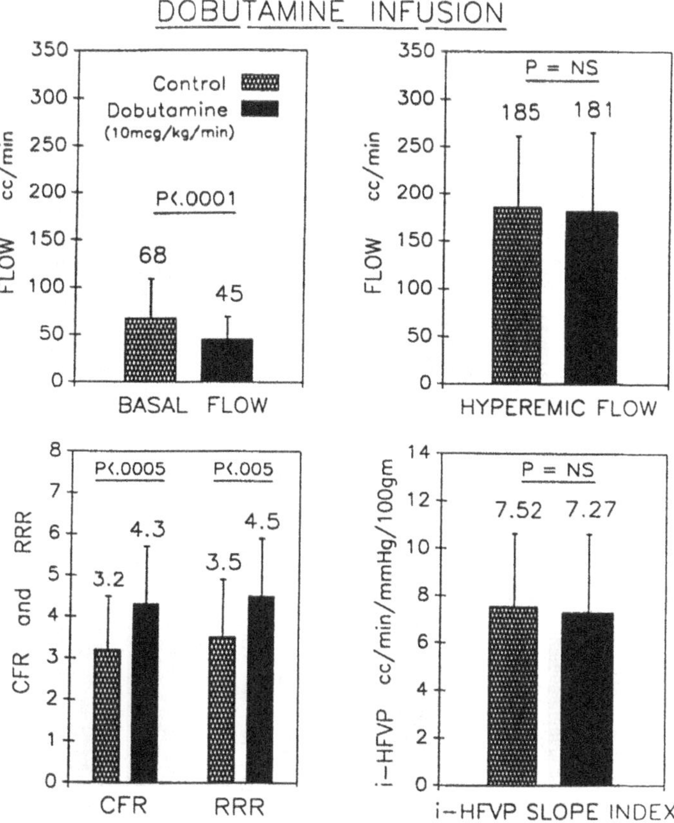

Figure 17.9. Effects of dobutamine infusion. Format is the same as in Figure 17.8. (Reproduced with permission from Reference 11.)

logically sound timing parameter. Moreover, because of the desire to make measurements analogous to coronary flow reserve, that is, the desire to compare hyperemic conditions to basal conditions, prior attempts were confounded by changes in vascular volume that occurred between basal and hyperemic states. Another problem to be dealt with was the change in flow and volume induced by contrast medium itself. Finally, the problem of videodensitometric calculations of contrast density, instead of contrast concentration, had to be overcome.

The conceptual leap taken by Pijls *et al.* was to recognize that these problems could be circumvented by performing all studies during maximal coronary hyperemia. This restriction provided assurance that the myocardial vascular bed attained its maximal volume and that this volume remained constant throughout the measurement period. Contrast material no longer was a factor in altering myocardial bed volume because the material could

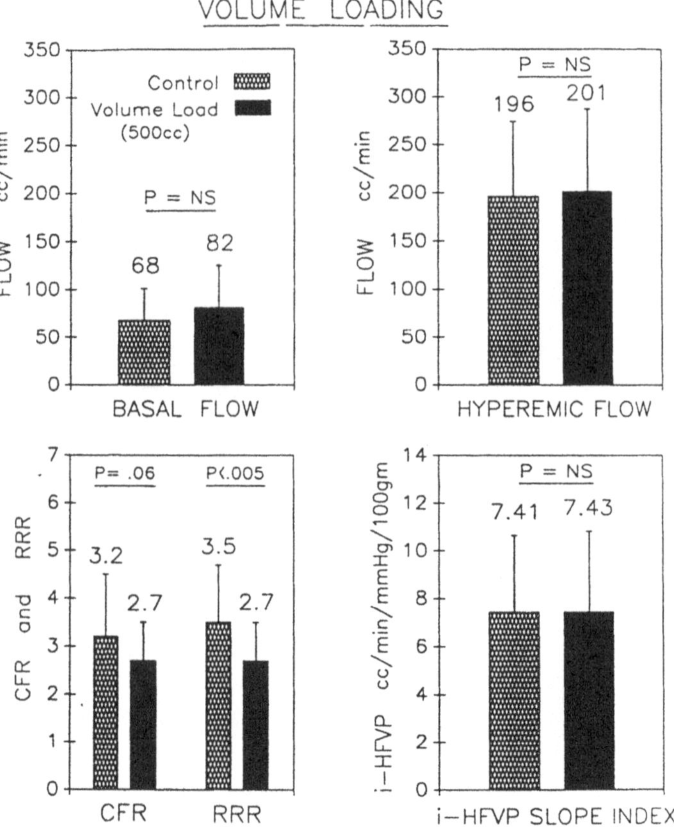

Figure 17.10. Effects of volume loading. Format is the same as in Figures 17.8 and 17.9. (Reproduced with permission from Reference 11.)

not induce any further increases once papaverine-induced maximal hyperemia had been achieved. Moreover, the videodensitometric problem was circumvented because contrast concentration and contrast density are linearly proportional when vascular volume is constant and maximal.

The exercise then boiled down to one of paying meticulous attention to generating and measuring time-density curves so that T_{mn} could be measured accurately and reliably. T_{mn} measurements were based on assuming a square-wave pulse injection of contrast material at the ostium of the coronary artery (time = 0 seconds) and then calculating the mean time of onset of a time-density curve (after determining the best gamma curve fit) detected in myocardial regions of interest.

The T_{mn} measurement, however, is of limited utility by itself. Its major value is as a means of assessing an intervention, such as angioplasty, within

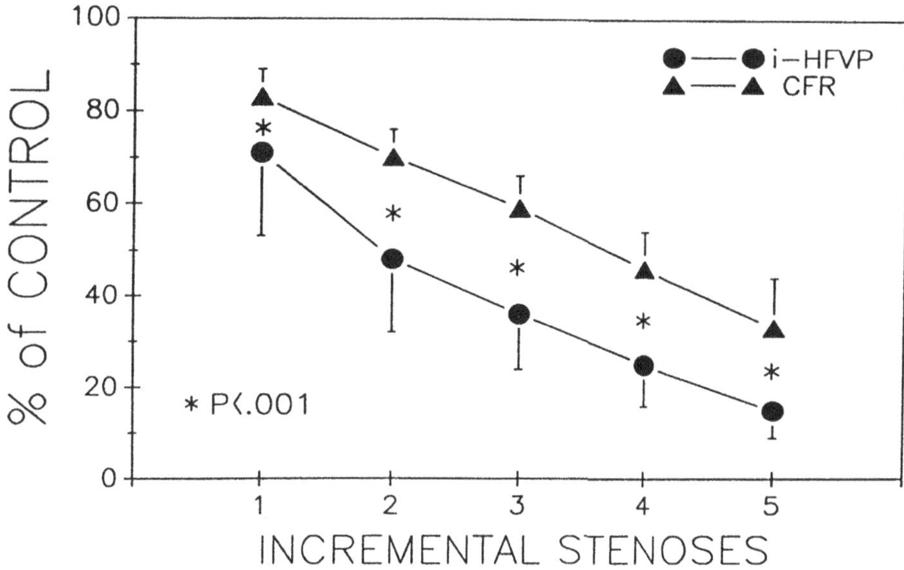

Figure 17.11. The percentage reductions in the i-HFVP and CFR indexes in the presence of incremental stenoses are shown for the entire data set. The i-HFVP is significantly more depressed for each stenosis than is the CFR. (Reproduced with permission from Reference 12.)

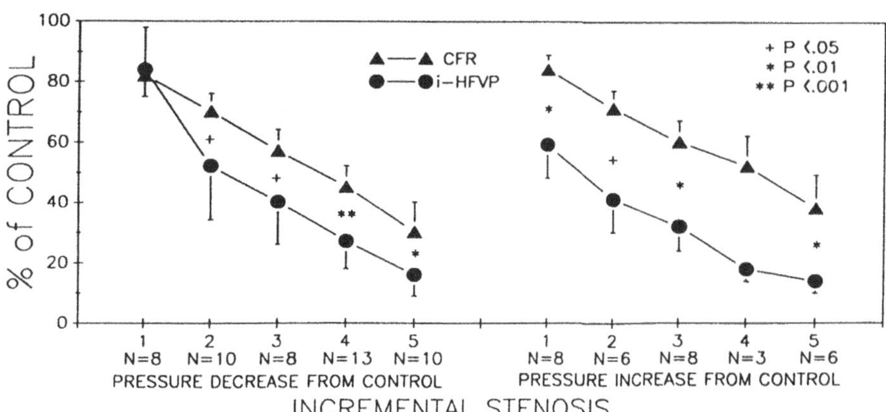

Figure 17.12. The percentage reductions in the i-HFVP and CFR are shown when mean aortic pressure during hyperemia was lower (left panel) or higher (right panel) than in the absence of a stenosis. These analyses demonstrate that part of the apparent 'sensitivity' of CFR for stenosis #1 can be ascribed to a lowered mean aortic pressure. In all other instances, the i-HFVP demonstrated greater percentage decreases in value. In the right hand panel, the inferiority of the CFR may be partially due to increased pressures which maintained the CFR values inappropriately high. (Reproduced with permission from Reference 12.)

a given patient. Accordingly, these investigators developed the concept of the Maximal Flow Ratio (MFR) defined as follows:

$$\text{MFR} = \frac{\text{T}_{\text{mn}} \text{ at condition 'a'}}{\text{T}_{\text{mn}} \text{ at condition 'b'}}$$

Conditions 'a' and 'b' could be, for example, before angioplasty and after angioplasty, respectively. Alternatively, 'a' and 'b' could be, diseased vessel and totally normal vessel, respectively. Other chapters in this book develop the theory and resulting applications of MFR more fully.

Pressure derived measurement

This method takes advantage of the fact that there is a direct relation between coronary pressure and flow if the resistances in the coronary circulation are constant (and minimal) as is the case during maximal arteriolar vasodilation. A theoretical model was developed for the different components of the coronary circulation and a set of equations was derived by which the relative maximum flow or fractional flow reserve in both the stenotic epicardial artery and the myocardial vascular bed, and the proportional contribution of coronary arterial and collateral flow to myocardial blood flow, are calculated from measurements of arterial, distal coronary, coronary wedge (during balloon occlusion) and central venous pressure during maximum arteriolar vasodilation [8]. This is an extension of the original component analysis model proposed by Gould *et al.* but which provided an incomplete characterization due to neglect of the collateral flow component [13].

This more comprehensive approach also encompasses the simple, and time honoured method of measuring translesional gradients. The authors discount the translesional gradient approach, however, by pointing out that prior attempts to relate transstenotic pressure gradients to the functional significance of a stenosis have been disappointing and the change in gradient after angioplasty is poorly correlated with success and adds little to the obvious, morphologic changes that can be detected easily after the procedure. The criticisms are based on the fact that prior gradients have been measured with bulky, angioplasty hardware that creates artifactual gradients. In addition, gradient measurements have generally been made in the basal state in which the gradient itself is determined primarily by the ambient flow. This ambient flow is in turn predominantly affected by distal coronary autoregulation. Since flow and pressure are related to each other by epicardial and myocardial vascular resistance, if the resistances are changing in response to myocardial oxygen demand, arterial pressure, contrast injections, and coronary vasomotion, then the pressure and flow parameters cannot be related to stenosis severity. However, if the resistances are known or at least remain constant, as is the case during maximal hyperemia, then there is a direct relation between the pressure gradients and the stenosis severity. Finally, even studies that related transstenotic pressure gradients, before and after an intervention, to the aortic pressure were limited because this approach fails to recognize that the stenosis is only one part of a complex, hydrodynamic system, other parts of which, especially collaterals, may also affect the influence of the stenosis on myocardial blood flow. Accordingly, the reduction of a stenotic gradient from one level to another may have entirely different significance in different patients even if the level of the gradient and the degree of fall in the gradient are identical.

Accordingly, this group developed a model to derive equations relating pressures to the regional distribution of maximum perfusion. Maximum flow through a stenotic artery is compared to what maximum flow would be in that same artery in the absence of that stenosis (i.e. if the pressure gradient across a stenosis were eliminated and equal to zero). Consequently, coronary flow reserve is expressed as a fraction of its normal, expected value in the same artery in the absence of a stenosis.

Other chapters demonstrate both the model and the equations.

Comparative advantages and limitations of new approaches to measuring coronary flow dynamics

Table 17.2 summarizes the differences among these three, new approaches. The PDM requires the most simple acquisition of data in the setting of angioplasty. Only mean pressure measurements are required. The need to measure venous (right atrial pressure) requires the minor, additional procedure of right heart catheterization. The calculations, however, are extensive and must be done either after the procedure or by personnel dedicated to the task during the procedure. This aspect could be automated fairly easily. The PIMMP technique, as originally described, requires meticulous attention to breath holding to avoid subtraction artifacts that will degrade the image and the parametric data it contains. The time period of acquisition must be relatively long to ensure recording of an adequate myocardial blush phase from which a time-density curve is derived and subjected to gamma curve fitting. However, the concept underlying PIMMP could be used with the Doppler velocimeter, thereby making this approach relatively simple in the catheterization laboratory. The i-HFVP may eventually be even simpler than the PDM approach if technological advances proceed as predicted. Software has already been developed that allows the pressure volume loops to be displayed on-line. The calculations are all automated. Currently, however, 'in-house' bioengineering is required to begin to measure this parameter by bringing digitized Doppler and pressure signals together. Even this accomplishes only an initial approximation of what was intended by the original index. That is, until ways of measuring or accounting for myocardial mass are available, the Doppler/pressure approach can be used only as a relative index within patients. Moreover, quantitative coronary angiography or endovascular echocardiography, to measure cross sectional area at the site of

Table 17.2. Comparative summary of three new approaches to measuring coronary dynamics.

Features	i-HFVP[a]	PIMMP[b]	PDM[c]
Simplicity	no	moderately	very
Quickness	potentially	no	moderately
Expense	? (recurring)	high (capital)	? (recurring)
Hemodynamic or load dependency	no	yes	somewhat
Reproducibility	good	good	pending
Sensitivity	good	pending	pending
Validated	yes	yes	partially
Characterization of stenoses	yes	yes	yes
Characterization of myocardial bed	'yes'	'yes'	yes
Characterization of collaterals	no	no	yes
Affected by collaterals	yes (overestimates)	yes (overestimates)	yes (underestimates)
Applicable to interventions within patients	yes	yes	yes
Applicable to routine cases	yes	yes	no
Index can be used to compare patients or beds	possible	possible	possible
Can help make a clinical decision before an intervention	possible	possible	no
Can help make a clinical decision after an intervention	yes	yes	yes

Notes
[a] Instantaneous hyperemic flow versus pressure slope index.
[b] Parametric imaging of maximal myocardial perfusion.
[c] Pressure derived measurements of fraction of maximal coronary flow or perfusion.

velocity measurements, are still required to convert the velocity signals to flow measurements.

There are very few catheterization laboratories that function at much less than a frenetic pace. At least a part of this pace is out of deference to patient comfort and safety. Accordingly, if any of these physiologically based methods are to become increasingly common in catheterization practices, they must be quick. In this regard, the i-HFVP and the PDM approaches are probably the best candidates since both require only brief data acquisitions and both can conceivably yield indexes that can be calculated on-line, during the procedure, by computer. The PIMMP can also yield results during the procedure but an operator must be dedicated to this task. The time required to train patients to hold their breath for prolonged periods is significant. Moreover, should movement artifacts occur, tedious repetitions of image runs will add substantially to the length of the procedure, the use of contrast material and the use of vasodilating agents.

Expense is of obvious importance and is becoming an increasingly important, limiting factor in cardiac practice. The PIMMP requires the expensive, initial capital expenditure for a digital cardiac imaging laboratory. Most laboratories now have this capability and, therefore, the ability to perform PIMMP may be considered a bonus since it is a capability of the system that would have been purchased for routine imaging anyway. The other methods will have lower initial capital expenses. Unlike the digital catheterization labaoratory, however, this capital expense has no justification or purpose other than to undertake the specific measurements that have been described. Moreover, recurring costs for the devices cannot be predicted at this time and may be out of keeping with routine clinical use. If the new technology is combined with clinically indicated devices (ie angioplasty devices and guiding catheters) then costs could conceivably be kept down and defrayed to a certain extent.

The i-HFVP slope index has been extensively studied in animals and appears to have virtually no significant hemodynamic or heart rate dependency. The PDM has not been extensively studied but, in theory, it should be relatively independent of hemodynamic and load changes because the method monitors these parameters to calculate the ratios. One of the major drawbacks of this procedure, however, is the need to measure coronary wedge pressure, ie distal coronary pressure during balloon occlusion. The real limitation here is not so much in obtaining this pressure but more so in ensuring that it is obtained during stable hemodynamic conditions. Since this pressure is typically measured only during the clinically indicated dilatation procedure, this single value is only valid for insertion into the theoretical equations if all other hemodynamic parameters remained constant. If hemodynamic changes have occurred between the time of initial coronary wedge measurements and follow-up gradient measurements or venous pressure measurements then the authors specify that coronary wedge pressures must be recalculated to conform to the mathematical theory upon which the original equations are based. On-going studies suggest that such recalculations yield new wedge pressures that correlate very well with wedge pressures that are actually measured (N. Pijls, pers. comm.). The PIMMP is dependent on perfusion pressure. This can be taken into account, in a fashion analogous to dividing maximal coronary flow by the ambient mean pressure to derive a maximal conductance value. This approach, however, has been shown to still be subject to hemodynamic dependency [2].

Based on available data, all the methods appear to be suitably sensitive to the presence of coronary stenoses but only the i-HFVP has been compared to other measures of coronary flow reserve. PIMMP has been compared to results of stress testing and quantitative angiography but neither of these comparisons directly substantiate a practical superiority of this flow index over other flow indexes. The PDM has not been compared yet to other directly measured indexes of flow reserve or other direct methods of assessing functional severity of a stenosis.

All of the methods have undergone animal validation studies. The concept of measuring coronary collateral flow by the PDM approach, however, has not yet been directly validated using standardized microsphere measurements. Moreover, it is not currently clear how well the theoretical equations would actually fair in measuring true blood flows in humans. Such a study could be done now that velocity (and flow) and pressure measurements can both be made in man. Reproducibility in man is good for the i-HFVP and the PIMMP but is unknown for the PDM.

The i-HFVP and the PIMMP both give information about the relative severity of a given stenosis in the context of the status of its subtended perfusion bed. That is, these approaches do not give information solely about the severity of the stenosis itself, results are affected by the status of the myocardial bed. The PDM approach can 'compartmentalize' or separate the contributions of the stenosis from that of the myocardial bed. Moreover, the latter approach can give an estimate of collateral flow. This estimate, however, reflects only the collateral flow that may occur during total occlusion of the vessel or stenosis being investigated. In other words, it gives an indication of the upper limit of collateral flow that may affect perfusion of a given arterial distribution but it does not allow one to measure the amount of collateral flow occurring in the natural setting. It should be noted that the assessment of myocardial reserve is also only valid as a ratio measurement. If, for example, the bed were diseased by diabetic arteriopathy, for example, the ratios before and after an intervention would be valid but these ratios would be based on subnormal reference flows. This is due to the fact that the pressure distal to stenoses and coronary wedge pressures are measured proximal to the myocardial bed which may have small vessel disease.

As specific measures of stenosis severity, the three approaches are also affected differently by the presence of collateral flow. The i-HFVP and the PIMMP will tend to give an overestimate of the deleterious effect of any given stenosis on actual myocardial perfusion if there is substantial collateral flow at the time of measurement. That is, these indexes, by virtue of reflecting coronary dynamics proximal to a stenosis, may suggest severe stenoses which, however, might not be appreciated by microsphere measures of coronary perfusion or clinical stress test results. Whether this is viewed as an advantage or disadvantage may be argued since one may not want to be prevented from dilating a lesion only because collateral flow appeared to be adequate. In contrast, the PDM approach may lead to an underestimation of the intrinsic severity of a given stenosis if the coronary wedge pressure and distal coronary pressure are sufficiently elevated by profuse collateral flow. In these circumstances, the translesional gradient would be falsely low because of a distal pressure that is maintained at a 'falsely' increased level due to profuse collateral flow. Finally, the PDM approach is valid only if maximal recruitable collateral flow remains constant during the procedure.

Because the PDM method requires total occlusion of the stenosis, it is applicable only to the angioplasty setting whereas the others can conceivably be applied in routine, diagnostic settings. As mentioned above, the wedge pressure measured at that specific point in time is only valid for insertion into the equations if it was measured during conditions that are constant both before and after the procedure. Otherwise, theoretical wedge pressures must be calculated for insertion into the PDM equations. All of these methods are applicable to interventions such as angioplasty or any other comparisons that one might want to undertake *within* patients. Comparisons from patient to patient, are also possible as long as the indexes are expressed as ratios. The same is true of the PIMMP but some data exists suggesting that the absolute value of T_{mn} can help differentiate the adequacy of blood flow in different beds and in different patients.

Although all of these methods can be used to gauge the efficacy of a given intervention, it is not clear whether these methods can be used to make a decision to proceed to angioplasty or any other intervention. However, the PDM concept requires coronary occlusion (ie balloon inflation) even for initial measurements. Therefore, the PDM concept cannot be used to make initial decisions as to whether to proceed or not. The translesional pressure gradient data may, within limits, be helpful in this process. There is some limited information suggesting that the initial T_{mn} obtained by PIMMP can distinguish between normal and abnormal flow states and hence this index may be somewhat useful in deciding whether to proceed. The i-HFVP normalized by bed weight is theoretically capable of identifying abnormal flow prior to a procedure and may therefore play a role in deciding on the advisability of an intervention provided that the impairement is due solely to the stenosis and not also due to problems in the small vessels of the myocardium (eg. diabetes, hypertrophy etc). In the absence of normalization by bed weight, its major role will be to assess interventions within patients.

Conclusion

As is evident from the introduction, the ability to measure absolute coronary blood flow and absolute myocardial perfusion, particularly during maximal hyperemia, would allow us to more directly gauge coronary disease, make therapeutic decisions and monitor the resultant effects. Imagination and ingenuity have provided us with numerous, simpler surrogates against which any new technology, such as the ones described herein, will have to be proven to be more valuable either overall or, at a minimum, in very well defined circumstances. The cardiac catheterization laboratory is a fairly well defined circumstance that, despite non-invasive pre-testing, continues to present us with patients with numerous confounding constellations of disease. Even after dilating a lesion that is unequivocally severe, the angioplaster is often faced with the decision as to whether other lesions are also hemodynamically significant and worthy of intervention. In addition, the hemodynamic results of lesions that are dilated are often far from clearly predictable from the resultant morphology. So a better means of monitoring and assessing the results would be helpful. Accordingly, it is quite practical to focus on developing methods that will improve the decision making process within the angioplasty laboratory. The three approaches described in this chapter may begin to help meet these needs. The combination of high fidelity micromanometry, Doppler velocimetry and either quantitative coronary angiography or, preferably, endolumenal echocardiography, allows us to begin to imagine the ability to measure absolute coronary blood flow in specified segments of the coronary tree in practical ways. If these modalities could be configured to accommodate the current practice and hardware of interventional cardiology, then major improvements in our understanding of coronary disease and our treatments will ensue. Patients will be thankful for this; economists might not!

References

1. Hoffman JIE. Maximal coronary flow and the concept of coronary vascular reserve. Circulation 1984; 70: 153–9.
2. Mancini GBJ, McGillem MJ, DeBoe SF, Gallagher KP. The diastolic hyperemic flow versus pressure relation: a new index of coronary stenosis severity and flow reserve. Circulation 1989; 80: 941–50.
3. Di Mario C, de Feyter PJ, Gil R, de Jaegere P, Strikwerda S, Serruys PW. Intracoronary blood flow velocity and transstenotic pressure gradient simultaneously assessed with sensor-tip Doppler and pressure guidewires [abstract]. Circulation 1992; 86 (4 suppl): I–122.
4. DiMario C, Meneveau N, Gil R *et al.* Beat to beat variability of the hyperemic coronary pressure/flow velocity relation in patients without significant coronary stenoses [abstract]. J Am Coll Cardiol 1993; 21 (Suppl A): 210A.
5. Pijls NH, Aengevaeren WR, Uijen GJ *et al.* Concept of maximal flow ratio for immediate evaluation of percutaneous transluminal coronary angioplasty result by videodensitometry. Circulation 1991; 83: 854–65.
6. Pijls NH, Uijen GJH, Hoevelaken A *et al.* Mean transit time for the assessment of myocardial perfusion by videodensitometry. Circulation 1990; 81: 1331–40.
7. Pijls NH, den Arend J, van Leeuwen K *et al.* Maximal myocaridal perfusion as a measure of the functional significance of coronary artery disease. In Reiber JHC, Serruys PW (eds): Advances in quantitative coronary arteriography. Dordrecht: Kluwer Academic Publishers 1993: 213–33.
8. Pijls NH, van Son JAM, Kirkeeide RL, deBruyne B, Gould KL. Experimental basis of determining maximum coronary, myocardial, and collateral blood flow by pressure measurements for assessing functional stenosis severity before and after percutaneous transluminal coronary angioplasty. Circulation 1993; 87: 1354–67.
9. Dole WP, Alexander GM, Campbell AB, Hixson EL, Bishop VS. Interpretation and physiological significance of diastolic coronary artery pressure-flow relationships in the canine coronary bed. Circ Res 1984; 55: 215–26.

10. Mancini GBJ, Cleary RM, DeBoe SF, Moore NB, Gallagher KP. The instantaneous hyperemic flow versus pressure slope index: microsphere validation of an alternative to measures of coronary reserve. Circulation 1991; 84: 862–70.
11. Cleary RM, Ayon D, Moore NB, DeBoe SF, Mancini GBJ. Tachycardia, contractility, and volume loading alter conventional indices of coronary flow reserve, but not the instantaneous hyperemic flow versus pressure slope index. J Am Coll Cardiol 1992; 20: 1261–9.
12. Cleary RM, Moore NB, DeBoe SF, Mancini GBJ. Sensitivity and reproducibility of the instantaneous hyperemic flow versus pressure slope index compared to coronary flow reserve. Am Heart J 1993. In press.
13. Gould KL, Kirkeeide RL, Buchi M. Coronary flow reserve as a physiologic measure of stenosis severity. J Am Coll Cardiol 1990; 15: 459–74.

PART FOUR

QCA in progression/regression of atherosclerotic disease

18. Towards complete assessment of progression/regression of coronary atherosclerosis: Implications for intervention trials

PIM J. DE FEYTER, CARLO DI MARIO, CEES J. SLAGER, PATRICK W. SERRUYS & JOS R.T.C. ROELANDT

Summary

Visual assessment of serial angiograms has always been the standard method to study progression/regression of coronary atherosclerosis. Visual assessment is subjective and suffers from the large intra- and interobserver variability. This stimulated the development of quantitative coronary angiography, employing computer based edge-finding detection techniques, which are currently applied and now considered as the new 'standard'.

However, angiography has its inherent limitations to assess progression/-regression mainly because the technique is 'indirect' as it provides a shadowgram of the contrast-filled lumen only.

Coronary atherosclerosis causes alterations of the coronary artery wall. In the earlier phases of atherosclerosis vascular remodelling preserves the original vascular lumen; only in later phases of the disease encroachment on the lumen takes place.

Intracoronary ultrasound imaging (ICUS) holds great promise to study progression/regression of coronary atherosclerosis. It is a 'direct' imaging technique and allows assessment of the arterial wall, components of the plaque including lipid content, fibrous tissue or calcification, and it allows quantification of the extent of the plaque. Thus ICUS provides insights into the underlying pathologic processes, during all stages of the coronary atherosclerosis. It may predict which lesion has potential for progression/ regression, and it may be used to monitor the effects of an intervention.

The functional significance of a coronary lesion can be assessed by applying the concept of coronary flow reserve. Measurement of coronary blood flow velocity with intracoronary Doppler-techniques (Flo-map wire or Doppler catheter) at baseline and during maximal vasodilation is currently possible in clinical practise.

Complete assessment of progression/regression with the application of quantitative coronary angiography, intracoronary ultrasound and intracoronary Doppler, three complementary techniques, is now possible and soon will be implemented in clinical practise.

J.H.C. Reiber and P.W. Serruys (eds): Progress in quantitative coronary arteriography, 295–305.

Introduction

During the recent years a large body of evidence has emerged that clearly demonstrates a link between cholesterol reduction, reduction in the frequency of clinical events and arrest or even regression in angiographic coronary artery disease severity [1–3].

Currently, pharmacotherapeutic modification of the atherosclerotic process has become a reality, and its effects on coronary atherosclerosis can be assessed by serial coronary angiography. However, newer techniques such as intracoronary ultrasound and intracoronary Doppler [4] theoretically have a greater potential to study these processes.

Endpoints from coronary angiography, intracoronary ultrasound and Doppler should be considered as surrogate endpoints as each one represents one aspect of a continuum of clinical and pathophysiological manifestations of disease. The continuum encompasses abnormalities ranging from lipid metabolism detected in serum samples, early 'prestenotic' sub-intimal thickening detected by intracoronary ultrasound, advanced coronary arteriosclerosis detected by coronary angiography and intracoronary ultrasound, or functional consequences assessed by intracoronary Doppler to clinical manifestations including angina pectoris, myocardial infarction and coronary death.

However, surrogate endpoints nowadays are becoming more and more acceptable to the community, since they provide significant information about the efficacy of an intervention. This information is obtained at considerable less costs because less patients need to be studied during a shorter intervention period.

In this review we will critically review the relative strengths and limitations of coronary angiography, intracoronary ultrasound and intracoronary Doppler to assess progression/regression of coronary atherosclerosis.

Quantitative coronary angiography

Serial angiographic studies designed to assess retardation of progression or regression of coronary artery disease have focused on changes of pre-existing lesions or on the development of new lesions [1–3]. The observed changes have been expressed in terms of changes of percent diameter stenosis or absolute measurement of the minimal luminal diameter (mm) of a stenosis. However, progression and possibly regression, of coronary atherosclerosis is a complex process that is not limited to focal areas of the coronary artery tree but frequently involves the entire arterial wall [5–7].

Therefore, to assess the effect of an intervention on progression and regression of coronary atherosclerosis, both focal and diffuse changes should be measured [4].

Visual interpretation of coronary angiograms has its limitations because assessment of stenosis severity is associated with: a) a large intra- and interobserver grading variability (8–37%) b) only relative stenosis measurements are provided and c) severity of diffuse atherosclerosis is difficult to estimate [4].

Quantitative coronary angiography allows assessment of both focal and diffuse atherosclerosis and provides us with a) relative measurements of diameter stenosis and area stenosis, b) absolute measurements, both from lesions and segments of the coronary tree including minimal luminal diameter stenosis (mm) and mean luminal diameter segment (mm).

Coronary angiography is an indirect technique and coronary atherosclerosis is detected only when luminal encroachment has taken place. Conceptually angiographical assessment of progression or regression should be viewed as an increment or decrement of volume of the atherosclerotic plaque intruding on the arterial lumen of the entire coronary tree. Progression is defined as the occurrence of a) increase of degree and extent of focal atherosclerosis b) development of a new lesion c) increase of degree and extent of diffuse atherosclerosis and d) the combination of a, b and c. This implies that we should measure changes in the luminal volume of the opacified coronary artery tree. However, the complex coronary anatomy, the varying course of the arteries in a three-dimensional space, and the cyclic changing caliber of the coronary arteries, further complicated by the beating heart, makes it impossible to measure the 'volume' of the coronary tree in man with current analytic angiographic techniques. A rather simplified two-dimensional approach is employed and the surface area of a coronary segment is calculated (Figure 18.1). The surface area is derived from the mean of the individual luminal diameters determined at many sampling points along the entire segment from proximal to distal multiplied by the length of the entire segment. Since the length of the entire segment is kept equal in a baseline and follow-up angiogram, this quantity is discarded from the equation. Progression/regression of focal or diffuse coronary atherosclerosis will result in a change in the individual luminal diameters at the site of disease and this will be reflected in a change of the mean luminal diameter. Therefore, the derived mean luminal diameter (average of all individual luminal diameters) can be considered as a measure that does assess, in a two-dimensional plane, either focal or diffuse coronary atherosclerotic processes. In addition, this method also identifies the minimal luminal diameter (focal atherosclerosis) of a coronary segment.

Another approach would be to assess the actual vessel area by the summation of all pixels between the contours; this has been implemented in the latest generation of quantitative angiographic analytic systems.

A series of measurements derived from quantitative coronary angiography can be used to assess progression or regression of coronary atherosclerosis. The mean luminal diameter (mm) is the most informative measurement, because it is able to assess progression/regression of both diffuse atherosclerotic disease and focal atherosclerotic disease.

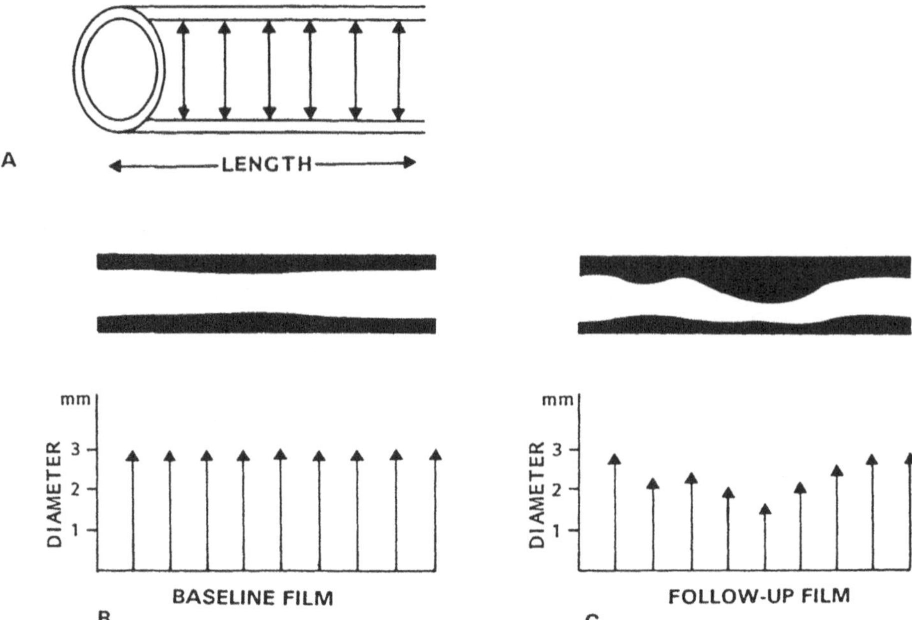

Figure 18.1. (A) Determination of individual luminal diameters at different sample points to derive at surface area. The average of all individual luminal diameters is the mean luminal diameter. Surface area = length × mean luminal diameter (width). The factor length in the equation can be discarded because length at baseline and follow-up is the same. (B) Determination of mean luminal diameter in baseline film. (C) Progression of disease changes the individual luminal diameters and thus on mean luminal diameter (decrease) in follow-up film. In addition this method also determines the minimal luminal diameter of a diseased coronary artery segment.

The absolute measurement, (minimal luminal diameter in mm) of lesions is extremely valuable to assess changes of focal atherosclerosis. Although relative measurements are subject to many drawbacks it may be useful to present these to meet the traditional clinical practice of grading stenoses as percent stenosis.

Angiographic assessment of progression/regression is limited because it assesses only the contour of the arterial lumen and thus the underlying pathologic process can be identified only by inference. This often causes underestimation of the severity and extent of coronary atherosclerosis when compared to post-mortem pathological studies [8–16]. Another problem is that the early stages of coronary atherosclerosis are associated with remodelling of the coronary artery.

Remodelling of the coronary artery, due to compensatory wall enlargement and medial thinning underneath the plaque, results in preservation of the normal lumen cross sectional area so that early stage coronary atherosclerosis is angiographically undetectable [17–21]. Also gradually proceeding diffuse

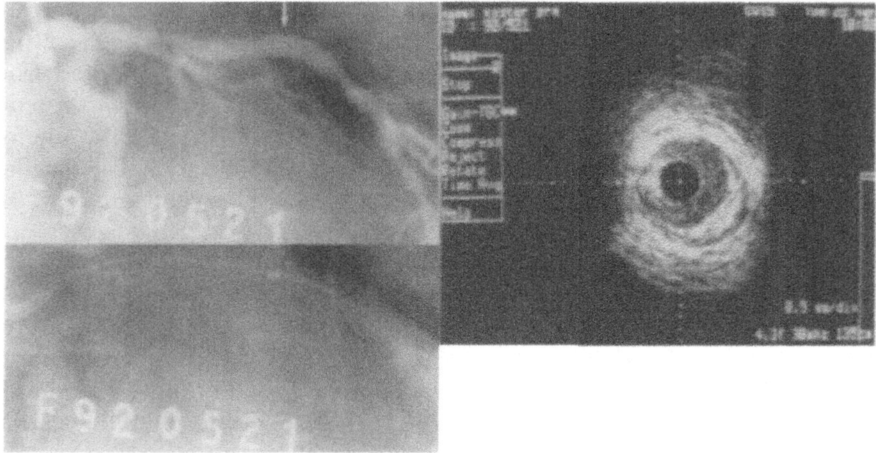

Figure 18.2. Left upper panel: coronary angiogram demonstrating normal contour of the vessel at the site of image acquisition (arrow). Left lower panel: intracoronary ultrasound device in coronary artery. Right panel: cross-sectional ultrasound image demonstrating preserved lumen, eccentric plaque between 2 and 6 o'clock separated from the adventitia by a dark echolucent medial layer.

atherosclerotic disease, causing a smooth narrowing of an entire vessel develops often unnoticed and is only suspected when it has advanced to a severe degree. Misinterpretation of regression is likely in case of 1) lysis of mural or occlusive thrombus, 2) relaxation of vasospasm (catheter induced; related to endothelial dysfunction) or 3) age related vasodilation.

Intracoronary ultrasound imaging

Unlike coronary angiography, intracoronary ultrasound imaging has the potential to image the coronary artery wall beyond the lumen and thus overcomes the problems encountered by coronary angiography. This ability permits *in vivo* inspection of the vessel wall and its pathology both in the early prestenotic phase of atherosclerosis and in its more advanced stages. The normal coronary artery generally has a three-layered appearance in the adults [22–27]. The bright inner layer represents a combination of the intima and internal elastic lamina. The media is poorly reflective of ultrasound and appears as a characteristic dark band. The adventitia is bright, forming an outer layer that is usually indistinguishable from the surrounding peri-adventitial tissue (Figure 18.2).

Imaging of the plaque permits quantitative analysis of the cross-sectional area of the plaque and gives information about the plaque composition because the variations in ultrasound backscatter permit to some extent the differentiation between various tissue components [23–31]. In general the plaques can be classified as soft, hard or calcified. Images obtained from fibromuscular tissue generally have a soft appearance compared with dense fibrous plaques, which produce bright echoes. Calcium produces an intense echo reflection and lack of penetration beyond the area of calcification ('shadowing'). Lipid-lakes in atheroma appear as echo-lucent areas within the plaque [32].

Intravascular ultrasound imaging has some apparent limitations.

Precise measurement of the plaque may be difficult if there is a) a strong reflection from a prominent internal elastic lumina causing 'blooming' of the interface echo, so that the plaque size is overestimated [33] b) thinning of the media underneath the plaque makes precise definition of border of plaque/media more difficult [34] c) calcium with shadowing behind the calcific deposits precludes identification of the exact depth of the plaque.

Until now the majority of ultrasound systems provide only two dimensional cross-sectional images acquired at areas of interest. Cross-sectional images do not provide information on longitudinal architecture and extent of the plaque. Other more complex techniques are necessary to produce that kind of information. Successful attempts have been made to reconstruct serially recorded cross-sectional images into a three-dimensional display [35–37]. The serial cross-sections are digitized and reconstructed in a stacked format along the length of the artery to yield sagittal and cylindrical display formats. The three-dimensional representation of the coronary artery lumen and atherosclerotic plaque provides very useful information to better understand plaque morphology.

Because ICUS is, in principle, an invasive technique using a catheter with finite physical dimension, only the proximal parts of the coronary tree can be studied and severe proximal coronary lesions cannot be crossed because the catheter may damage the plaque. Extreme tortuosity of the coronary vessel may hamper appropriate placement of the catheter.

Serial interrogation requires precise repetition of the sites where the initial images were obtained. Determination and standardization of anatomical landmarks in the coronary tree are needed and 3–dimensional reconstruction techniques may be instrumental in this regard in the future.

It appears that intracoronary ultrasound imaging has a great potential as a new diagnostic tool and as a research tool to study the pathobiology of atherosclerosis. Intracoronary ultrasound imaging offers the opportunity to acquire information of vessel wall, atherosclerotic plaque and vessel wall dynamics in living patients. It can differentiate lipid plaques, potentially amenable to regression with lipid lowering interventions from fibro-calcific plaques which are less likely to regress. It allows 'monitoring' of progression/regression interventions of selected areas and may provide information about the pathophysiological processes underlying regression.

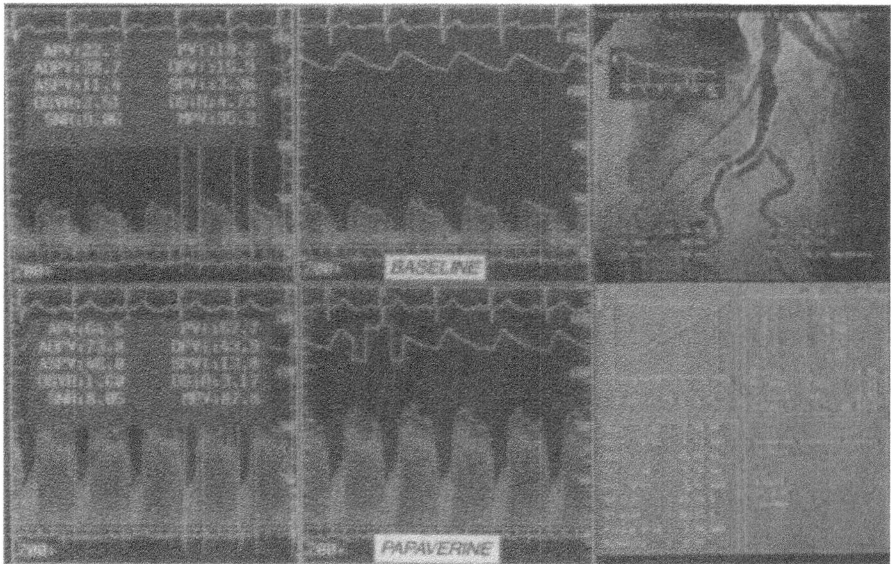

Figure 18.3. Example of a hemodynamic non-significant lesion (34%) demonstrating an increase in coronary blood flow velocity of approximately × CBF = ±3 (baseline velocity = 23 cm/s, papaverine induced maximal coronary blood flow velocity 65 cm/s).

Intracoronary doppler

The physiological significance of a coronary stenosis can be assessed by its effect on the coronary blood flow reserve capacity, assuming the fact that physiological significant obstructive lesions should decrease the vasodilator reserve [38–42].

Coronary blood flow reserve is the ratio between maximum coronary blood flow to resting coronary blood flow. A ratio of 4 to 5 is found in normal situations. Maximum coronary blood flow is obtained for instance by intracoronary injection of papaverine, inducing maximal dilatation of the distal coronary vasculature. Coronary flow reserve begins to decrease at 40% to 50% diameter stenosis.

A new intracoronary guide-wire technique based on the Doppler principle is now available to assess the physiological significance of a stenosis in terms of coronary flow reserve. It is possible to measure intracoronary blood flow velocity without disturbing the flow pattern, using a guide wire with Doppler sampling located at the tip (diameter: 0.46 mm; Cardiometrics) [43, 44]. The coronary reserve is determined by calculating the ratio between the maximal flow velocity to resting flow velocity (Figure 18.3). The effects of progression

Table 18.1. Significance of parameters to assess progression/regression of coronary atherosclerosis: proximal epicardial vessels and distal coronary vascular bed.

Technique Parameter lumen	Prox. epicardial vessels		Combination of diffuse and focal atherosclerosis	Distal
	Diffuse atherosclerosis	Focal atherosclerosis		Coronary vascular bed
Angiography				
Mean luminal diameter per vessel segment (mm)	+	±	++	–
Minimal luminal diameter (mm)	±	+	+	–
Diameter stenosis%	–	+	±	–
ICUS				
Lumen	+	±	+	–
Wall	++	++	+++	–
Components plaque	++	++	+++	–
Doppler				
Flow	+	++	++	++

Table 18.2. Strengths and limitations of angiography, ICUS and intracoronary Doppler to assess progression/regression of coronary atherosclerosis.

	Angiography	ICUS	Doppler
Coronary tree:			
Proximal vessel	+	+	+
Distal vessel	+	–	+
Distal coronary bed	–	–	+
Lumen	+	+	–
Wall: components	–	+	–
Plaque:			
Components	–	+	–
Quantification	±	+	–
Topography	±	+	–
Coronary blood flow	±	–	+
Thrombus	±	±	–
Vasodynamics	+	+	–

or regression including the distal coronary bed is reflected in the change of the coronary blood flow reserve.

A lipid altering intervention trial, using a comprehensive life style change, was associated with a 6% improvement of the coronary flow reserve which was assessed using positron emission tomography [45]. Functional improvement was also demonstrated in the Lipid Research Clinics Coronary Primary

Prevention Trial in which cholestyramine reduced the frequency of an abnormal stress electrocardiogram by 25% [46].

However, a major problem in assessing the effect of a coronary stenosis on coronary blood flow is that myocardial perfusion is the integrated response of the entire coronary vascular system consisting of several components including stenosis geometry, characteristics of epicardial vessel, endothelial function, distal vascular bed, myocardium, collateral circulation, aortic pressure, coronary vascular tone and the effectiveness of the coronary vasodilator stimulus.

The interpretation of changes in the coronary flow reserve can not exclusively be related to changes in the severity of an epicardial coronary artery stenosis but may rather reflect the overall effect of an intervention on the coronary circulation.

Conclusion

Serial quantitative coronary angiography is a powerful tool, widely available to assess progression/regression of coronary atherosclerosis. However, angiography is limited because it is an indirect 'luminographic' technique. Intravascular ultrasound provides a direct imaging technique and allows demonstration of actual regression of plaque or modification of specific components of plaque (lipids versus fibrocalcific components) in selected segments. Intracoronary Doppler provides functional assessment of coronary artery lesions. The strengths and limitations of the techniques and the significance of the derived parameters are tabulated in Table 18.1 and Table 18.2. It appears that all three techniques provide different information, which is complementary and necessary for complete assessment of progression/regression of coronary atherosclerosis.

References

1. Davies MJ, Krikler DM, Katz D. Atherosclerosis: inhibition or regression as therapeutic possibilities. Br Heart J 1991; 65: 302–10.
2. Vos J, de Feyter PJ, Simoons ML, Tijssen JG, Deckers JW. Retardation and arrest of progression or regression of coronary artery disease: a review. Prog Cardiovasc Dis 1993; 35: 435–54.
3. Thompson GR. Progression and regression of coronary artery disease. Curr Opin Lipidol 1992; 3: 263–7.
4. de Feyter PJ, Serruys PW, Davies MJ, Richardson P, Lubsen J, Oliver MF. Quantitative coronary angiography to measure progression or regression of coronary atherosclerosis. Value, limitations, and implications for clinical trials. Circulation 1991; 84: 412–23.
5. Vlodaver Z, Edwards JE. Pathology of coronary atherosclerosis. Prog Cardiovasc Dis 1971; 14: 256–74.
6. Marcus ML, Harrison DG, White CW, McPherson DD, Wilson RF, Kerber RE. Assessing

the physiologic significance of coronary obstructions in patients: importance of diffuse undetected atherosclerosis. Prog Cardiovasc Dis 1988; 31: 39–56.
7. Waller BF. Topography of atherosclerotic coronary artery disease. Clin Cardiol 1990; 13: 435–42.
8. Marcus ML, Armstrong ML, Heistad DD, Eastham CL, Mark AL. Comparison of three methods of evaluating coronary obstructive lesions: postmortem arteriography, pathologic examination and measurement of regional myocardial perfusion during maximal vasodilation. Am J Cardiol 1982; 49: 1699–706.
9. Schwartz JN, Kong Y, Hackel DB, Bartel AG. Comparison of angiographic and postmortem finds in patients with coronary artery disease. Am J Cardiol 1975; 36: 174–8.
10. Hutchins GM, Bulkley GH, Ridolfi RL, Griffith LS, Lohr FT, Piasio MA. Correlation of coronary arteriograms and left ventriculograms with postmortem studies. Circulation 1977; 56: 32–7.
11. Thomas AC, Davies MJ, Dilly S, Dilly N, Franc F. Potential errors in the estimation of coronary arterial stenosis from clinical arteriography with reference to the shape of the coronary arterial lumen. Br Heart J 1986; 55: 129–39.
12. Arnett EN, Isner JM, Redwood DR *et al.* Coronary artery narrowing in coronary heart disease: comparison of cineangiographic and necropsy findings. Ann Intern Med 1979; 91: 350–6.
13. Kemp HG, Evans H, Elliott WC, Gorlin R. Diagnostic accuracy of selective coronary cinearteriography. Circulation 1967; 36: 526–33.
14. Vlodaver Z, Frech R, Van Tassel RA, Edwards JE. Correlation of the antemortem coronary arteriogram and the postmortem specimen. Circulation 1973; 47: 162–9.
15. Grondin CM, Dyrda I, Pasternac A, Campeau L, Bourassa MG, Lespérance J. Discrepancies between cineangiographic and postmortem findings in patients with coronary artery disease and recent myocardial revascularization. Circulation 1974; 49: 703–8.
16. Isner JM, Kishel J, Kent KM, Ronan JA Jr, Ross AM, Roberts WC. Accuracy of angiographic determination of left main coronary artery narrowing. Angiographic histologic correlative analysis in 28 patients. Circulation 1981; 63: 1056–64.
17. Glagov S, Weisenberg E, Zarins CK, Stankunavicius R, Kolettis GJ. Compensatory enlargement of human atherosclerotic coronary arteries. N Engl J Med 1987; 316: 1371–5.
18. Zarins CK, Weisenberg E, Kolettis G, Stankunavicius R, Glagov S. Differential enlargement of artery segments in response to enlarging atherosclerotic plaques. J Vasc Surg 1988; 7: 386–94.
19. Stiel GM, Stiel LS, Schofer J, Donath K, Mathey DG. Impact of compensatory enlargement of atherosclerotic coronary arteries on angiographic assessement of coronary artery disease. Circulation 1989; 80: 1603–9.
20. McPherson DD, Sirna SJ, Hiratzka LF *et al.* Coronary arterial remodeling studied by high-frequency epicardial echocardiography: an early compensatory mechanism in patients with obstructive coronary atherosclerosis. J Am Coll Cardiol 1991; 17: 79–86.
21. Isner JM, Donaldson RF, Fortin AH, Tischler A, Clarke RH. Attenuation of the media of coronary arteries in advanced atherosclerosis. Am J Cardiol 1986; 58: 937–9.
22. Yock PG, Johnson EL, Linker DT. Intravascular ultrasound: development and clinical potential. Am J Card Imaging 1988; 2: 185–93.
23. Gussenhoven EJ, Essed CE, Lancée CT *et al.* Arterial wall characteristics determined by intravascular ultrasound imaging: an *in vitro* study. J Am Coll Cardiol 1989; 14: 947–52.
24. Mallery JA, Tobis JM, Griffith J *et al.* Assessment of normal and atherosclerotic arterial wall thickness with an intravascular ultrasound imaging catheter. Am Heart J 1990; 119: 1392–400.
25. Coy KM, Maurer G, Siegel RJ. Intravascular ultrasound imaging: a current perspective. J Am Coll Cardiol 1991; 18: 1811–23.
26. Nissen SE, Gurley JC, Grines CL *et al.* Intravascular ultrasound assessment of lumen size and wall morphology in normal subjects and patients with coronary artery disease. Circulation 1991; 84: 1087–99.

27. Fitzgerald PJ, St. Goar FG, Connolly AJ *et al.* Intravascular ultrasound imaging of coronary arteries. Is three layers the norm? Circulation 1992; 86: 154–8.
28. Tobis JM, Mallery JA, Gessert J *et al.* Intravascular ultrasound cross-sectional arterial imaging before and after balloon angioplasty *in vitro*. Circulation 1989; 80: 873–82.
29. Nishimura RA, Edwards WD, Warnes CA *et al.* Intravascular ultrasound imaging: *in vitro* validation and pathologic correlation. J Am Coll Cardiol 1990; 16: 145–54.
30. Hodgson JM, Reddy KG, Suneja R, Nair RN, Lesnefsky EJ, Sheehan HM. Intracoronary ultrasound imaging: correlation of plaque morphology with angiography, clinical syndrome and procedural results in patients undergoing coronary angioplasty. J Am Coll Cardiol 1993; 21: 35–44.
31. Di Mario C, The SH, Madretsma S *et al.* Detection and characterization of vascular lesions by intravascular ultrasound: an *in vitro* study correlated with histology. J Am Soc Echocardiogr 1992; 5: 135–46.
32. Potkin BN, Bartorelli AL, Gessert JM *et al.* Coronary artery imaging with intravascular high-frequency ultrasound. Circulation 1990; 81: 1575–85.
33. Yock PG, Fitzgerald PJ, Linker DT, Angelsen BAJ. Intravascular ultrasound guidance for catheter-based coronary interventions. J Am Coll Cardiol 1991; 17 (Suppl B): 39B–45B.
34. Gussenhoven EJ, Frietman PAV, The SHK *et al.* Assessment of medial thinning in atherosclerosis by intravascular ultrasound. Am J Cardiol 1991; 68: 1625–32.
35. Kitney RL, Moura L, Straughan K. 3–D visualization of arterial structures using ultrasound and Voxel modelling. Int J Card Imaging 1989; 4: 135–43.
36. Rosenfield K, Losordo DW, Ramaswamy K *et al.* Three-dimensional reconstruction of human coronary and peripheral arteries from images recorded during two-dimensional intravascular ultrasound examination. Circulation 1991; 84: 1938–56.
37. Coy KM, Park JC, Fishbein MC *et al.* *In vitro* validation of three-dimensional intravascular ultrasound for the evaluation of arterial injury after balloon angioplasty. J Am Coll Cardiol 1992; 20: 692–700.
38. Klocke FJ. Measurements of coronary blood flow and degree of stenosis: current clinical implications and continuing uncertainties. J Am Coll Cardiol 1983; 1: 31–41.
39. Kirkeeide RL, Gould KL, Parsel L. Assessment of coronary stenoses by myocardial perfusion imaging during pharmacologic coronary vasodilation. VII. Validition of coronary flow reserve as a single integrated functional measure of stenosis severity reflecting all its geometric dimensions. J Am Coll Cardiol 1986; 7: 103–13.
40. Gould KL, Kirkeeide RL, Buchi M. Coronary flow reserve as a physiologic measure of stenosis severity. J Am Coll Cardiol 1990; 15: 459–74.
41. Klocke FJ. Measurements of coronary blood flow reserve: defining pathophysiology versus making decisions about patient care. Circulation 1987; 76: 1183–9.
42. Hoffman JIE. A critical view of coronary reserve. Circulation 1987; 75 (suppl I): I6–I11.
43. Emanuelsson H, Dohnal M, Lamm C, Tenerz L. Initial experiences with a miniaturized pressure transducer during coronary angioplasty. Cathet Cardiovasc Diagn 1991; 24: 137–43.
44. Doucette JW, Corl PD, Payne HM *et al.* Validation of a Doppler guide wire for intravascular measurement of coronary artery flow velocity. Circulation 1992; 85: 1899–911.
45. Ornish D, Brown SE, Scherwitz LW *et al.* Can lifestyle changes reverse coronary heart disease? The Lifestyle Heart Trial. Lancet 1990; 336: 129–33.
46. The Lipid Research Clinics Coronary Prevention Trial results. 1. Reduction in incidence of coronary heart disease. JAMA 1984; 251: 351–64.

19. Are qualitative features of coronary artery lesions useful in predicting progression?

JACQUES LESPÉRANCE, GILLES HUDON, PIERRE THÉROUX & DAVID WATERS

Summary

Morphologic characterization of coronary artery lesions can provide useful information on clinical stability, pathophysiologic mechanisms and prognosis, beyond that provided by the traditional interpretation of coronary angiography in terms of lesion severity and number of diseased arteries. Thus, more numerous lesions, defined by a higher extent score, are associated with a more progressive disease and a worse prognosis. Lesions of only moderate severity, but with a geometry favoring flow separation carry a higher risk of thrombotic occlusion and myocardial infarction. More severe lesions occlude more, but often without symptoms. The acute process is characterized by a complex plaque with eccentricity, steep inflow angle, ulcerations and with filling defects by partially or completely occluding thrombi. Subsequent remodeling leads to lesion progression with edge irregularities. A residual thrombus is associated with a higher risk of recurrent coronary events and also of procedural complications during angioplasty.

Introduction

The extent and severity of coronary atherosclerosis are assessed clinically by coronary arteriography and the results are usually expressed in terms of number of diseased vessels with 50% or more diameter stenosis. Many studies have shown that cardiac mortality increases with the number of diseased vessels [1]. Diameter stenoses less than 50% are ordinarily not severe enough to cause myocardial ischemia and thus are not treated with coronary angioplasty or coronary bypass surgery. Yet, coronary occlusion at lesions in this range cause a substantial proportion of myocardial infarctions [2].

The morphologic features of coronary lesions are usually ignored in the clinical classification of coronary disease. This is so for several reasons. First, the clinical significance of different morphologic features and their prognostic importance has not been defined as explicitly as have other measurements. Also, different descriptors of morphologic characteristics exist in the literature and the assessment of lesion morphology is both subjective and associated with a high degree of interobserver variability.

J.H.C. Reiber and P.W. Serruys (eds): Progress in quantitative coronary arteriography, 307–324.

Levin *et al.* compared the post-mortem angiographic and pathologic features of coronary artery lesions [3]. Stenoses with irregular borders or intraluminal lucencies at angiography, corresponded on histologic sections to plaque rupture, plaque hemorrhage, and superimposed partially occluding, or recanalized thrombus. Conversely, stenoses with smooth borders, an hourglass configuration and no intraluminal lucencies at arteriography, had no 'complicated' histology. These results suggest that post-mortem angiography is quite sensitive and specific for the detection of the complex lesion. By extrapolation, the accuracy of coronary arteriography in living patients can be assumed to be similar.

This chapter illustrates specific plaque features useful to evaluate the diagnosis, pathophysiology and prognosis of coronary artery disease. For this purpose, selected angiographic images are described in their clinical context.

Plaque morphology

The angiographic morphology of the *complex lesions* may include one or more of the following features.

1. *Eccentricity*

Eccentricity refers to lesions with a lumen lying in the outer quarter of the main lumen diameter of the artery [4]. Eccentricity per se has little significance when the edges of the lesion are smooth [5]. However, eccentric lesions with abrupt or overhanging edges or with steep inflow or outflow angles, are often associated with acute coronary syndromes (Figures 19.1B, 19.2C, 19.2E, 19.4 and 19.5A). The inflow angle is defined by the angle formed by the main axis of the vessel and a line from the proximal border of the lesion to its maximal narrowing [4, 6]. Steep lesions have an angle of less than 135°.

2. *Irregularities*

The endoluminal edges of the lesions can be smooth and regular, or coarse with roughening and a so-called saw-tooth appearance [4, 5]. Irregular lesions often lack definition because of hazy margins [6]. The lesions illustrated in Figures 19.1B, 19.2B and 19.8 are coarse and irregular and the lesions in Figures 19.2A and 19.6B, smooth. Irregular lesions may represent a partially resorbed thrombus or healing ulcerations and remodeling. Their incidence in patients with stable angina is less than 4%. In one study it was 1.5% [7] and in another 3.5% [4]. The definition of irregularity is partly subjective.

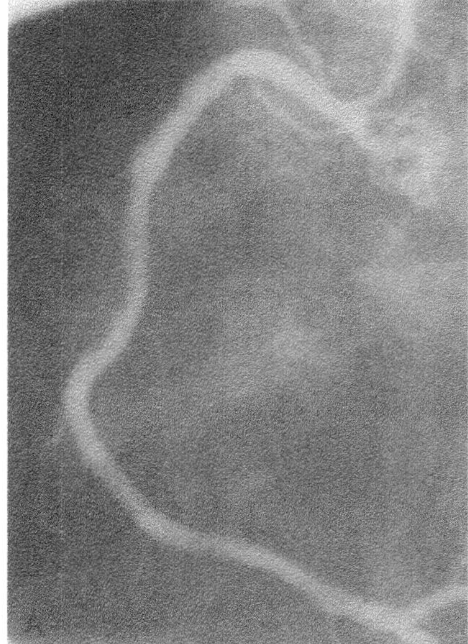

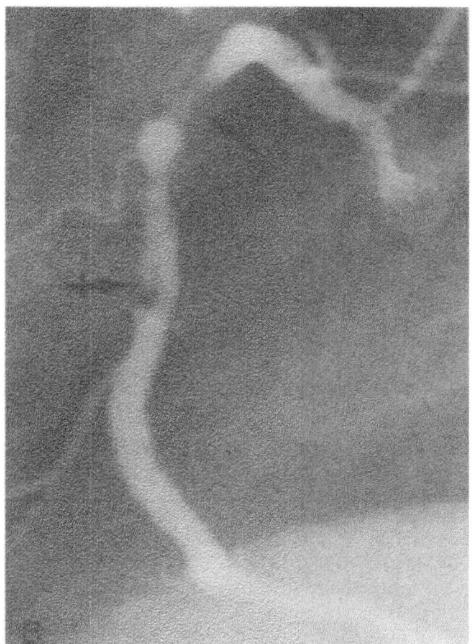

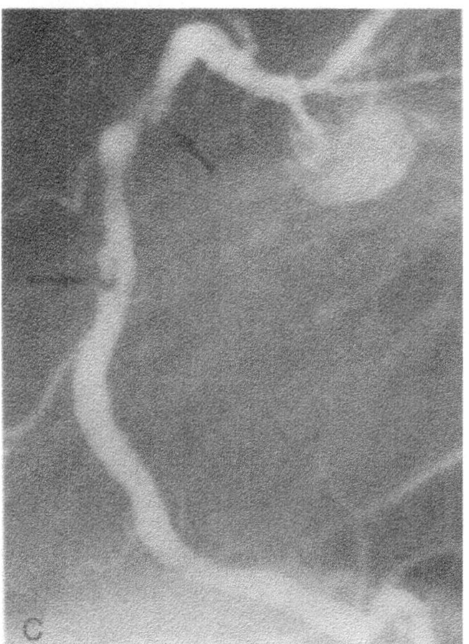

Figure 19.1. Non-severe lesion of the right coronary artery progressing to a complex lesion. (A) Right coronary angiogram (RCA) in a 48–year-old white male with stable angina. Minimal narrowings can be seen on the proximal and mid-segments of the right dominant coronary artery. The contrast left ventriculogram was then normal. (B) Four and a half years later, the patient sustained an acute inferior wall myocardial infarction. RCA angiogram 2 hours after the initiation of thrombolytic therapy showed two complex lesions. The proximal stenosis has hazy ill-defined margins, representing a mural thrombus. It contains a small, poorly visualized ulceration in its distal portion. Note that the lesion is not eccentric and does not have overhanging abrupt angles. The more distal lesion is eccentric with a deep ulceration of its proximal portion, parallel to the vessel wall (→). The left Ventriculogram showed severe hypokinesia of the inferior wall. (C) A control RCA angiogram obtained 6 days later showed better definition of the margins of the proximal lesion which contains a well-defined ulceration probably the result of resorption of a previous intraluminal thrombus (→). The more distal lesion is unchanged (→).

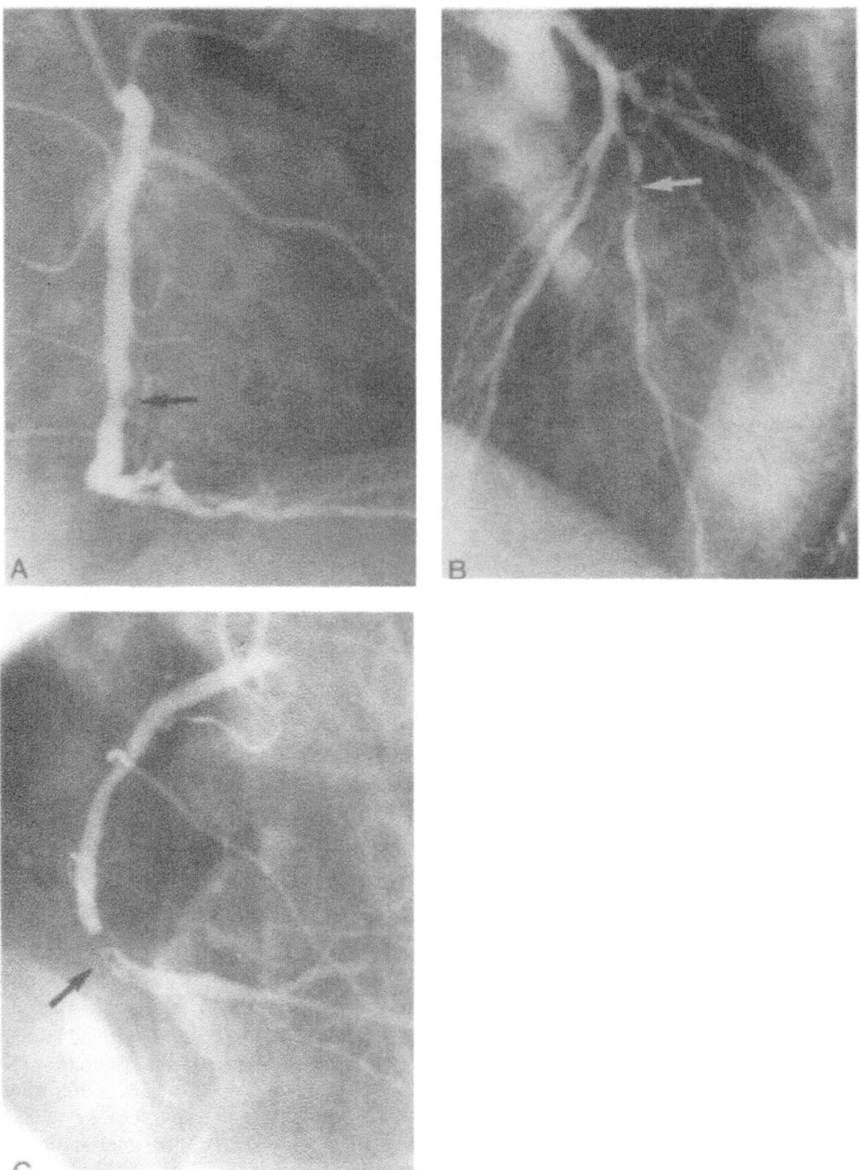

Figure 19.2A–C. A moderately severe non-complex lesion progressing to near-complete occlusion. (A) RCA angiogram in a 62–year-old white male admitted for stable angina: multiple but mild narrowings can be seen in the proximal and mid-segments of the right coronary artery. The smooth, eccentric 40% stenosis on mid-RCA (→) segment has an inflow angle measured at 145°, thus greater than the ≤135° criterion for an abrupt proximal face as proposed by Davies [6]. (B) The LCA angiogram reveals an eccentric and possibly ulcerated 70% diameter stenosis superimposed on a proximally irregular first diagonal branch (→) supplying a large territory, a

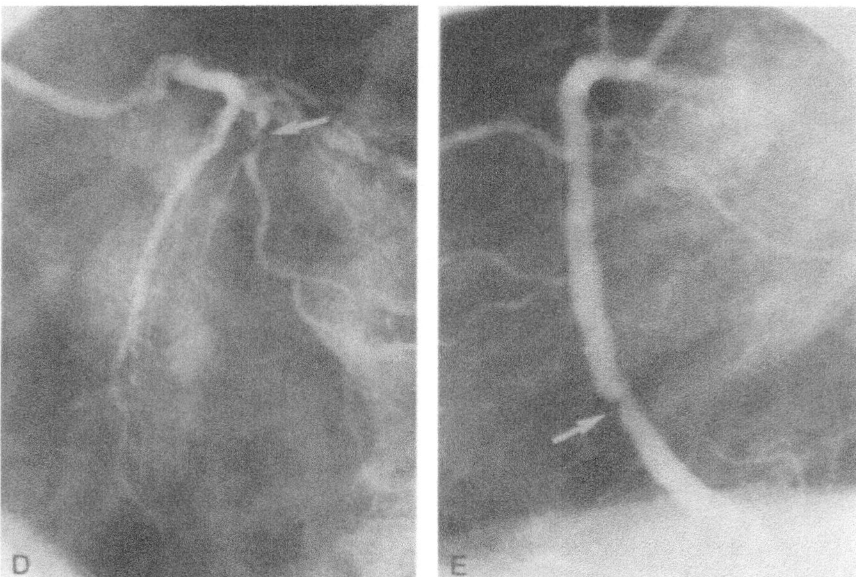

Figure 19.2D,E A moderately severe non-complex lesion progressing to near-complete occlusion. (D) The LCA angiogram showed no progression of the previously severe and ulcerated stenosis of the first diagonal branch (→). (E) Control RCA angiogram obtained 6 days after myocardial infarction and thrombolytic therapy showed restoration of a TIMI-3 antegrade flow. The distal filling defects had completely disappeared. A short, eccentric 40–50% diameter stenosis persists (→).

3. *Ulceration*

Ulcerations correspond to contrast-medium-opacified craters within the area of a stenosis. They presumably are the consequence of plaque rupture. Figures 19.1B, 19.1C, 19.6A and 19.2B are examples of ulcerations of different shapes and sizes. Their aspect may vary with time in the same patient in relation to the degree of filling of the rupture by the thrombus and healing with plaque remodeling following the acute event. An index of ulcerations was defined by Wilson *et al.* [8] as the ratio of the diameter of the least severe stenosis divided by the maximum intralesional diameter (Figure 19.10). This

---

lesion considered at high risk. (C) The patient was admitted 2.5 months later for an acute inferior wall infarction. The RCA showed a rapid progression of the 40% stenosis to an 80% with appearance of a complex morphology including eccentricity, acute inflow angle almost perpendicular to the long axis of the vessel and endoluminal distal filling defects. These aspects are characteristic of a large thrombus (→). The flow is delayed with only partial distal opacification (TIMI grade 2).

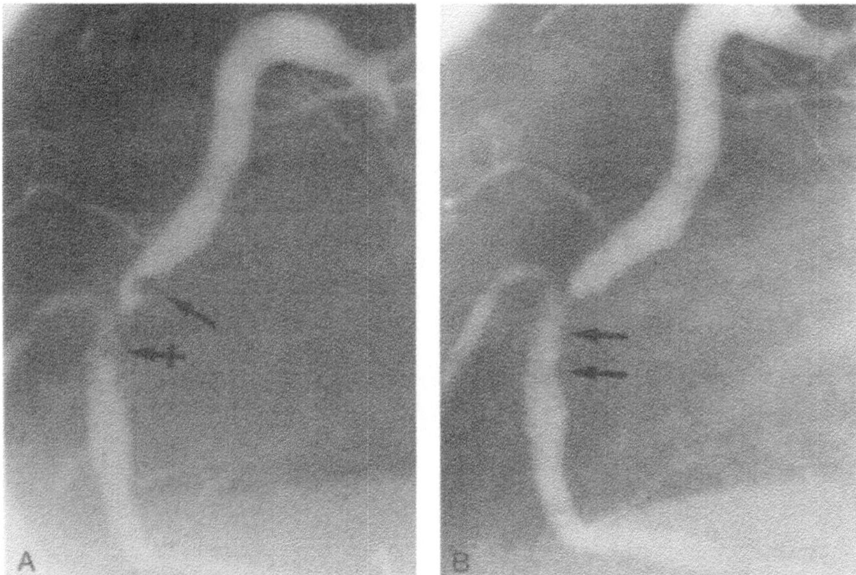

Figure 19.3. Presence of a division branch as a risk factor for thrombosis. (A) RCA obtained within 2 hours of the onset of chest pain in a 43–year-old white male with an acute inferior myocardial wall infarction: an intraluminal filling defect with angular borders, proximal to a concentric 70% lumen diameter stenosis (+→) of the mid-segment of the RCA is present. This narrowing strongly suggesting a mural thrombus (→), is immediately proximal to a large acute marginal branch. Numerous poorly defined small intraluminal filling defects are present distal to the stenosis. (B) RCA angiogram of the same patients 6 days after thrombolytic therapy: the endoluminal filling defects have completely disappeared, and the severity of the stenosis has not changed. Note the discrete mural irregularities distal to the stenosis (→).

ratio was independent of the severity of the stenosis and allowed separation of patients with stable and unstable coronary artery disease. Davies *et al.* [6] modified this index, as the ratio of the maximal to the minimal intralesional diameter (Figure 19.10) and used this as a predictor of early clinical instability following thrombolytic therapy.

4. *Filling defects*

Filling defects are defined as intraluminal radiotranslucent images, sub-opacified as compared to the adjacent lumen. The filling defects are of various sizes, usually ovoid (Figure 19.4) or polypoid in shape (Figure 19.2C). They are attached to the underlying plaque; they may be completely (Figures 19.5B and 19.7A) or partly occlusive (Figures 19.2C and 19.4). When smooth and well delineated by the contrast media, they are pathognomonic of intraluminal thrombi (Figures 19.2C and 19.4). Occlusive thrombi usually show a convex upstream aspect (Figure 19.5B). Older thrombi may have the

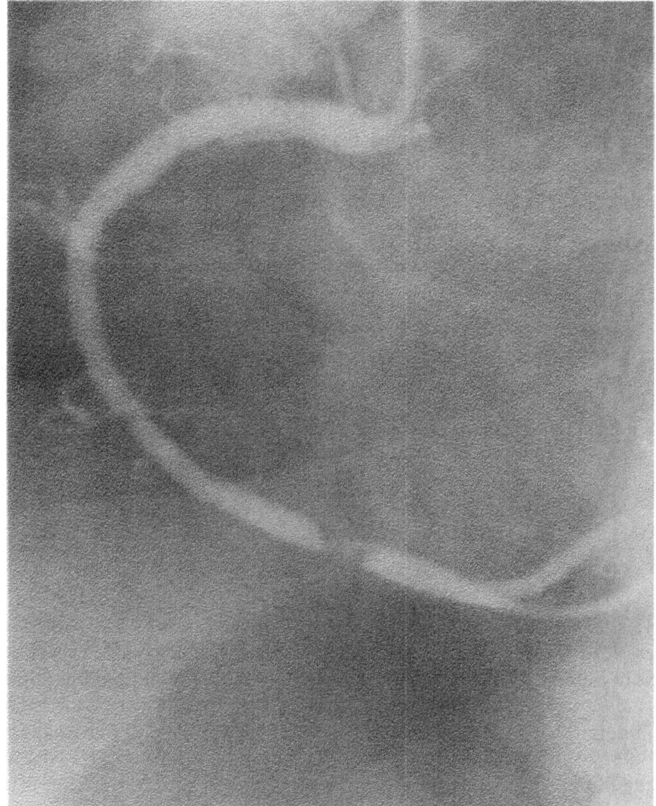

Figure 19.4. Right coronary angiogram obtained in a 56–year-old patient admitted for *unstable angina*. The figure demonstrates a smooth, eccentric severe (75%) stenosis of the distal RCA with abrupt, steep inflow angle (120°), and a well-circumscribed endoluminal filling defect just distal to the stenosis. This aspect is characteristic of a thrombus forming on a complex plaque.

appearance of adherent intraluminal mass with irregular or angular borders creating a very eccentric lumen (Figure 19.3A). More chronic obstruction usually tapers smoothly to supply a terminal side branch.

5. *Contrast medium stagnation*

Stagnation can be manifested by contrast medium impregnation of the clot (Figure 19.5B) but more often by contrast media stagnation proximal to the thrombus (Figure 19.7B) [9]. The proximal blood stagnation sets the stage for upstream extension of the thrombus and chronic vessel obstruction.

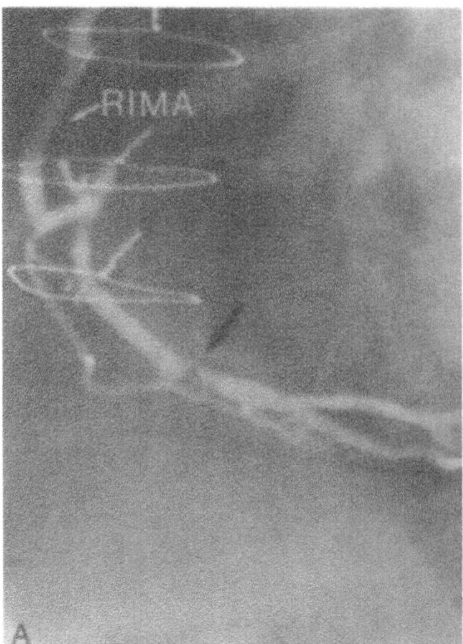

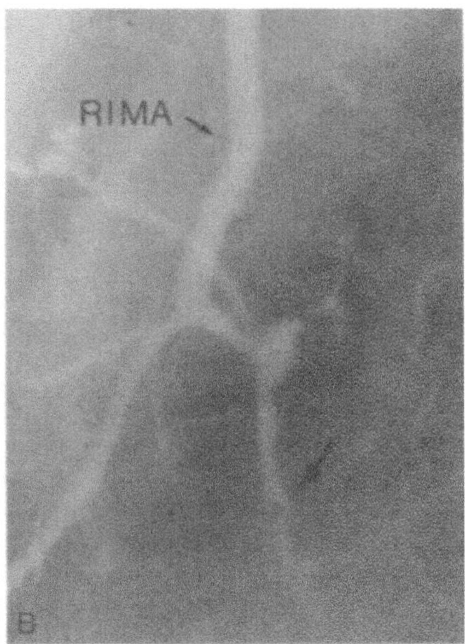

Figure 19.5. Lesion morphology in unstable angina culminating to myocardial infarction. (A) Contrast injection of a right internal mammary artery (RIMA) grafted on the marginal branch of a distal right dominant RCA 8 years previously, in a 63-year-old patient admitted for unstable angina. A very eccentric lesion (→) can be seen in the distal third of the native artery, with a 75% lumen diameter obstruction. The lesion is discrete, abrupt and has steep inflow and outflow angles but regular contours; no thrombus can be seen at this time. (B) Angiogram repeated 6 days later, after the onset of an acute Q-wave myocardial infarction. The distal right coronary artery is now completely occluded at the site of the previous narrowing by an endoluminal filling defect surrounded with dye impregnation. This defect has an upstream convex shape, characteristic of a thrombus. Wall motion abnormalities had now appeared in postero-lateral and diaphragmatic left ventricular segments.

6. *Multiple irregularities*

Multiple irregularities are defined by the presence of 3 of more adjacent stenoses or by diffuse narrowing between 2 close stenoses (Figure 19.8) [4, 5]. Healing and remodeling of ulcerated plaques usually account for this aspect. Multiple irregularities should be differentiated from diffuse atherosclerosis illustrated in Figure 19.9.

---

patient? *Bottom.* The angiograms shown in C and D were obtained 4 years later, shortly after an acute Q-wave inferior wall myocardial infarction. The distal right coronary artery is now completely occluded (→) at the site of the previously moderately stenotic but ulcerated lesion. The 60% and 80% stenoses of the LCA have surprisingly remained unchanged whereas the stenosis on the proximal left circumflex artery has progressed from 30% to 60% lumen diameter reduction.

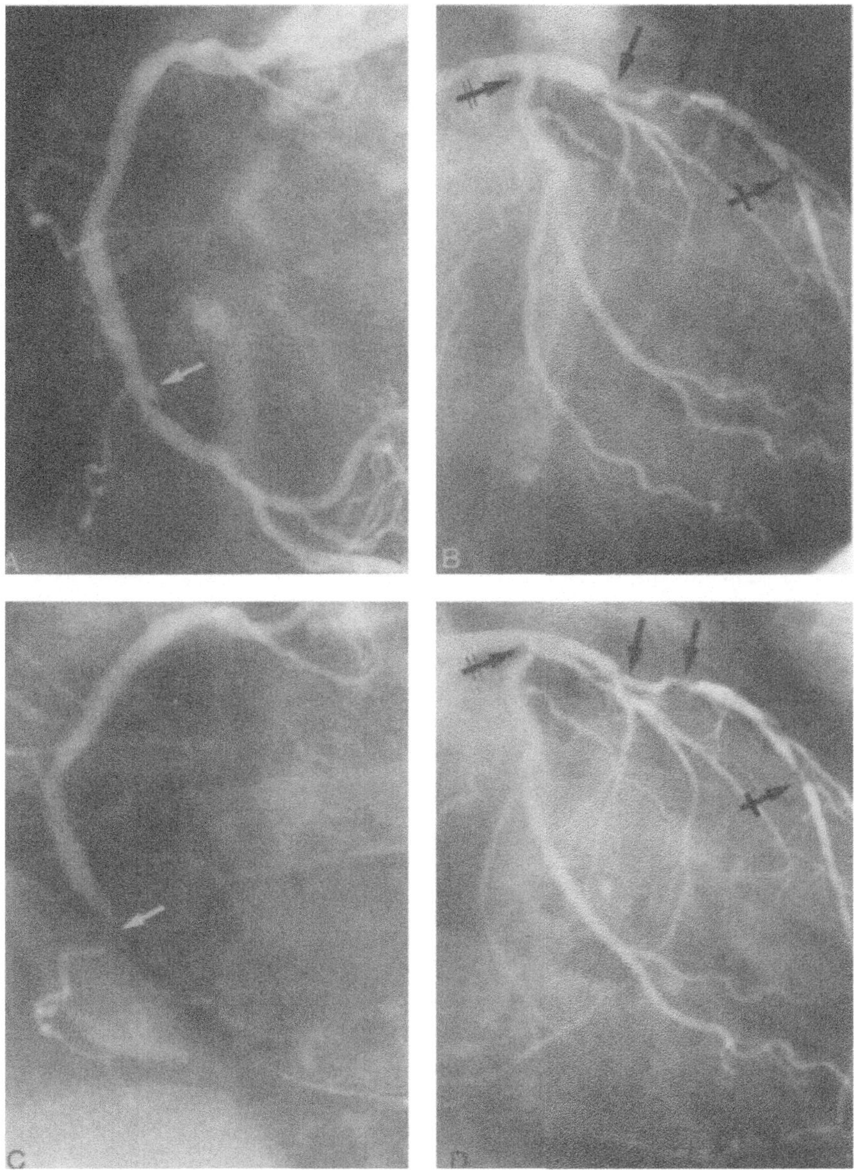

Figure 19.6. Lesion morphology in unstable angina progressing to myocardial infarction. *Top*. RCA (A) and LCA (B) coronary angiograms obtained 3 days after a non-Q-wave inferior wall myocardial infarction. The right coronary angiogram demonstrates a lesion of moderate severity (50% lumen diameter reduction) with an ulceration (→) and a side branch. It can be postulated that this lesion transiently developed a thrombus which has resolved. The left angiogram showed a 60% lumen diameter stenosis on the proximal left anterior descending artery (LAD) (→) and an 80% stenosis on its midportion (+→). A 30% narrowing on the proximal left circumflex artery is also seen (+→). What were the lesions at risk of progression in the following years in this

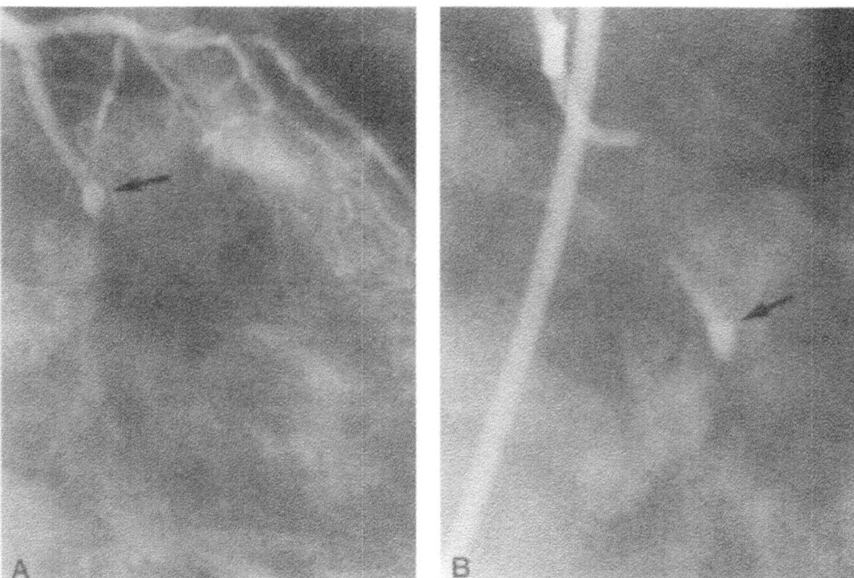

Figure 19.7. Dye stagnation in acute myocardial infarction. (A) An abrupt cutoff of the left circumflex coronary artery in the acute phase of myocardial infarction. This lesion typically represents an occlusive thrombus (→). (B) Stagnation of the contrast medium proximal to the site of the abrupt occlusion (→). In more chronic obstruction, the occlusion tapered smoothly just distal to a terminal side branch assuming runoff of the dye.

Quantification of complex morphology

Wilson [8] was first to try to quantify morphology to overcome the limitation of subjective interpretation. Later, Kalbfleisch *et al.* have developed an analysis involving 5 morphometric parameters, 4 derived from the normalized curvature signature and one based on the concept of fractal analysis [10]. Excellent intraobserver and interobserver reproducibility was reported for each parameter, and all were independent of the degree of stenosis. Such methods of analysis may prove to be useful in the future.

Extent of disease

Lesion severity

The traditional interpretation of the coronary angiogram consists in the identification of the diseased segments and of the severity of the stenoses. These descriptors influence therapy. More proximal stenoses and more severe

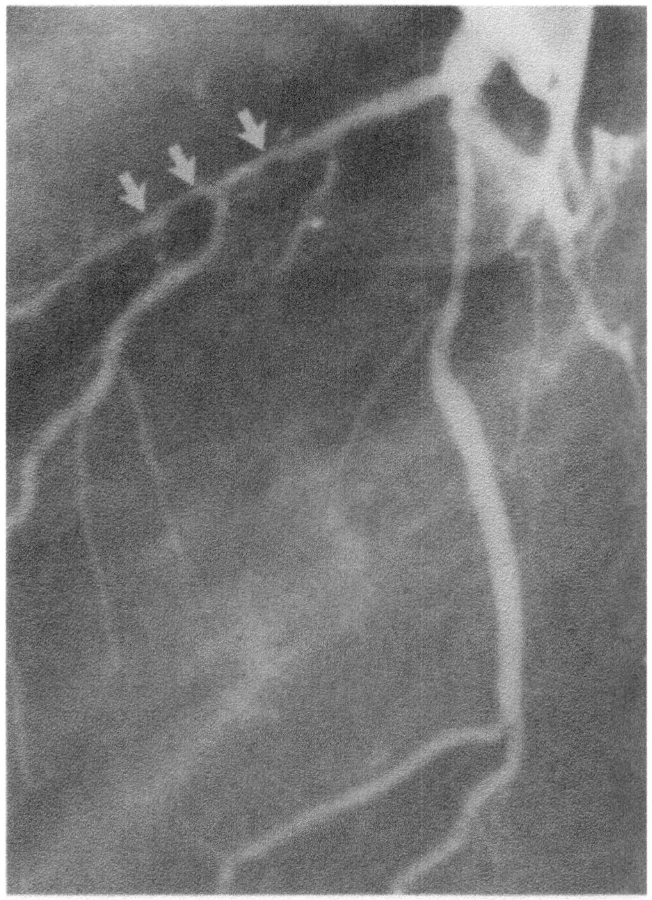

Figure 19.8. Stenosis with multiple irregularities. LCA angiogram in a 50-year-old white male showing severe diffuse disease with multiple irregularities of the proximal and mid-segments of the LAD (→). Contrast left ventricular angiography showed moderate hypokinesis of the antero-lateral wall.

stenoses, with 50% or more lumen diameter reduction, are often oriented to angioplasty or bypass surgery.

Number of lesions

Various indices have been proposed for a global evaluation of extent and severity of disease. Most epidemiologic studies have however retained the number of diseased vessels as the predictor of prognosis. Recently, an extent score of disease has been used to study progression of coronary artery disease and the risk of an acute coronary artery event [11]. This extent score can be

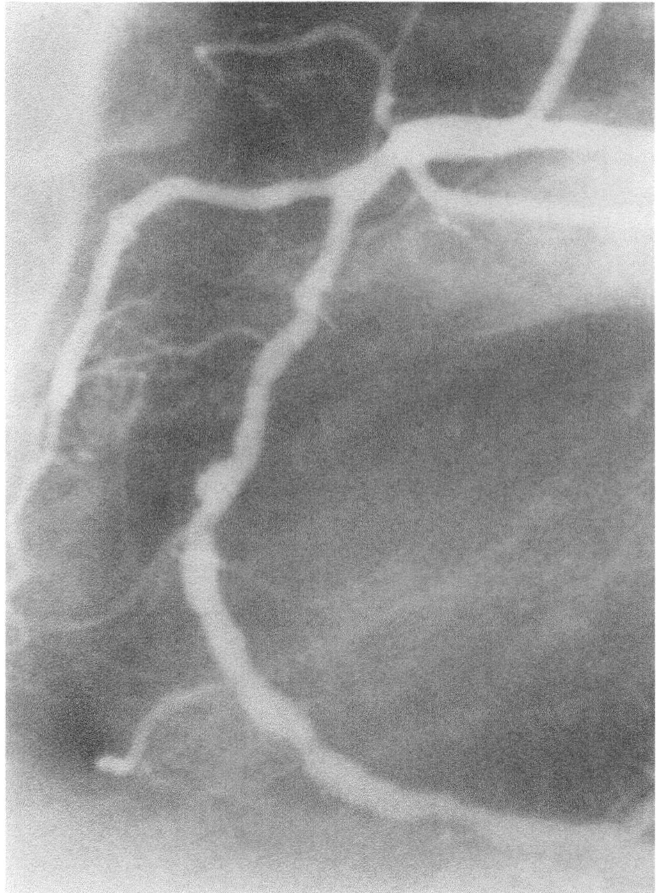

Figure 19.9. LCA angiogram in a 55-year-old white male showing diffuse atherosclerotic coronary artery disease of the dominant RCA with normal CLV. This aspect should be differentiated from plaque ulceration and from stenoses with multiple irregularities.

assessed as the simple mathematical addition of all segments with minimal stenosis or more. An extent score of 4 or more is associated with a greater risk of subsequent progression and occlusion. Figure 19.6 is an example of a patient with a high extent score.

Angiographic morphology preceding the acute event

Lesion severity

The risk of progression to total occlusion increases with the severity of the stenosis. In a prospective 2–year follow-up of 335 patients, it was less than

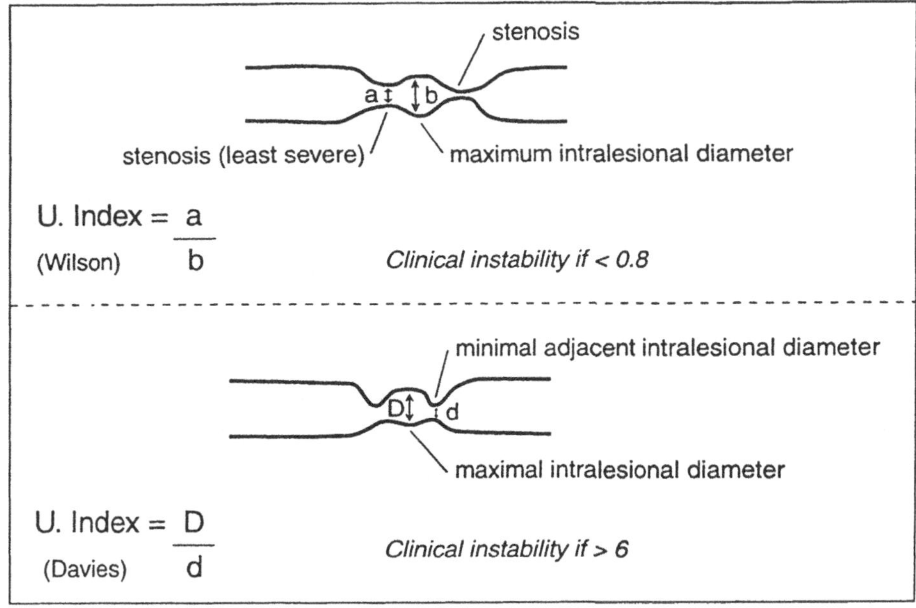

Figure 19.10. Two related methods for quantifying the degree of ulceration. The indices derived can be useful to identify unstable and higher risk patients.

1% for stenoses smaller than 40% and more than 20% for stenosis greater than 70% (Figure 19.11 top) [7]. Interestingly, only 22% of new occlusions were associated with myocardial infarction. Occlusions leading to myocardial infarction were associated with less severe initial stenosis. Occlusion of more severe stenoses resulted sometimes in unstable angina, more severe angina or were often asymptomatic (Figure 19.12). Examples of non-severe stenosis with subsequent thrombus formation and myocardial infarction are shown in Figures 19.1, 19.2 and 19.6. Figure 19.6 more specifically shows thrombus formation on a moderate stenosis of the right coronary artery, whereas the most severe stenoses on the left coronary angiogram remained unchanged.

Lesion morphology

The lesions associated with a higher risk of acute coronary syndrome in addition of being of modest severity, present morphologic features that favor flow separation and turbulence: they possess steeper inflow and outflow angles often with a division branch in their vicinity (Figures 19.3, 19.5A and 19.6A) [2]. The lesions may also be longer, irregular, and may occur at sites of an angulation or bending of 45° or more [4].

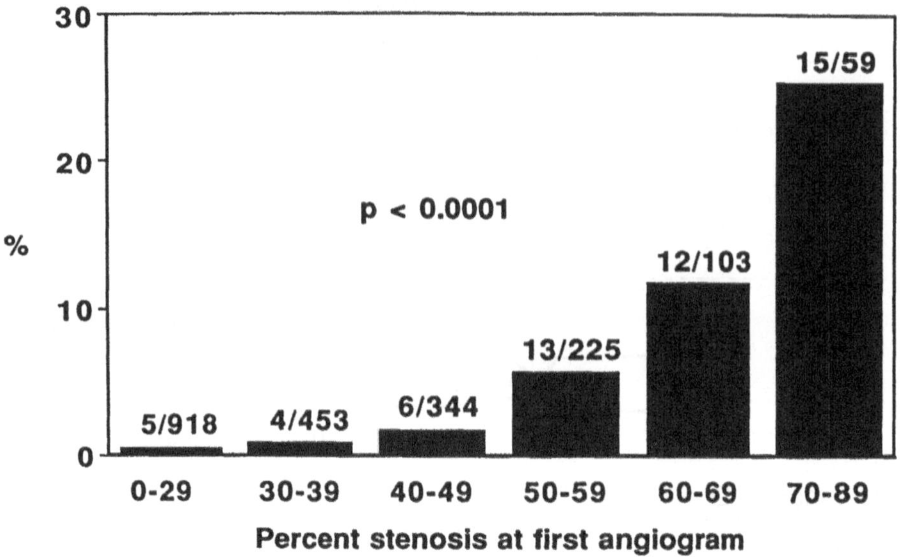

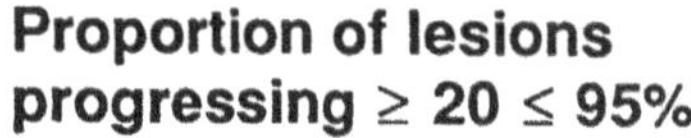

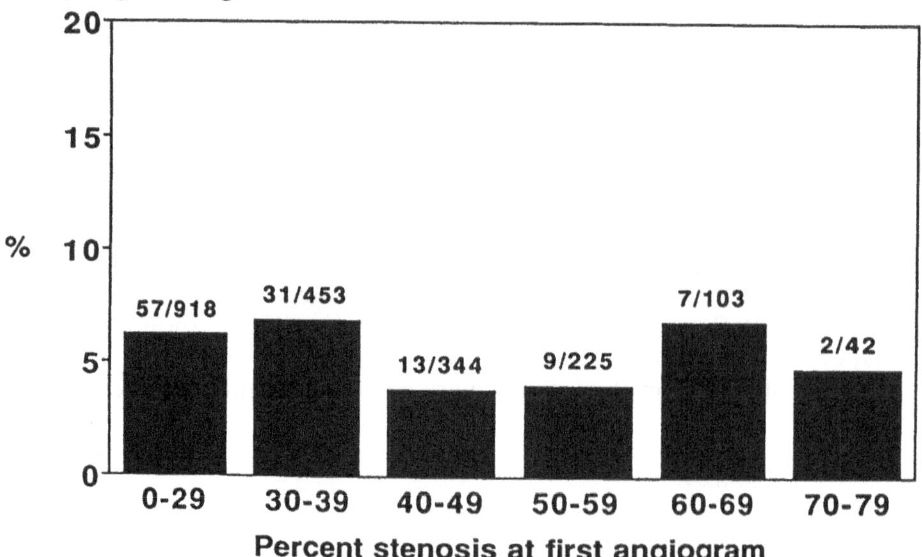

Figure 19.11. Progression to occlusion is more frequent with more severe initial stenoses (top). Progression, excluding occlusion is however independent of the initial degree of stenosis (bottom).

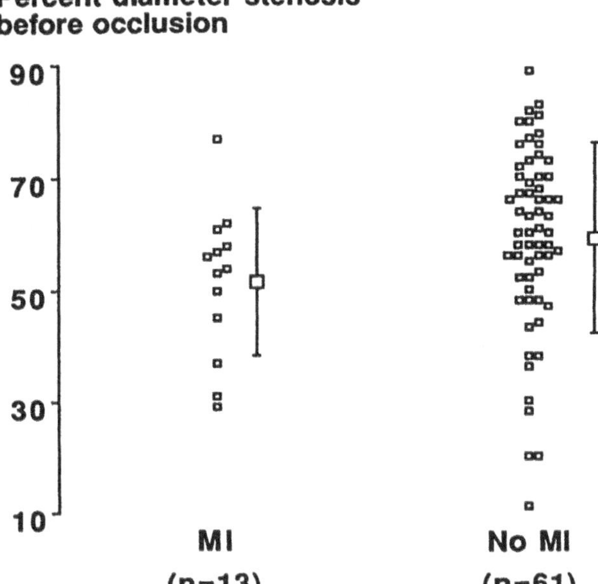

Figure 19.12. The new coronary occlusions after a follow-up of 2 years in a prospective angiographic trial were associated with myocardial infarction when the initial stenosis was less severe. More severe stenoses occluded more often but without creating a myocardial infarction. In only one lesion with an initial stenosis greater than 70% was the occlusion associated with a myocardial infarction.

Extent score

Progression without occlusion as opposed to progression to occlusion is not related to the initial severity of the stenosis and occurs as frequently in less severe as in more severe stenosis (Figure 19.11 bottom). Such progression can be independently predicted by the extent of coronary artery disease as assessed by the extent score [11]. A higher score thus marks not only more extensive but also more active disease. Progression may occur more frequently in larger >2 mm) arteries, in a proximal or mid-artery position and in the right coronary artery [12]. Progression in serial angiograms should be recognized since it is associated with an impaired prognosis [13, 14]. Table 19.1 summarizes the variable correlation of some of the morphologic features in the prediction of coronary disease progression.

Table 19.1. Morphologic features predictive of coronary disease progression.

	Positive correlation	Negative correlation
Steep inflow angle	Taeymans [2] Ambrose [5]	Davies [6] Ellis [4]
Eccentricity	Ellis (borderline significance, $p < 0.06$) [4]	Kalbfleisch [10] Davies [6] Taeymans [2]
Luminal irregularities	Ellis [4] Waters [7]	Taeymans [2]
Branch point	Ellis [4] Taeymans [2]	Davies [6]
Length (tubular)	Ellis [4]	Davies [6] Taeymans [2]
Bend point > 45°	Ellis [4]	Davies [6]
Site proximal, or mid-artery position and right coronary artery	Jost [12]	
Size > 2 mm	Jost [12]	
Extent score: ⩾4 lesions of ⩽75%	Moise [11] Waters [13]	

Lesion characteristics during the acute phase

Unstable angina

Unstable angina marks progression of the severity of the lesions [15], usually caused by an intracoronary thrombus only partially obstructing (Figure 19.4) [5]. Ambrose *et al.* classified the coronary artery lesions into (1) concentric, with symmetric narrowing and smooth or only slightly irregular borders (Figures 19.3A and 19.6B), (2) type I eccentric, with asymmetric stenosis but broad base and smooth borders (Figure 19.2A), (3) type II eccentric with the asymmetry forming an angulated intraluminal obstruction with a narrow base due to one or more overhanging edges (Figures 19.1B, 19.4 and 19.5) or borders that are irregular or ulcerated (Figures 19.1B and 19.6), and (4) multiple irregularities (Figure 19.8). Concentric, type I eccentric and multiple irregularities are found in patients with stable angina and type II eccentric in patients with unstable angina [5]. The TIMI-3A study characterized the culprit lesion within 24 hours after unstable angina or non-Q-wave MI in 306 patients. An absence of flow (TIMI 0) was found in 18% of patients. An apparent thrombus was present 35% and a possible thrombus in 40%. The plaque was ulcerated in 12% and the lumen eccentric in 39% [16].

Acute Q-wave myocardial infarction

An occlusive thrombus is almost invariably found in acute myocardial infarction with ST segment elevation. In the initial description by De Wood et al, an occlusive thrombus was observed in 84% of patients catheterized within 6 hours after onset of symptoms [17]. The typical angiographic aspect is shown in Figures 19.2C, 19.5B and 19.7A. Following thrombus lysis, the underlying plaque shows residual intraluminal thrombus (Figure 19.3A) and sometimes plaque rupture (Figure 19.1B). The severity and characteristics of the underlying plaque can be better appreciated later after complete resorption of the thrombus (Figures 19.1C, 19.2E and 19.3B).

Angiographic morphology after the event

The presence of a complex lesion in patients with an acute coronary syndrome predicts more in-hospital coronary events (Figures 19.5 and 19.6) and also a higher risk of acute thrombosis complicating balloon angioplasty. Acute procedural occlusion in a consecutive series of 1423 angioplasties from the Thoraxcenter, was independently predicted by unstable angina, multivessel disease and the presence of a complex lesion [18]. The ulceration index calculated after thrombolytic therapy predicted early clinical instability [6]. The presence of a residual thrombus after thrombolysis was also predictive of reocclusion 3 months after balloon angioplasty [19]. A decrease in the ulceration index commonly occurs during heparin therapy in the days following infarction. Nakagawa *et al.* used serial angiography to document the resorption of thrombus and remodeling of the mural architecture that occurs over 1 month with rigorous anticoagulation [20].

Much remains to be learned about the angiographic anatomy of the plaque and a need for some form of quantification exists. Our understanding of the pathophysiologic process will be accelerated by the additional information provided by angioscopy and by intravascular ultrasound.

References

1. Mock MB, Ringqvist I, Fisher LD *et al.* Survival of medically treated patients in the Coronary Artery Surgery Study (CASS) registry. Circulation 1982; 66: 562–8.
2. Taeymans Y, Théroux P, Lespérance J, Waters D. Quantitative angiographic morphology of the coronary artery lesions at risk of thrombotic occlusion. Circulation 1992; 85: 78–85.
3. Levin DC, Fallon JT. Significance of the angiographic morphology of localized coronary stenoses: histopathologic correlations. Circulation 1982; 66: 316–20.
4. Ellis S, Alderman EL, Cain K, Wright A, Bourassa M, Fisher L. Morphology of left anterior descending coronary territory lesions as a predictor of anterior myocardial infarction: a CASS Registry Study. J Am Coll Cardiol 1989; 13: 1481–91.

5. Ambrose JA, Winters SL, Stern A *et al.* Angiographic morphology and the pathogenesis of unstable angina pectoris. J Am Coll Cardiol 1985; 5: 609–16.
6. Davies SW, Marchant B, Lyons JP *et al.* Irregular coronary lesion morphology after thrombolysis predicts early clinical instability. J Am Coll Cardiol 1991; 18: 669–74.
7. Waters D, Lespérance J, Hudon G. Progression of coronary atherosclerosis: a prospective, quantitative angiographic study [abstract]. Circulation 1990; 82 (4 Suppl): III-251.
8. Wilson RF, Holida MD, White CW. Quantitative angiographic morphology of coronary stenoses leading to myocardial infarction or unstable angina. Circulation 1986; 73: 286–93.
9. Freeman MR, Williams AE, Chisholm RJ, Armstrong PW. Intracoronary thrombus and complex morphology in unstable angina. Relation to timing of angiography and in-hospital cardiac events. Circulation 1989; 80: 17–23.
10. Kalbfleisch SJ, McGillem MJ, Simon SB, DeBoe SF, Pinto IMF, Mancini GBJ. Automated quantitation of indexes of coronary lesion complexity. Comparison between patients with stable and unstable angina. Circulation 1990; 82: 439–47.
11. Moise A, Théroux P, Taeymans Y *et al.* Clinical and angiographic factors associated with progression of coronary artery disease. J Am Coll Cardiol 1984; 3: 659–67.
12. Jost S, Deckers JW, Nikutta P *et al.* Progression of coronary artery disease is dependent on anatomic location and diameter. The INTACT investigators. J Am Coll Cardiol 1993; 21: 1339–46.
13. Waters D, Lespérance J, Craven TE, Hudon G, Gillam LD. Advantages and limitations of serial coronary arteriography for the assessment of progression and regression of coronary atherosclerosis. Implications for clinical trials. Circulation 1993; 87 (3 Suppl): II-38-47.
14. Buchwald H, Matts JP, Fitch LL, Stamler J. Clinical prognostic significance of serial changes in coronary arteriograms: 10-year data from the Program on the Surgical Control of the Hyperlipidemias (POSCH) [abstract]. Circulation 1991; 84 (4 Suppl): II-287.
15. Moise A, Théroux P, Taeymans Y *et al.* Unstable angina and progression of coronary atherosclerosis. N Engl J Med 1983; 309: 685–9.
16. Early effects of tissue-type plasminogen activators added to conventional therapy on the culprit coronary lesion in patients presenting with ischemic cardiac pain at rest. Results of the Thrombolysis in Myocardial Ischemia (TIMI IIIA) trial. Circulation 1993; 87: 38–52.
17. DeWood MA, Spores J, Notske R *et al.* Prevalence of total coronary occlusion during the early hours of transmural myocardial infarction. N Engl J Med 1980; 303: 897–902.
18. de Feyter PJ, van den Brand M, Jaarman GJ, van Domburg R, Serruys PW, Suryapranata H. Acute coronary artery occlusion during and after percutaneous transluminal coronary angioplasty. Frequency, prediction, clinical course, management, and follow-up. Circulation 1991; 83: 927–36.
19. de Guise P, Théroux P, Bonan R, Lévy G, Côté G, Crépeau J. Re-thrombosis after successful thrombolysis and angioplasty in acute myocardial infarction [abstract]. J Am Coll Cardiol 1988; 11 Suppl A: 192A.
20. Nakagawa S, Hanada Y, Koiwaya Y, Tanaka K. Angiographic features in the infarct-related artery after intracoronary urokinase followed by prolonged anticoagulation. Role of ruptured atheromatous plaque and adherent thrombus in acute myocardial infarction. Circulation 1988; 78: 1335–44.

PART FIVE

QCA in recanalization techniques

20. Laser overview

ANDREAS BAUMBACH, KARL K. HAASE &
KARL R. KARSCH

Summary

The use of laser irradiation in the setting of coronary angioplasty has concentrated on pulsed excimer laser systems. Acute results and complications have been reported to multicenter registries in the US and Europe. All clinical studies documented the safety and feasibility of coronary excimer laser angioplasty. As demonstrated in these registries, the acute results are comparable to conventional balloon angioplasty. The primary use of excimer laser angioplasty for specific complex lesion morphology (long lesions, ostial lesions, calcified stenoses, total occlusions, saphenous vein grafts, and after unsuccessful balloon dilatation) is suggested by two of the ongoing multicenter registries. However, these indications await approval by randomized clinical trials. Fatal complications of laser angioplasty are correlated to high-risk patients. The results suggest that perforations are more frequently seen at vessel branch points, in total occlusions and female patients. It is of major importance that the size of the catheter needs to be adjusted to the vessel diameter. The incidence of restenosis is 47 to 56%, thus a reduction of restenosis could not be achieved using the current technology.

Future developments include the use of systems with a reduced extent of pressure wave formation and vapor bubble expansion and smart lasers with the ability to identifiy the target tissue using laser spectroscopy.

Introduction

The use of percutaneous transluminal coronary angioplasty has gained widespread acceptance as a symptomatic treatment for obstructive coronary artery disease. Within 14 years of clinical application, balloon technology and operator skill have reached a tremendous quality and the indications for PTCA were extended to patients with multivessel disease and complex lesion morphology. Initial drawbacks of the method in the treatment of complicated lesions [1] were reduced, and recent reports of the results document a high success rate for most of the target lesions [2]. Nevertheless, in an effort to further optimize the results achieved with the percutaneous approach to a narrowed or occluded coronary artery, an arsenal of new devices was developed, and the operators are confrontated with various technologies, promising improved outcome for specific indications. However, while acute

J.H.C. Reiber and P.W. Serruys (eds): Progress in quantitative coronary arteriography, 327–338.

results are favorable, the major limitation of coronary angioplasty remains the incidence of restenosis, reducing the long-term efficacy of this treatment to approximately 50%. In this chapter we want to focus on a technology, which was initially designed to improve both, acute results and long-term efficacy of coronary angioplasty. We will summarize the experimental and clinical results achieved with different laser systems and comment on current experimental investigations and their impact on the future development of clinical laser applications.

Laser systems

When laser irradiation is used in the setting of percutaneous transluminal coronary angioplasty, the major advantage of this technique is thought to be a reduction of the atherosclerotic plaque with only minimal injury to the adjacent vessel wall structures [3, 4]. As opposed to a mandatory fissuring and cracking of the plaque and overdistension of the arterial wall using conventional PTCA [5–7], the new method may have the theoretical potential of reducing complications, and, probably as a result of reduced injury, resulting in a reduction of restenosis [8].

Initial experience was achieved with continuous wave laser systems, which used heat as a major mechanism of stenosis reduction. Hot tip lasers had a metal tip, which was irradiated by a laser source, thus avoiding direct laser irradiation of tissue. The heated tip leads to a coagulation of the plaque material [9]. Other systems were designed to apply laser irradiation directly to the target tissue and reduce the atherosclerotic plaque by coagulation [9, 10]. However, the use of heat in the coronary artery turned out to be associated with high complication rates, especially vasospasm and perforations [10–13]. Thus, the clincial investigations with continuous wave lasers were not further extended.

The profile of pulsed excimer laser irradiation was attractive for clinical use for several reasons: Excimer lasers emit ultraviolet light, which is absorbed by proteins, not by water [14]. Ablation of plaque material can be achieved with minimal thermal injury to adjacent tissue structures [3]. The ablation process is precisely limited to the fiber area in contact with the tissue and the low ablation depth of 10–20 μm per pulse prevents extensive ablation into deeper vessel wall layers. Three systems are available for clinical use. All three are xenon-chloride excimer lasers with a wavelength of 308 nm. There are differences in pulsewidth and catheter design. The technique of laser angioplasty and the laser systems have been described in detail elsewhere [15–17].

Holmium lasers were thought to be a promising alternative to excimer laser systems. Holmium light is absorbed in water, ablation of tissue follows the vaporisation of the water molecules bound in the target tissue structures. The ablation depth of a holmium laser pulse is up to 100 fold higher as compared to an excimer laser pulse in soft, fibrous and calcified plaque [18]. However, experimental investigations *in-vivo*, comparing the histologic results and the proliferative response to holmium and excimer laser irradiation in the rabbit carotid artery showed an extensive tissue damage followed by holmium laser treatment. Dissections, thermal injury and destruction of cell nuclei in the media were frequent observations [19]. Although a clinical trial on holmium laser coronary angioplasty is still running, no published data on the clinical experience are available so far.

Acute results

Initial clinical results with excimer laser angioplasty were reported for all systems [15–17] and documented safety and feasibility of the procedure. The first experience with the Technolas system (Max 10, Technolas, Munich) was achieved with a prototype catheter system [15]. Although the improvement of catheter and system parameters resulted in an improved success rate [20], the number of patients treated with this system was limited. Larger patient cohorts were treated with the AIS (Pulsewidth >180 ns, Advanced Interventional Systems, Irvine, CA) and Spectranetics (Pulsewidth 135 ns, Spectranetics Inc., Colorado Springs, CO) excimer lasers. The results have been reported to multicenter databases for both systems by the investigators in the US and to the European Coronary Excimer Laser Angioplasty Registry by several centers in Europe.

An analysis of lesions not ideal for balloon dilatation was published by Cook *et al.* on 100 patients undergoing excimer laser angioplasty [21]. They reported a success rate of 86% on a subgroup of 10 tubular stenoses, 29 diffuse lesions, 18 chronic total occlusions, and eight ostial lesions. Bittl *et al.* [22] documented favorable success rates for a subgroup of 6 lesion types, which they entitled the "alpha class" of lesions: saphenous vein graft lesions, long lesions, ostial lesions, calcified stenoses, total occlusions, and unsuccessful balloon dilatation. This analysis was performed on 764 patients of the Spectranetics registry. The FDA gave approval for the system for these 6 indications. However, since the comparison of the laser results relies on historical data for the results of conventional balloon dilatation, these results warrant verification in controlled trials.

The European Coronary Excimer Laser Angioplasty Registry was initiated in 1990 to assess information on acute results, complications, and longterm efficacy of the procedure. The registry is coordinated by a steering committee in association with the European Society of Cardiology, which had approved the registry protocol. Participation in the registry is solely voluntary. Patient selection and laser intervention was performed depending on the discretion of the individual investigator. All patients must be candidates for conventional PTCA. There are no additional inclusion or exclusion criteria. However, advice was given to restrict the treatment of complicated lesions to experi-

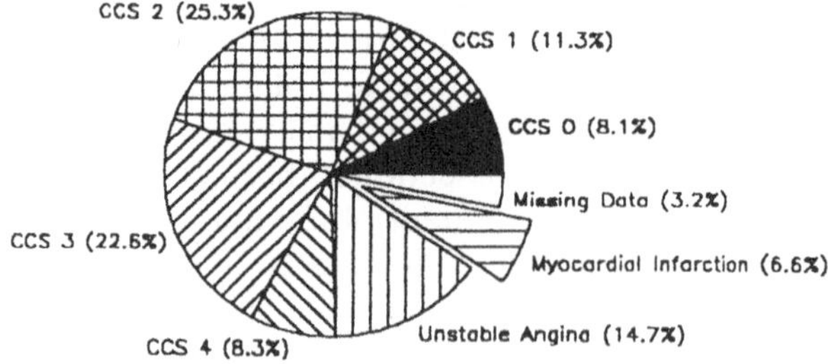

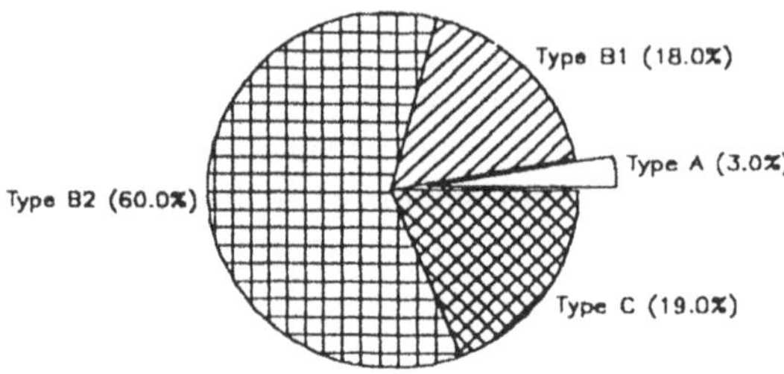

Figure 20.1. Frequency of symptoms and lesion types in the population of the European Coronary excimer Laser Angioplasty Registry.

enced operators and to avoid treatment of acute ischemic syndromes. Quantitative coronary analysis (QCA) was performed in a central core-lab (Deutsches Herzzentrum Berlin). Data on 477 lesions treated in 470 patients are available from 11 centers in Europe. The number of patients per center varied between 2 and 159. The symptom classification according to the Canadian Cardiovascular Function Score [23] and acute ischemic syndroms and the distribution of the lesion types according to the classification of the AHA/ACC task force [24] in the modification of Ellis *et al.* [1] is illustrated in Figure 20.1. One obvious difference to the US trials is, that the trend toward treatment of complex lesions and saphenous vein grafts is more dominant in the US multicenter populations.

Failure of laser angioplasty occurred in 57 interventions (11.9%). The reason for laser failure was inability to cross the lesion despite energy delivery (N:37, 65%), to reach the lesion with the laser catheter (N:11, 19%), to place the guide wire (N:3, 5%), to select the target vessel with the guide catheter (N:1, 2%), due to guide catheter backup (N:1, 2%), or due to laser system failure (N:4, 7%). Analysis of the angiographic data in failed laser procedures revealed a higher incidence of failure in long segmental lesions, lesions located in vessel bends, total occlusions and lesions in segments distal to vessel tortuosities. In the logistic regression analysis, long segmental

Table 20.1. Complications of coronary excimer laser angioplasty. Results from the European Coronary Excimer Laser Angioplasty Registry.

N:477 minor complications	Observed following laser	%	Observed following PTCA[a]
Vasospasm	64	13.4%	11
Thrombus formation	23	4.8%	14
Embolization	2	0.4%	1
Minor dissection	70	14.7%	88
Severe dissection	19	4.0%	19
Acute closure	37	7.8%	13
Extravasation of dye	8	1.7%	0
Severe perforation	1	0.2%	1
Major complications	N	%	
Myocardial infarction	10	2.1%	
CABG	9	1.9%	
Death	7	1.5%	

[a] Includes interventions with observation of the same complication post laser.
[b] CABG: coronary artery bypass grafting during the hospitalization.

lesions, occlusions and severe prestenotic vessel tortuosity were independent risk factors for laser failure. Using conventional balloon angioplasty procedural success was achieved in 41/57 cases following laser failure.

Stand alone laser angioplasty was performed in 83 interventions (17.4%). Additional balloon angioplasty was performed following laser angioplasty to improve the angiographic result in 277 interventions and due to complications in 60 interventions (not including interventions following laser failure). In 6 interventions a stent was implanted as a bail-out procedure. Procedural success was achieved in 76/83 stand-alone interventions, and in 308/337 combined laser and balloon interventions. The overall procedural success therefore was 89.1%. An analysis of procedural success revealed a higher success rate in single discrete lesions and reduced success was associated with the presence of thrombus and calcification in the multivariate analysis. The complications of the procedure are given in Table 20.1. Fatal complications occurred in 4/100 patients (4%) treated for unstable angina pectoris or myocardial infarction and in 3/370 patients (0.8%) with stable angina pectoris.

QCA was performed on 317 interventions. The lumen achieved by laser angioplasty showed a correlation to the catheter size used (Figure 20.2). Additional balloon angioplasty resulted in a significant luminal increase (Figure 20.3). Therefore, larger size catheters or catheters with an eccentric and steerable design are neccessary to achieve larger luminal increase and to reduce the need for additional balloon angioplasty.

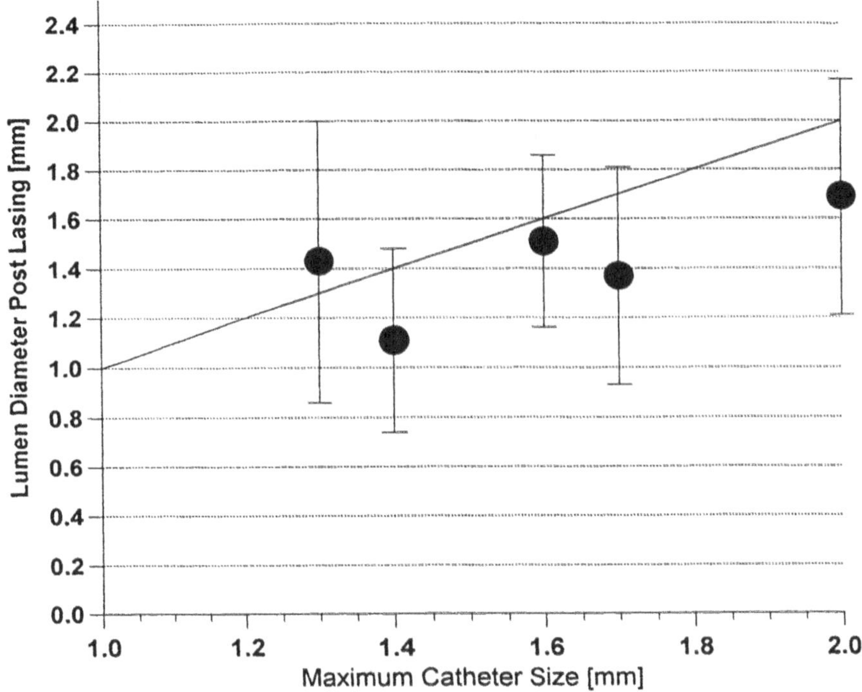

Figure 20.2. Catheter size and lumen diameter after excimer laser irradiation. Results of QCA analysis.

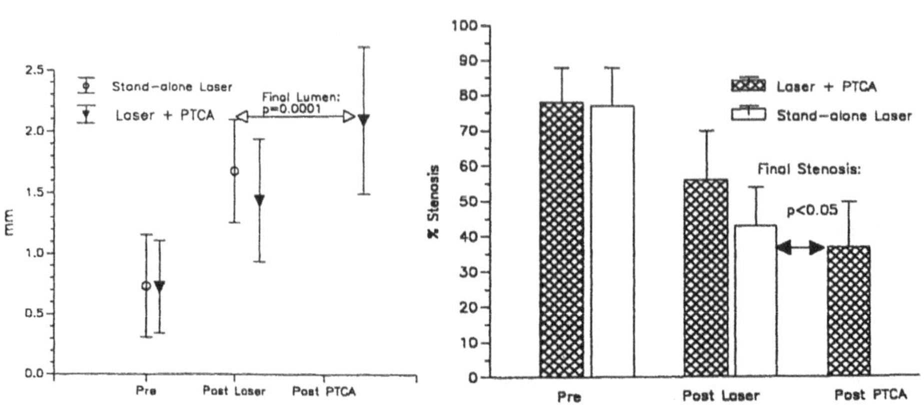

Figure 20.3. Lumen diameter and percent stenosis before treatment, following laser angioplasty and following additional balloon angioplasty.

Complications

Analyses performed on complications of excimer laser angioplasty revealed a correlation of larger catheter size and higher energy densities with the incidence of dissections [25]. Vessel wall dissection is the most frequently observed overall and laser-related complication. Due to the mechanism of the procedure, dissection is an almost inevitable consequence of balloon dilatation [6, 7, 26], although angiography reveals dissections after PTCA in only 14–32% of cases [27, 28]. This rate is comparable to that found in the laser studies. However, the initial expectations based upon the different mechanism of stenosis reduction using excimer laser irradiation suggested a reduced vessel injury. In early clinical studies, mechanical side effects and ineffective ablation was thought to be responsible for observed side effects [15]. However, the development of newer devices with reduced mechanical dead space at the catheter tip and the transmission of high energy densities via fibers with increased ablation efficacy did not result in the expected reduction of dissections [29]. Thus, the clinical observations suggest that intimal dissection may be a direct result of laser irradiation. This is substantiated by recent experimental findings of vapor bubble formation [30] and pressure waves [31], which are associated with the ablation process following excimer laser irradiation.

The demand for larger laser catheters is therefore limited by the considerations on laser induced vessel trauma. A recently published paper by Bittl *et al.* [32] found a higher incidence of perforations in interventions performed with a catheter size which was equivalent to the vessel diameter. A safety margin of 1 mm was proposed to reduce the risk of perforations. The incidence of complications was increased in lesions located at vessel branch points [22, 32]. Further specific lesion morphologic parameters were also found to be a risk factor for dissections and perforations in an extensive analysis of laser complications [25]. Two morphological variables were associated with a higher incidence of dissections: lesion length of more than 10 mm and presence of a side branch. Obviously, the ostium of a side branch at the lesion site represents a possible location for laser irradiation into the normal vascular wall, if the laser catheter is not strictly coaxially positioned. Especially in these situations, ablation into the media may occur and induce dissection. Longer lesions may just have a higher statistical chance of dissection by neccessitating longer irradiation times. Perforations were found to occur more frequently in female patients, total occlusions and lesions at vessel branch points [25, 32]. The higher incidence of perforations in occlusions and branch points may be due to an increased risk of laser irradiation into deeper vessel wall layers, because coaxial alignment of the laser catheter is difficult under these conditions. The angle of the channel created is determined by the alignment of the catheter to the vessel wall. If ablation deep into the medial layer occurs, the created channel most probably has an oblique direction through the wall. Although acoustic side effects [31] and vapor bubble expansion [30] in deeper wall layers remain to be investigated, scattering of tissue is likely to occur. Thus, whether extravasation of contrast media after laser irradiation represents an oblique direct channel or a complex dissection with scattering of medial and adventitial tissue remains open to question. It is of importance that balloon angioplasty can resolve the extravasation in many cases [29, 33, 34], probably by simply compressing the vessel wall.

However, the overall complication rate of coronary excimer laser angioplasty compares with the results of conventional balloon dilatation [2, 27]. The incidence of vasospasm is low in the patient cohorts, which are almost routinely treated with laser and additional balloon angioplasty. Vessel closure following laser and balloon angioplasty also shows an incidence comparable to conventional balloon dilatation [35]. The incidence of fatal complications is related to the treatment of patients with a high risk for percutaneous interventions.

Longterm success

The data available on the longterm success of coronary excimer laser angioplasty suggest, that the incidence of restenosis is not reduced with the current laser technology.

Initial reports showed an incidence of restenosis of 42% [15]. However, the longterm results achieved with an improved technology did not show a significant improvement. Bittl and Sanborn [36] reported on a cohort of 200 patients with a clinical 6 months follow-up in 98.5% and an angiographic follow-up in 83.1%. Restenosis defined as a reduction of the lumen diameter of more than 50% was found in 47.6% of patients. Follow-up angiography is available on 114 patients in the European Coronary Excimer Laser Angioplasty Registry. QCA-Analysis documented a restenosis rate of 56%. The incidence of restenosis was higher in a small subgroup of patients after standalone laser angioplasty (69%; N:18), as compared with patients who were treated with laser and additional balloon angioplasty (50%, N:44). However, the difference did not show statistical significance.

Experimental results and future clinical applications

Recent experimental findings demonstrated rapidly expanding vapor bubbles, which occur immediately after laser ablation. On the way of least resistance this bubble probably seeks the cleavage plane between plaque and media [30, 37], causing intimal dissection. Furthermore, shock waves resulting in barotrauma of vessel wall structures adjacent to the ablation site occur routinely following the ablation process [31, 38]. Since excimer laser irradiation is absorbed in blood, contact of fiber with blood during irradiation results in pressure wave formation as well.

Recently, a method of flushing the coronary artery with saline infusion during excimer laser irradiation has been introduced [39] and a clinical study was designed. By lowering the concentration of blood in front of the catheter tip, the authors aim at reducing the extent of pressure wave formation. Another method of reducing the amount of pressure waves generated per laser pulse, is realized in the SELCA (Smooth Excimer Laser Coronary Angioplasty) system. The fiber area at the catheter tip is divided into 8 to 12 fiber bundles. Each bundle is separately irradiated. This results in a reduced area at the tip, which emits the laser light one at a time. As a consequence, the volume of the resulting mass explosion is reduced and the peak pressures measured lateral to the catheter tip are reduced approximately 8-fold as compared to a conventional front firing excimer laser system. Initial experimental results proved the efficacy of the system. The etch rates were documented to be comparable to conventional systems [9]. An *in-vivo* study showed a reduced response of the rabbit carotid artery in terms of smooth muscle cell proliferation as compared to conventional excimer laser treatment [40]. Initial results of the human application are promising; however, the limited number of patients treated with this innovative technology does not yet allow for precise and sufficient interpretation.

A possible and promising future approach in laser technology is the use of spectroscopy as a tool to identify the target tissue [41]. Provided the ability to distinguish atherosclerotic from normal arterial tissue by their characteristic fluorescence spectra, remote spectroscopy through optical fibers can be incorporated into a 'smart' laser angioplasty system. By detecting the presence of atherosclosis, and by signalling completion of plaque ablation, fluorescence spectroscopy could guide selective laser ablation of atherosclerotic plaques. This guidance capability could result in safe and effective laser angioplasty systems.

Conclusion

The clinical results documented the safety and feasibility of the method. Indications for the primary use of laser angioplasty have to be determined in randomized trials. However, the incidence of restenosis is not reduced by laser angioplasty using the current technology.

Despite these interim results, it has to be stated that there is an enormous potential for considerable improvements. Laser angioplasty represents a complex technology which is in the state of development. The capacity of systems with reduced pressure wave formation and with the ability to detect the target tissue await further experimental and clinical studies.

References

1. Ellis SG, Vandormael MG, Cowley MJ, DiSciascio G, Deligonul U, Topol EJ. Coronary morphologic and clinical determinants of procedural outcome with angioplasty for multivessel coronary disease. Implications for patient selection.Multivessel Angioplasty Prognosis Study Group. Circulation 1990; 82: 1193–202.
2. Myler RK, Shaw RE, Stertzer SH *et al.* Lesion morphology and coronary angioplasty: current experience and analysis. J Am Coll Cardiol 1992; 19: 1641–52.
3. Grundfest WS, Litvack F, Forrester JR *et al.* Laser ablation of human atherosclerotic plaque without adjacent tissue injury. J Am Coll Cardiol 1985; 5: 929–33.
4. Isner JM, Gal D, Steg PG *et al.* Percutaneous, *in vivo* excimer laser angioplasty: results in two experimental animal models. Lasers Surg Med 1988; 8: 223–32.
5. Waller BF. Pathology of new interventions used in the treatment of coronary heart disease. Curr Probl Cardiol 1986; 11: 665–760.
6. Steele PM, Chesebro JH, Stanson AW *et al.* Balloon angioplasty. Natural history of the pathophysiological response to injury in a pig model. Circ Res 1985; 57: 105–12.
7. Waller BF. "Crackers, breakers, stretchers, drillers, scrapers, shavers, burners, welders and melters" – the future treatment of atherosclerotic coronary artery disease? A clinical-morphologic assessment. J Am Coll Cardiol 1989; 13: 969–87.
8. Hanke H, Haase KK, Hanke S *et al.* Morphological changes and smooth muscle cell proliferation after experimental excimer laser treatment. Circulation 1991; 83: 1380–9.
9. Sanborn TA, Faxon DP, Haudenschild CC, Ryan TJ. Experimental angioplasty: circumferential distribution of laser thermal energy with a laser probe. J Am Coll Cardiol 1985; 5: 934–8.
10. Sanborn TA, Faxon DP, Kellet MA, Ryan TJ. Percutaneous coronary laser thermal angioplasty. J Am Coll Cardiol 1986; 8: 1437–40.
11. Lee G, Seckinger D, Chan MC, Embi A *et al.* Potential complications of coronary laser angioplasty. Am Heart J 1984; 108: 1577–9.
12. Consigny PM, Teitelbaum GP, Gardiner GA Jr, Kerns WD. Effects of laser thermal angioplasty on arterial contractions and mechanics. Cardiovasc Intervent Radiol 1989; 12: 83–7.
13. Gal D, Steg PG, Rongione AJ, DeJesus ST, Clarke RH, Isner JM. Vascular spasm complicates continuous wave but not pulsed laser irradiation. Am Heart J 1989; 118: 934–41.
14. Haller JD, Srinivasan R. Laser-tissue interactions in laser angioplasty. In Karsch KR, Haase KK (eds): Coronary laser angioplasty: an update. Darmstadt: Steinkopff Verlag 1991: 19–24.
15. Karsch KR, Haase KK, Voelker W, Baumbach A, Mauser M, Seipel L. Percutaneous coronary excimer laser angioplasty in patients with stable and unstable angina pectoris Acute results and incidence of restenosis during 6 month follow-up. Circulation 1990; 81: 1849–59.
16. Litvack F, Eigler NL, Margolis JR *et al.* Percutaneous excimer laser coronary angioplasty. Am J Cardiol 1990; 66: 1027–32.
17. Sanborn TA, Torre SR, Sharma SK *et al.* Percutaneous coronary excimer laser-assisted balloon angioplasty: initial clinical and quantitative angiographic results in 50 patients. J Am Coll Cardiol 1991; 17: 94–9.
18. Haase KK, Baumbach A, Wehrmann M *et al.* Potential use of Holmium lasers for angioplasty: evaluation of a new solid state laser for ablation of atherosclerotic plaque. Lasers Surg Med 1991; 11: 232–7.
19. Hassenstein S, Hanke H, Kamenz J *et al.* Vascular injury and time course of smooth muscle cell proliferation after experimental holmium laser angioplasty. Circulation 1992; 86: 1575–83.
20. Baumbach A, Haase KK, Karsch KR. Improved results of coronary excimer laser angioplasty by the use of advanced transmission devices. Lasers Med Sci 1991; 6: 317–21.

21. Cook SL, Eigler NL, Shefer A, Goldenberg T, Forrester JR, Litvack F. Percutaneous excimer laser coronary angioplasty of lesions not ideal for balloon angioplasty. Circulation 1991; 84: 632–43.
22. Bittl JA, Sanborn TA, Tcheng JE, Siegel RJ, Ellis SG. Clinical success, complications and restenosis rates with excimer laser coronary angioplasty. The Percutaneous Excimer Laser Coronary Angioplasty Registry. Am J Cardiol 1992; 70: 1533–9.
23. Campeau L. Grading of angina pectoris [letter]. Circulation 1976; 54: 522–3.
24. Guidelines for percutaneous transluminal coronary angioplasty: a report of the American College of Cardiology/American Heart Association Task Force on Assessment of Diagnostic and Therapeutic Cardiovascular Procedures (Subcommittee on Percutaneous Transluminal Coronary Angioplasty). J Am Coll Cardiol 1988; 12: 529–45.
25. Baumbach A, Bittl JA, Fleck E *et al.* Acute complications of coronary excimer laser angioplasty: a detailed analysis of multicenter results. J Am Coll Cardiol 1994; in press.
26. Waller BF, Orr CM, Pinkerton CA, Van Tassel J, Peters T, Slack JD. Coronary balloon angioplasty dissections: "the good, the bad and the ugly". J Am Coll Cardiol 1992; 20: 701–6.
27. Dorros G, Cowley MJ, Simpson J *et al.* Percutaneous transluminal coronary angioplasty: report of complications from the National Heart, Lung, and Blood Institute PTCA registry. Circulation 1983; 67: 723–30.
28. Hermans WRM, Rensing BJ, Foley DP *et al.* Therapeutic dissection after successful coronary balloon angioplasty: no influence on restenosis or on clinical outcome in 693 patients. The MERCATOR Study Group (Multicenter European Research Trial with Cilazapril after Angioplasty to prevent Transluminal Coronary Obstruction and Restenosis). J Am Coll Cardiol 1992; 20: 767–80.
29. Haase KK, Baumbach A, Hanke H, Voelker W, Mauser M, Karsch KR. Success rate and incidence of restenosis following coronary excimer laser angioplasty: results of a single center experience. J Intervent Cardiol 1992; 5: 15–23.
30. Van Leeuwen TG, Van Erven L, Meertens JH, Motamedi M, Post MJ, Borst C. Origin of arterial wall dissections induced by pulsed excimer and mid-infrared laser ablation in the pig. J Am Coll Cardiol 1992; 19: 1610–8.
31. Haase KK, Hanke H, Baumbach A *et al.* Occurrence, extent and implications of pressure waves during excimer laser ablation of normal arterial wall and atherosclerotic plaque. Lasers Surg Med 1993; 13: 263–70.
32. Bittl JA, Ryan TJ, Keaney JF Jr *et al.* Coronary artery perforation during excimer laser angioplasty. The Percutaneous Excimer Laser Coronary Angioplasty Registry. J Am Coll Cardiol 1993; 21: 1158–65.
33. Haase KK, Baumbach A, Voelker W, Kühlkamp V, Karsch KR. Gefäßwandperforation nach koronarer Excimer-Laser-Angioplastie. Z Kardiol 1991; 80: 230–3.
34. Parker JD, Ganz P, Selwyn AP, Bittl JA. Successful treatment of an excimer laser-associated coronary artery perforation with the stack perfusion catheter. Cathet Cardiovasc Diagn 1991; 22: 118–23.
35. Detre KM, Holmes DR Jr, Holubkov R *et al.* Incidence and consequences of periprocedural occlusion. The 1985–1986 National Heart, Lung, and Blood Institute Percutaneous Transluminal Coronary Angioplasty Registry. Circulation 1990; 82: 739–50.
36. Bittl JA, Sanborn TA. Excimer laser-facilitated coronary angioplasty. Relative risk analysis of acute and follow-up results in 200 patients. Circulation 1992; 86: 71–80.
37. Isner JM, Pickering JG, Mosseri M. Laser-induced dissections: pathogenesis and implications for therapy. J Am Coll Cardiol 1992; 19: 1619–21.
38. Tomaru T, Geschwind HJ, Boussignac G, Lange F, Tahk SJ. Characteristics of shock waves induced by pulsed lasers and their effects on arterial tissue: comparison of excimer, pulsed dye, and holmium YAG lasers. Am Heart J 1992; 123: 896–904.
39. Tcheng JE, Phillips HR, Wells LD, Golobic RA, Power JA, Deckelbaum LI. A new technique for reducing pressure pulse phenomena during coronary excimer laser angioplasty [Abstract]. J Am Coll Cardiol 1993; 21 (Suppl A): 386A.

40. Oberhoff M, Hassenstein S, Hanke H *et al.* Smooth excimer laser coronary angioplasty (SELCA) – initial experimental results [Abstract]. Circulation 1992; 86 (4 Suppl): I–800.
41. Deckelbaum LI, Lam JK, Cabin HS, Clubb KS, Long MB. Discrimination of normal and atherosclerotic aorta by laser-induced fluorescence. Lasers Surg Med 1987; 7: 330–5.

21. Coronary atherectomy devices

JEFFREY J. POPMA, YA CHIEN CHUANG, GARY S. MINTZ, LUELLA T. LEWIS & MARTIN B. LEON [1]

Summary

New angioplasty devices have been developed to surmount the limitations of standard balloon angioplasty in complex lesion subsets. Two categories of new angioplasty devices have been used: 1) those that extract, ablate, or excise atherosclerotic plaque (atherectomy/ablative devices); and 2) those that mechanically or physiologically scaffold the inner arterial lumen (stents, low stress or thermal angioplasty). This review summarizes the procedural outcome in 1170 patients (1438 lesions) undergoing coronary or saphenous vein graft atherectomy using three clinically available atherectomy devices (directional, rotational, and extraction atherectomy). It is suggested that better initial angiographic results can be obtained with these new devices than with standard balloon angioplasty, due to their effect on lesion compliance and reduction in the magnitude of elastic recoil. Intravascular ultrasound studies have demonstrated that these changes in lesion compliance occur in the absence of complete plaque removal, lending credence to the suggestion that complex (rigid and elastic) lesions can be managed with partial plaque debulking using atherectomy devices followed by balloon dilatation to maximize lumen dimensions. Importantly, the final angiographic result (% diameter stenosis or minimal lumen diameter) appears to be an important predictor of ultimate clinical outcome after new device angioplasty.

Introduction

Over the past 8 years, a variety of new angioplasty devices have been introduced as alternative methods of coronary revascularization in patients with coronary lesions deemed high-risk for standard balloon angioplasty [1, 2]. These new devices may be broadly classified as falling into two categories: 1) those that extract, ablate, or excise atherosclerotic plaque (e.g., directional, rotational, or extraction atherectomy or excimer laser angioplasty); and 2) those that mechanically or physiologically scaffold the inner arterial lumen, thereby reducing elastic recoil (stent, thermal balloon angioplasty). As the experience with new angioplasty devices has evolved, it has become

---

[1] Supported by a Research Grant from the Cardiology Research Foundation.

J.H.C. Reiber and P.W. Serruys (eds): Progress in quantitative coronary arteriography, 339–351.

apparent that no one alternative device will serve as a panacea for all coronary lesions, although *each* new device may yield a particular benefit in one or more high-risk lesion subsets. Accordingly, based on early nonrandomized experience, a lesion-specific approach for new device selection has been proposed [3], but has yet to undergo prospective study. Further recommendations for *generalized* clinical use of these new devices will be derived from well-designed, randomized studies involving standard balloon angioplasty and alternative modalities.

Atherectomy devices have been the most widely used of these alternative angioplasty strategies; 3 atherectomy devices (i.e., directional, rotational, and extraction) have been approved for marketing in the United States by the Food and Drug Administration. Unlike balloon angioplasty, which improves coronary lumen dimensions by stretching and tearing the atherosclerotic plaque [4], atherectomy devices exert their beneficial effect on the coronary lumen by partially extracting, ablating or excising atherosclerotic plaque. Notably, clinical and intravascular ultrasound studies have suggested that actual plaque removal contributes only partially to the final angiographic result obtained with atherectomy devices [5–7]; often, a significant amount of mechanical 'dottering' and balloon dilatation also occur. Given the varying mechanisms and outcomes associated with the use of contemporary atherectomy devices, this chapter has three specific purposes: 1) to review the procedural results, complications and late clinical outcome of 1170 patients (1438 lesions) treated with coronary or saphenous vein graft atherectomy at the Washington Hospital Center over the past 2 years; 2) to discuss the effect of partial plaque removal on lesion compliance and the immediate angiographic result after atherectomy; and 3) to evaluate the potential impact of plaque removal on the late outcome after atherectomy.

Directional coronary atherectomy

Since its initial clinical evaluation in 1986 [8], directional coronary atherectomy has been used in >100,000 patients worldwide. The directional atherectomy catheter (Devices for Vascular Intervention, Redwood City, CA) contains a cylindrical cutter with a unilateral balloon mounted opposite a 9 mm cutting window. After the unilateral balloon has been inflated to 10–40 psi, a motor drive unit rotates the cutting blade at 2000 rpm which is advanced forward and allows resection of biopsy-sized (10–25 mg) fragments of atherosclerotic plaque. A flexible distal nose cone stores the resected atherosclerotic plaque, which is subsequently removed for histologic examination. The principal advantage of this method of atherectomy is its capacity to directionally excise bulky atherosclerotic plaque, potentially avoiding balloon-induced barotrauma and vessel disruption. Its major disadvantage is that it requires the use of large guiding (10 Fr) and atherectomy (5–7 Fr) catheters, which also have the potential to cause traumatic arterial injury (dissection, perforation), particularly in those patients with peripheral vascular disease or smaller (<2.5 mm) coronary or graft vessels.

Nonrandomized single center [9, 10] and randomized multicenter [11, 12] series have reported procedural success rates ranging from 82% to 95% after directional coronary atherectomy. Although these procedural success rates are comparable to [12], or slightly better than [11], those obtained with balloon angioplasty in matched non-complex lesions, the role of directional atherectomy in high-risk lesions (ostial lesions, intimal flaps, focal dissections, saphenous vein graft stenoses) has not been tested in randomized studies. Importantly, when evaluating procedural outcome after directional atherectomy, the 2 components of procedural success – *angiographic success* (final% diameter stenosis <50%) and the development of post procedural *complications* (death, myocardial infarction, and coronary bypass operation) – should be carefully examined. In 2 randomized series of directional atherectomy and balloon angioplasty, angiographic success rates were *higher* for those patients treated with directional atherectomy than balloon angioplasty [11, 12]. However, major peri-procedural complications occurred more often in patients undergoing directional atherectomy in one series [12]; compared with patients treated with balloon angioplasty, patients treated with directional atherectomy had higher rates of myocardial infarction (6% versus 3%; $p = 0.035$), due both to abrupt closure (7% versus 3%) and to isolated enzymatic evidence of myocardial necrosis using creatinine phosphokinase MB levels (19% versus 8%; $p < 0.001$).

These randomized studies of balloon angioplasty and directional atherectomy have also compared the effect of the 2 techniques on the occurrence of restenosis [11, 12]. In one series, 1012 patients were randomly assigned to directional atherectomy (N = 512) or balloon angioplasty (N = 500) [12]. Angiographic follow-up was obtained in 90% of 959 successfully-treated patients; angiographic restenosis (≥50% follow-up diameter stenosis) occurred in 57% of patients treated with balloon angioplasty and 50% of patients treated with directional atherectomy ($p = 0.06$). Importantly, the minimal lumen diameter immediately after the procedure was the most important predictor of the follow-up minimal lumen diameter ($p < 0.001$). Other independent predictors of late angiographic outcome included vessel size ($p < 0.001$), presence of diabetes mellitus ($p < 0.001$), and left anterior descending artery location ($p = 0.02$) [12]. Although the need for repeat revascularization was similar in the 2 groups, the cumulative occurrence of myocardial infarction was significantly higher in patients treated with directional atherectomy (7.6% versus 4.4% for patients treated with balloon angioplasty; $p = 0.04$). In the Canadian Coronary Atherectomy Trial, 274 patients were randomly assigned to treatment with directional atherectomy (N = 138) or balloon angioplasty (N = 136) of the proximal left anterior descending artery. Angiographic restenosis (≥50% follow-up diameter stenosis) occurred in 46% of patients treated with directional atherectomy and in 43% of patients treated with balloon angioplasty (p = 0.71). Clinical outcomes were not significantly different between the two groups.

A 'conservative' atherectomy approach was used by protocol design in both of these studies; the 29% [12] and 26% [11] residual diameter stenoses after directional atherectomy may have had an important influence on the overall procedural outcomes and rates of angiographic restenosis in patients treated with directional atherectomy. Lower residual diameter stenoses (6–18%) and major complications (2–4%) after directional atherectomy have been reported in other single [9, 10] and multicenter [13] reports using an 'aggressive' approach to atherectomy. Adjunct balloon angioplasty was performed, if needed, to optimize the final angiographic result or treat angiographic complications. A critical question remaining is whether a favorable (<15%) residual diameter stenosis after directional atherectomy can be routinely achieved without incurring more frequent complications due to oversized devices and aggressive plaque removal.

Given these results, directional atherectomy should be reserved for those lesions deemed 'high-risk' for complications using standard balloon angioplasty. In our series of 492 lesions treated with directional atherectomy, 94% had one or more adverse morphologic features using the modified criteria [14] of the American College of Cardiology/American Heart Association (Table 21.1); 76% lesions were eccentric, 25% were ostial in location, and 21% had mild-to-moderate calcification. Despite the overall lesion complexity, a 15% residual diameter stenosis and 2.51 ± 0.59 mm minimal lumen diameter were obtained. Adjunct balloon angioplasty was performed in nearly half of the cases, generally to improve the final angiographic result (Table 21.2). Overall procedural success was obtained in 92% of patients treated with directional atherectomy (Table 21.3). Major complications were infrequent (4.2%) and included death (1.2%), Q-wave myocardial infarction (0.5%), and emergency coronary bypass surgery (3.3%). Importantly, over 75% of patients were free from a major cardiac event during the 1 year follow-up period.

Rotational coronary atherectomy

Rotational coronary atherectomy (Heart Technologies, Bellevue, WA) exerts its beneficial effect on the coronary lumen by ablating fibrocalcific plaque into microparticles, 80% of which are <5 μm in diameter and pass into the distal microcirculation. A 310 cm 0.009" stainless steel wire with a radioopaque platinum spring tip 0.014" in diameter is advanced into the distal vessel prior to advancement of the rotational atherectomy burr. The rotational atherectomy burr, which ranges in size from 1.25 mm to 2.5 mm and contains miniature diamond chips, rotates at 150,000 to 200,000 rpm. A high speed, compressed gas turbine connected to saline infusion lubricates and cools the system as the burr is advanced over the 0.009" wire and across the stenosis. The differential forward cutting of the rotational atherectomy burr

Table 21.1. Angiographic findings in 1438 lesions treated with coronary atherectomy.

	Directional atherectomy N = 492 (%)	Rotational atherectomy N = 813 (%)	Extractional atherectomy N = 133 (%)
Lesion location			
Right coronary artery	105 (21)	223 (27)	13 (10)
Left anterior descending	239 (49)	407 (50)	13 (10)
Left circumflex	87 (18)	181 (22)	3 (2)
Saphenous Vein Graft	61 (12)	2 (0.2)	104 (78)
ACC/AHACriteria*			
Type A	28 (6)	29 (4)	3 (2)
Type B1	124 (27)	112 (14)	12 (10)
Type B2	297 (63)	600 (75)	45 (36)
Type C	18 (4)	55 (7)	66 (52)
Ostial location*	121 (25)	178 (22)	25 (19)
Restenotic lesion*	107 (25)	253 (34)	17 (14)
Length (mm)*	7.38 ± 4.22	7.42 ± 5.88	10.59 ± 6.60
Eccentricity*	354 (76)	520 (65)	75 (59)
Calcification*	97 (21)	573 (72)	16 (13)
Angulation ≥45°*	65 (14)	227 (29)	9 (7)
Total occlusion*	4 (1)	22 (3)	15 (12)
Degenerated Vein Graft*	10 (2)	0 (0)	65 (51)
Thrombus*	16 (3)	12 (2)	59 (47)

* Percent, mean, and standard deviations did not include missing data.
ACC/AHA = modified American College of Cardiology/American Heart Association criteria [14].

Table 21.2. Quantitative results in 1438 lesions treated with coronary atherectomy.

	Directional atherectomy N = 492	Rotational atherectomy N = 813	Extraction atherectomy N = 133
Reference diameter (mm)[a]	2.95 ± 0.53	2.41 ± 0.48	3.13 ± 0.60
Minimal lumen diameter (mm)[a]			
Pre	0.88 ± 0.41	0.68 ± 0.36	0.74 ± 0.52
Post-device	2.27 ± 0.58	1.37 ± 0.41	1.58 ± 0.69
Final	2.51 ± 0.59	1.82 ± 0.45	2.16 ± 0.70
Percent diameter stenosis[a]			
Pre	70 ± 14	72 ± 14	76 ± 16
Post-device	25 ± 17	42 ± 15	49 ± 21
Final	15 ± 16	24 ± 15	29 ± 21
Acute gain (mm)[a]	1.63 ± 0.65	1.14 ± 0.49	1.43 ± 0.77
% Adjunct balloon[a]	210 (45)	677 (85)	103 (81)
Mean balloon:artery ratio[a]	1.08 ± 0.17	1.03 ± 0.17	1.03 ± 0.18
% Stretch[b,a]	70 ± 23	63 ± 22	66 ± 21
% Recoil[c,a]	11 ± 17	12 ± 14	16 ± 16
Angiographic success (%)[a]	444 (96)	755 (97)	114 (91)

[a] Percent, mean, and standard deviation did not include missing data.
[b] Stretch = (minimal diameter [balloon] – pre-minimal diameter [lumen])/reference diameter.
[c] Recoil = (minimal diameter [balloon] – post-minimal diameter [lumen])/reference diameter.

Table 21.3. Early (in-hospital) and late (1 year) procedural outcome in 1170 patients treated with coronary or Saphenous Vein Graft atherectomy.

	Directional atherectomy N (%)	Rotational atherectomy N (%)	Extraction atherectomy N (%)
Procedural outcome	N = 426	N = 639	N = 105
Procedural success	392 (92)	600 (94)	89 (85)
Major somplications	18 (4.2)	24 (3.8)	7 (6.7)
Death	5 (1.2)	6 (0.9)	3 (2.9)
Q-wave myocardial infarction	2 (0.5)	7 (1.1)	3 (2.9)
Coronary bypass operation	14 (3.3)	17 (2.7)	2 (1.9)
Other complications			
Non Q-wave infarction	41 (9.6)	52 (8.1)	18 (17)
Recurrent ischemia*	28 (7.3)	30 (4.8)	13 (13)
Out-of-lab abrupt closure*	8 (2.1)	11 (1.7)	3 (3.1)
Hierarchical late clinical outcome	N = 349	N = 558	N = 73
Death	4 (1.1)	6 (1.1)	6 (8.2)
Q-wave myocardial infarction	4 (1.1)	7 (1.3)	1 (1.4)
Coronary bypass operation	22 (6.3)	49 (8.8)	4 (5.5)
Repeat coronary angioplasty	55 (15.8)	95 (17.0)	13 (17.8)
Target lesion revascularization	N = 405	N = 701	N = 93
Any	92 (22.7)	174 (24.8)	21 (22.6)
Coronary bypass operation	28 (6.9)	57 (8.1)	6 (6.5)
Repeat coronary angioplasty	65 (16.0)	119 (17.6)	16 (17.2)

* Percent calculations did not include missing data.

results in ablation of the diseased plaque, leaving the normal, uninvolved arterial wall intact. The principle of rotational atherectomy is based upon the observation that elastic tissue (normal vessel wall) moves away from the diamond chipped burr while inelastic tissue (calcified, fibrous or fatty tissue) is fractured into microparticles. The high rotational speeds displace frictional components in an orthogonal vector which markedly enhances burr and catheter axial movement over the guidewire.

To date, there has been no randomized series of rotational atherectomy and balloon angioplasty to compare the procedural success rates in patients with complex coronary lesions. In the absence of these data, rotational atherectomy should be reserved for those lesions in which a suboptimal result might be expected using standard balloon angioplasty. In our experience of 813 lesions treated with rotational atherectomy, 96% had one or more adverse lesion characteristics (Table 21.1). Lesions were often calcified (72%), eccentric (65%), angulated (29%), or ostial in location (22%). Although angulated, *de novo* and bifurcation lesions and lesions located in vessels with proximal tortuosity may be at increased risk for procedural complications using rotational atherectomy, overall procedural results were still acceptable in many high-risk lesion subsets [15]. High rates of procedural success were obtained in calcified lesions (95%), eccentric lesions (94%), lesions ≥10 mm in length (95%), *de novo* lesions (94%) and angulated lesions (91%). In our series, major complications were uncommon (3.8%) and included death (0.9%), Q-wave myocardial infarction (1.1%), and coronary bypass operation (2.7%) (Table 21.3). Angiographic complications ('no reflow', abrupt closure, vasospasm, distal microparticulate embolization) may occur more often (8–10%), but can generally be treated with intracoronary nitrates, verapamil, and adjunct balloon dilatation.

Angiographic restenosis (≥50% follow-up diameter stenosis) occurs in approximately 50% of patients after rotational atherectomy [16–18]. Despite these relatively high rates of lumen re-narrowing, nearly 72% of patients remained free of major late (1 year) clinical events (Table 21.3). In 701 successfully treated lesions, coronary bypass surgery was performed in 57 (8.1%) patients and repeat coronary angioplasty was needed in 119 (17.6%). Multivariable predictors of target lesion revascularization included male gender (odds ratio [OR] = 1.82, $p < 0.005$), recent myocardial infarction (OR = 1.92; $p < 0.05$), and the final post-procedural% diameter stenosis (OR = 1.27, $p < 0.005$).

Transluminal extraction atherectomy

The transluminal extraction atherectomy catheter (InterVentional Technologies, San Diego, CA) was approved for marketing by the Food and Drug Administration Device Panel in June 1993. The extraction atherectomy catheter is comprised of a open, conical-shaped cutter attached to a motor driven torque tube which rotates at 750 rpms. Atheromatous plaque is cut into macroparticulate debris and removed via using continuous vacuum suction. The transluminal extraction catheter is available in catheter sizes ranging from 1.8–2.5 mm in diameter. Given the large diameter of many saphenous vein grafts treated with this device (>3.0 mm), adjunct balloon angioplasty is frequently (81%) required to maximize the final lumen dimensions.

Similar to other atherectomy devices, transluminal extraction atherectomy has been limited to lesions deemed high-risk for complications using standard balloon angioplasty. In our series, 98% of lesions had one or more high-risk characteristics (Table 21.1). We currently target our use of extraction atherectomy for the treatment of degenerated saphenous vein grafts (51%) and for those native vessel and saphenous vein graft lesions that contain significant amounts of thrombus (47%).

Procedural success rates >90% have been reported in a multicenter Registry of 1141 patients undergoing extraction atherectomy of less complex lesion subsets [19]. Major complications included acute occlusion, embolus, or dissection (1.3%), coronary bypass surgery (2.3%), in-hospital death (2.2%), and vessel perforation (1%). In our series of 105 patients with complex lesions treated with extraction atherectomy, an overall procedural success rate of 85% was obtained; major complications occurred in 6.7% of patients, including death (2.9%), Q-wave myocardial infarction (2.9%), and coronary bypass operation (1.9%) (Table 21.3). Notably, other complications may also occur after extraction atherectomy of these high-risk lesions [20]. Distal embolization has been reported in 14% of patients undergoing extraction atherectomy of saphenous vein graft lesions [20]. Unlike rotational atherectomy, distal embolization after extraction atherectomy is associated with significant periprocedural morbidity and mortality [20]. Distal embolization has been related to the use of adjunct balloon dilatation of friable grafts, and some have suggested the deferment of adjunct balloon angioplasty until the lumen surface has had sufficient time to heal.

Angiographic restenosis (≥50% follow-up diameter stenosis) has been reported in 55% of lesions treated in one multicenter series of extraction atherectomy [21]. Major late clinical events occurred in 33% of patients after extraction atherectomy in our experience (Table 21.3); these events included death (8.2%), Q-wave myocardial infarction (1.4%), coronary bypass operation (5.5%), and repeat coronary angioplasty (18%) (Table 21.3).

Effect of atherectomy on lesion compliance and initial angiographic results

Lesion compliance may be an important determinant of the initial angiographic result after atherectomy. Rigid lesions, typically resistant to complete balloon expansion unless high-pressure inflations are performed, may limit the initial angiographic result, particularly in fibrocalcific and ostial lesions. Conversely, elastic lesions may also inhibit the initial angiographic result through an excessive degree of elastic recoil, which reduces the maximal lumen dimension obtained with complete balloon inflation by 20–30%. In our series of 1438 lesions treated with coronary atherectomy, elastic recoil was lower after directional (11%) and rotational (12%) atherectomy than after extraction atherectomy (16%); although randomized data is lacking, these rates of elastic recoil are lower than those reported after balloon angioplasty (21%), using similar definitions [22]. Importantly, the magnitude of elastic recoil is directly related to the immediate post-procedural angiographic result after new device angioplasty (Figure 21.1). Intravascular ultrasound has suggested that these changes in lesion compliance may occur even though a significant amount of residual atherosclerotic plaque remains after atherectomy [5, 6, 23, 24]. Alterations in lesion compliance resulting from atherectomy would lend mechanistic support to several nonrandomized [25] and randomized series [11, 12] which have demonstrated that a lower initial residual% diameter stenosis can be obtained with some atherectomy devices than can be achieved in comparable lesions treated with standard balloon angioplasty.

Although the degree of late lumen loss is directly related to the immediate gain in lumen diameter, it has been suggested that the final lumen diameter achieved immediately after the procedure is the major clinical determinate of the late angiographic result [26]. The immediate angiographic result may

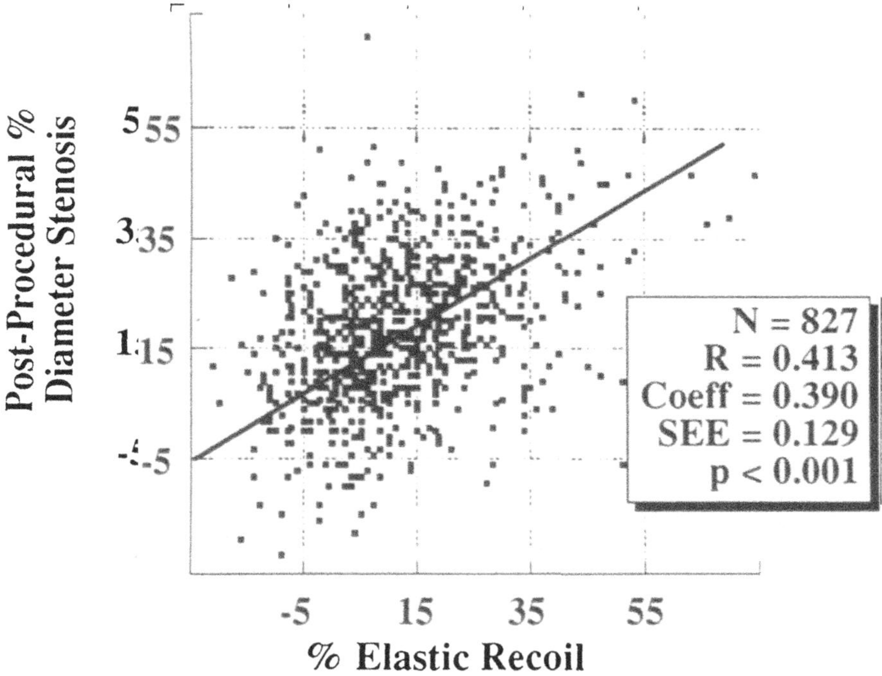

Figure 21.1. Direct relation between% elastic recoil ([minimal balloon diameter – minimal lumen diameter]/reference vessel diameter × 100) and post-procedural% diameter stenosis after new device angioplasty. SEE = standard error of the estimate. Modified from Reference 3 with permission.

also be an important determinant of late clinical outcome [27]. In a series of 1451 patients treated with new angioplasty devices, multivariable predictors of late (1 year) target lesion revascularization included male gender (OR: = 1.53; $p < 0.005$), LAD location (OR = 1.43, $p < 0.005$) and the final% diameter stenosis (OR = 1.14, $p < 0.005$). Based upon these factors, predictive models for late target lesion revascularization can be constructed (Figure 21.2).

Effect of plaque removal on late angiographic outcome

Despite the demonstration that the post-procedural residual lumen diameter is the single most important determinant of late angiographic outcome after balloon and new device angioplasty [26], it is not currently known whether the *amount of plaque removed* or simply the *final lumen dimension* primarily affects late angiographic outcome, given the limitations of angiography in assessing plaque burden. These factors have important clinical implications when a 'suboptimal' (>30% residual stenosis) angiographic result is obtained

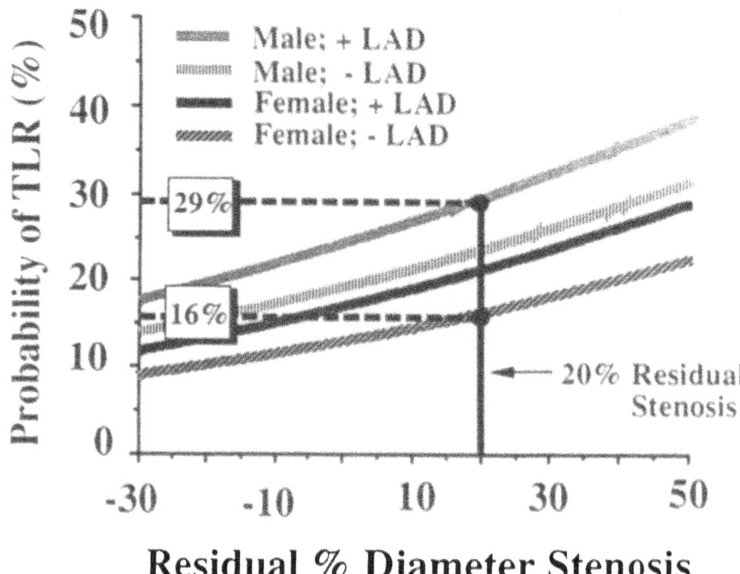

Figure 21.2. Predictive model for target lesion revascularization (TLR) (coronary bypass surgery or repeat coronary angioplasty) based upon late (9 month) outcome in 1451 patients (1729 lesions) undergoing successful new device angioplasty. Multivariable predictors for TLR included male gender (odds ratio [OR] = 1.53), left anterior descending artery (LAD) lesion location (OR = 1.43) and the final% diameter stenosis (OR = 1.14). A predictive model was constructed to estimate the probability of TLR based upon gender, LAD lesion location, and the final% diameter stenosis (see curves). Based upon this model, a 20% residual stenosis obtained in a man undergoing new device angioplasty of the LAD was associated with a 29% incidence of late TLR while a 20% residual stenosis in a woman undergoing non-LAD new device angioplasty was associated with a 16% incidence of late TLR.

after initial atherectomy. If the primary determinant of late angiographic outcome is the amount plaque removed, then more aggressive atherectomy would be recommended in the event of a residual stenosis. However, the aggressive use of larger devices, higher inflation pressures (directional atherectomy) and longer ablative runs (rotational atherectomy) may potentially be associated with an attendant risk of increased complications (e.g., dissections, perforation, and 'no reflow'). Conversely, if the primary determinant of late outcome is simply the final lumen diameter, irrespective of the amount of plaque removed, then adjunct balloon dilatation would be the preferred approach to maximize the final lumen diameter, while obviating the potential risk of complications due to aggressive atherectomy.

Further insights into the prognostic importance of the residual plaque burden after coronary atherectomy may be provided by intravascular ultrasound. Preliminary results from a series of 217 patients (255 lesions) undergoing pre- and post-procedural intravascular ultrasound after new device angioplasty in whom late (6 month) angiographic outcome was available suggested that the residual plaque burden (OR = 2.09; 95% confidence interval [CI] = 1.46–3.01; $p < 0.001$) and presence of fibrosis within the target lesion (OR = 2.26; 95% CI = 1.11–4.60; $p < 0.05$) were independent predictors for late angiographic restenosis (≥50% follow-up diameter stenosis) (GS Mintz, unpubl. data). These observations suggest that the extent of plaque removal may be an important independent factor in determining late angiographic outcome. Prospective confirmation of these preliminary observations will require intravascular ultrasound studies in larger numbers of consecutively treated patients after coronary atherectomy.

To determine the influence of residual plaque burden on late (6 month) angiographic restenosis after directional atherectomy, the *O*ptimal *A*therectomy *R*estenosis *S*tudy (OARS) was begun in October, 1993 at 4 clinical centers in the United States. In this protocol, 200 patients will undergo optimal atherectomy (target quantitative residual% diameter stenosis <15%) using 'aggressive' atherectomy or 'conservative' atherectomy with adjunct balloon dilatation to maximize the final angiographic result. Intravascular ultrasound will be obtained pre- and post-atherectomy and after adjunct balloon dilatation, if required. Using blinded ultrasound and quantitative angiographic readings, the independent contributions of the residual plaque burden and final lumen dimensions on the late angiographic outcome will be determined. These findings will formulate the basis for the strategic approach used in a larger 40 center study, the *B*alloon angioplasty versus *O*ptimal *A*therectomy *T*rial (BOAT), designed to compare the frequency of angiographic and clinical restenosis after balloon angioplasty and 'optimal' atherectomy; BOAT is scheduled to begin recruitment in the United States and Europe in early 1994.

Future directions in the use of coronary atherectomy

Over the next several years, the use of atherectomy devices in patients with symptomatic coronary artery disease will continue to undergo marked evolution. Results from randomized studies and contemporary registries (e.g., New Approaches to Coronary Intervention [NACI] Registry) will allow further refinement of the patients and lesions optimally treated with new devices. Second generation devices may improve the efficacy profiles of atherectomy catheters and reduce the incidence of untoward complications. The expanded use of intravascular ultrasound, either contained within the atherectomy device (e.g., ultrasound guided directional atherectomy) or obtained serially after atherectomy using designated ultrasound catheters, may allow more precise localization of the residual plaque and more directed, complete, and safe plaque removal and ablation. Determination of the importance of the residual plaque burden may also enhance the strategic use of atherectomy in conjunction with balloon angioplasty. Without question, while the current techniques of coronary atherectomy are in their infancy, these methods represent an exciting advance in the treatment of patients with symptomatic coronary artery disease.

References

1. Topol EJ. Promises and pitfalls of new devices for coronary artery disease. Circulation 1991; 83: 689–94.
2. King SB 3rd. Role of new technology in balloon angioplasty. Circulation 1991; 84: 2574–9.
3. Popma J, Leon M. A lesion-specific approach to new device angioplasty. In Topol EJ (ed): A textbook of interventional cardiology. Philadelphia: Saunders. 1994: 973–85.
4. Waller BF. "Crackers, breakers, stretchers, drillers, scrapers, shavers, burners, welders, and melters" – the future treatment of atherosclerotic coronary artery disease? A clinical-morphologic assessment. J Am Coll Cardiol 1989; 13: 969–87.
5. Kovach JA, Mintz GS, Pichard AD *et al.* Sequential intravascular ultrasound characterization of the mechanisms of rotational atherectomy and adjunct balloon angioplasty. J Am Coll Cardiol 1993; 22: 1024–32.
6. Popma JJ, Leon MB, Mintz GS *et al.* Results of coronary angioplasty using the transluminal extraction catheter. Am J Cardiol 1992; 70: 1526–32.
7. Safian RD, Gelbfish JS, Erny RE, Schnitt SJ, Schmidt DA, Baim DS. Coronary atherectomy. Clinical, angiographic, and histological findings and observations regarding potential mechanisms. Circulation 1990; 82: 69–79.
8. Popma JJ, Topol EJ, Hinohara T *et al.* Abrupt vessel closure after directional coronary atherectomy. The U.S. Directional Atherectomy Investigator Group. J Am Coll Cardiol 1992; 19: 1372–9.
9. Fishman RF, Kuntz RE, Carrozza JP Jr *et al.* Long-term results of directional coronary atherectomy: predictors of restenosis. J Am Coll Cardiol 1992; 20: 1101–10.
10. Popma JJ, Mintz GS, Satler LF *et al.* Clinical and angiographic outcome after directional coronary atherectomy: A qualitative and quantitative analysis using coronary arteriography and intravascular ultrasound. Am J Cardiol 1993; 72: 55E–64E.
11. Adelman AG, Cohen EA, Kimball BP *et al.* A comparison of directional atherectomy with balloon angioplasty for lesions of the left anterior descending coronary artery. N Engl J Med 1993; 329: 228–33.
12. Topol EJ, Leya F, Pinkerton CA *et al.* A comparison of directional atherectomy with coronary angioplasty in patients with coronary artery disease. The CAVEAT Study Group. N Engl J Med 1993; 329: 221–7.
13. Kent KM, Williams DO, King SB 3rd *et al.* Acute procedural and angiographic outcome in the angiopeptin for the prevention of restenosis after directional coronary atherectomy trial [abstract]. Circulation 1993; 88 (4 Pt 2): I546.
14. Ellis SG, Vandormael MG, Cowley MJ *et al.* Coronary morphologic and clinical determinants of procedural outcome with angioplasty for multivessel coronary disease. Implication for patient selection. Multivessel Angioplasty Prognosis Study Group. Circulation 1990; 82: 1193–202.
15. Popma JJ, Satler LF, Pichard AD *et al.* Clinical and angiographic predictors of procedural outcome after rotational coronary atherectomy in complex lesions [abstract]. J Am Coll Cardiol 1993; 21 (2 Suppl A): 228A.
16. Teirstein PS, Warth DC, Haq N *et al.* High speed rotational coronary atherectomy for patients with diffuse coronary artery disease. J Am Coll Cardiol 1991; 18: 1694–701.
17. Safian RD, Niazi KA, Strzelecki M *et al.* Detailed angiographic analysis of high-speed mechanical rotational atherectomy in human coronary arteries. Circulation 1993; 88: 961–8.

18. Popma JJ, Satler LF, Pichard AD *et al.* A quantitative analysis of factors affecting late angiographic outcome after rotational coronary atherectomy [abstract]. J Am Coll Cardiol 1993; 21 (2 Suppl A): 31A.
19. Sutton JM, Gitlin JB, Casale PN. Major complications after TEC atherectomy: preliminary analysis derived from the Multicenter Registry experience [abstract]. Circulation 1992; 86 (Suppl I): I456.
20. Hong MK, Popma JJ, Pichard AD *et al.* The clinical significance of distal embolization after transluminal extraction atherectomy in diffusely diseased saphenous vein grafts. Am Heart J. In press.
21. Popma JJ, O'Neill WW, Kramer B *et al.* A quantitative analysis of late angiographic outcome after transluminal extraction-endarterectomy [abstract]. Circulation 1992; 86 (Suppl. I): I457.
22. Hermans WR, Rensing BJ, Strauss BH, Serruys PW. Methodological problems related to the quantitative assessment of stretch, elastic recoil, and balloon-artery ratio. Cathet Cardiovasc Diagn 1992; 25: 174–85.
23. Mintz GS, Potkin BN, Keren G *et al.* Intravascular ultrasound evaluation of the effect of rotational atherectomy in obstructive atherosclerotic coronary artery disease. Circulation 1992; 86: 1383–93.
24. Mintz GS, Pichard AD, Popma JJ, Kent KM, Satler LF, Leon MB. Preliminary experience with adjunct directional coronary atherectomy after high-speed rotational atherectomy in the treatment of calcific coronary artery disease. Am J Cardiol 1993; 71: 799–804.
25. Muller DW, Ellis SG, Debowey DL, Topol EJ. Quantitative angiographic comparison of the immediate success of coronary angioplasty, coronary atherectomy and endoluminal stenting. Am J Cardiol 1990; 66: 938–42.
26. Kuntz RE, Gibson CM, Nobuyoshi M, Baim DS. Generalized model of restenosis after conventional balloon angioplasty, stenting, and directional atherectomy. J Am Coll Cardiol 1993; 21: 15–25.
27. Popma JJ, Chuang YC, Sweet LC, Syed R, Leon, MB. Clinical and angiographic predictors of target lesion revascularization after new device angioplasty: importance of obtaining a low residual stenosis [abstract]. Circulation 1993, 88 (4 pt 2): I150.

22. Rotational atherectomy – An overview

EUGÈNE P. McFADDEN, JEAN-MARC LABLANCHE, CHRISTOPHE BAUTERS, PHILIPPE QUANDALLE & MICHEL E. BERTRAND

Summary

Percutaneous transluminal rotational atherectomy is a novel treatment modality for the treatment of obstructive epicardial coronary atherosclerosis. This technic, which was introduced in an attempt to overcome some of the limitations of traditional balloon angioplasty, employs a burr coated with diamond chips that is introduced into the coronary artery; the burr which rotates at speeds of up to 200,000 revolutions per minute removes atheroma by grinding it into tiny particles that are dispersed into the distal coronary bed. In this chapter, we summarize the experience to date with high speed rotational atherectomy as a treatment for coronary disease. We discuss the complications unique to the technic; we describe the insights into the mechanisms of rotational atherectomy obtained with quantitative angiographic technics, and examine the future role of the technic as a stand-alone procedure or as an adjunct to balloon angioplasty.

Introduction

Since the initial description of the technic by Andreas Grüntzig in 1977, percutaneous transluminal coronary balloon angioplasty has become a widely performed treatment for obstructive atherosclerotic coronary disease [1]. Initially reserved for single, discrete, proximal, noncalcified stenoses, increased operator experience coupled with improvements in balloon technology have allowed its application in more complex situations. It quickly became apparent that lesions treated by coronary angioplasty often recurred [2]. The rate of recurrence varies widely in reported studies, predominantly due to the differing definitions of restenosis employed. In our institution, where follow-up angiography at 6 months is recommended to all patients with an initially successful procedure, angiographic restenosis after balloon angioplasty, defined as a recurrent stenosis of more than 50% at the dilated site measured by quantitative coronary angiography, occurs in 42.6% of patients and at 38% of lesions [3]. The other major limitations of balloon angioplasty are the inability to dilate certain types of lesion with standard balloon equipment. Uncomplicated failure has been reported at up to 4.7% of lesions [4]; it is particularly common with lesions that are heavily calcified, where even inflations at high pressure may fail to dilate; other lesions,

J.H.C. Reiber and P.W. Serruys (eds): Progress in quantitative coronary arteriography, 353–366.

particularly those in ostial locations are prone to immediate elastic recoil, despite a satisfactory initial result. Finally, the occurrence of acute closure after balloon angioplasty, albeit rare, remains a problem.

In response to these limitations, cardiologists sought to develop alternative technics of percutaneous revascularisation. These technics primarily differed from balloon angioplasty in that they were designed to physically remove atheromatous plaque. It was hoped that this different mechanism might facilitate the treatment of lesions where standard balloon angioplasty had produced disappointing primary results and would perhaps lead to a reduction in the rate of restenosis. Directional coronary atherectomy and transluminal extraction coronary atherectomy were developed to produce an improvement in lumen diameter by direct mechanical removal of atherosclerotic material from the vessel wall [5, 6]. High speed rotational coronary atherectomy has a different and unique mechanism; it removes plaque by abrading the atherosclerotic material producing millions of tiny particles that are dispersed into the distal coronary circulation [7]. In this chapter we discuss the technic of high speed rotational atherectomy with Rotablator™, we analyze the results reported to date, and attempt to define the present role of rotational atherectomy in the treatment of coronary disease.

Technique of rotational atherectomy

The Rotablator™ (HeartTechnology Inc, Bellevue, Washington, USA) consists of an abrasive tip welded to a long flexible drive shaft tracking along a central flexible guide wire. The abrasive tip is an elliptically shaped burr, available in various sizes (1.0 to 2.5 mm in diameter) whose distal portion is coated with diamond chips 30 to 50 microns in diameter. Rotational energy is transmitted by a compressed air motor which drives the flexible helical shaft at speeds up to 190,000 revolutions per minute.

The number of revolutions per minute is measured by a fiberoptic light probe and displayed on a control panel. The speed of rotation and the speed of advancement of the burr are controlled by the operator. During rotation, saline solution irrigates the catheter sheath to lubricate and cool the rotating parts. The burr and the drive shaft move freely over a central coaxial guide wire (0.009 inches in diameter, 3 meters in length), with a flexible radioopaque platinum distal part (20 mm long), which does not rotate with the burr during abrasion. The wire and the abrasive tip can be advanced independently, which allows the wire to be placed in a safe distal location before the burr is advanced into the diseased artery.

All patients are pretreated with aspirin and a calcium antagonist. A sheath is inserted into the femoral artery under local anesthesia and a standard 8F or 9F guiding catheter, depending on the size of the burr, is advanced to the ostium of the coronary artery. Following the intracoronary injection of isosorbide dinitrate (0.5 to 1 mg), a baseline angiogram is performed in three projections and heparin (10,000 IU) is given intravenously.

Rotary ablation begins with the placement of the special guide wire across the lesion to a safe distal vessel location. The small caliber of the wire may sometimes make this more difficult than with standard guidewires; it is occasionally necessary to cross the stenosis with a conventional over-the wire balloon system, which is subsequently exchanged for the Rotablator guidewire. The burr and the drive shaft are then manually advanced over the guide wire to the site of the lesion, and rotation is begun. When an adequate speed of rotation (175,000 revolutions per minute) has been achieved the abrasive tip is advanced gently over the guide wire. If resistance is encountered the tip is moved backwards and forwards to maintain a high speed of rotation. Several slow passes are usually required to achieve maximum plaque removal. Typical results of the procedure are shown in Figure 22.1.

The periprocedural complications encountered during rotational atherectomy differ somewhat from those seen during traditional balloon angioplasty. Diffuse spasm at the site of atherectomy and in the distal vessel was common during the early experience with the technic; prophylactic administration of large doses of intracoronary vasodilators, repeated during the procedure if required, have largely eliminated the problem. An infrequent problem that may be difficult to manage is the occurrence of myocardial ischemia, after technically successful rotational atherectomy, with a widely patent epicardial vessel. This mechanism is incompletely understood but presumably relates to diffuse spasm of vessels too small to be seen angiographically, due either to the high frequency vibrations produced by the rotating burr or to obstruction of these vessels by material embolized during atherectomy. It usually responds to intracoronary administration of nitrates or of calcium antagonists. Finally, transient atrioventricular block that usually lasts for less than a minute, is relatively common; it most frequently occurs during treatment of lesions in dominant right or circumflex coronary arteries, although we have also observed this phenomenon during treatment of left anterior descending lesions. The mechanism appears to relate to a microcavitatory effect produced by the spinning burr or to embolization of microscopic particles [8].

Rotational atherectomy: The global experience

As of January 1993, the results obtained with high speed rotational atherectomy at 2488 lesions in 2018 patients have been entered into the International Registry. This represents the cumulative experience of 14 centres. The mean age of the patients, 72% of whom were men, was 62.6 years. Forty-six percent of the patients had stable angina; 41% had unstable angina and 13% were asymptomatic. Eighteen percent of patients had previously undergone coronary artery bypass surgery, 41% had prior myocardial infarction, and

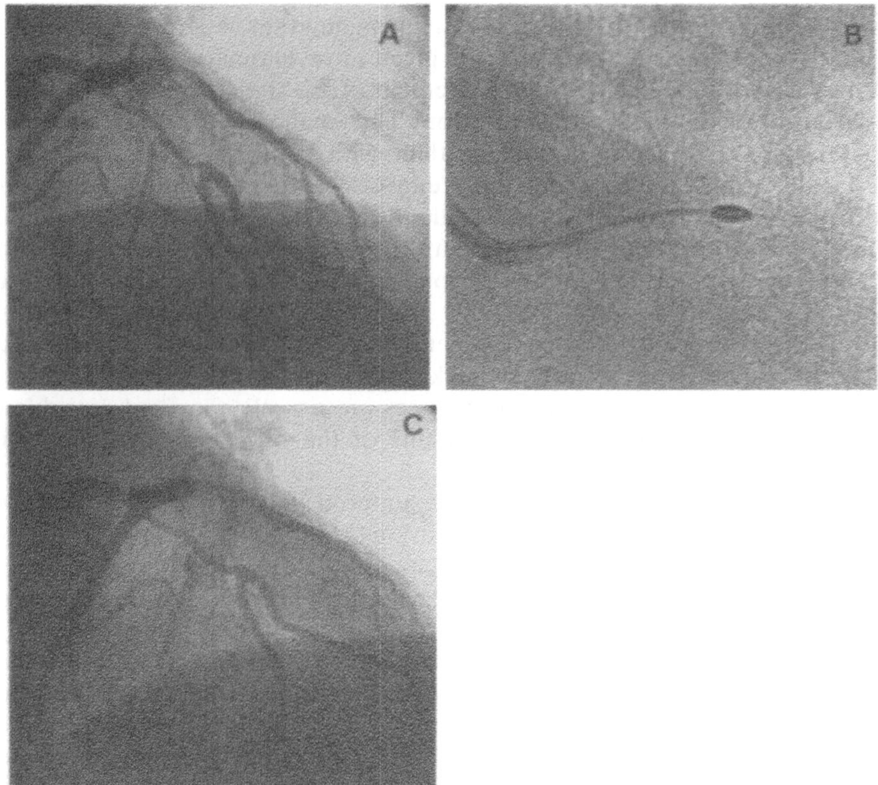

Figure 22.1. An example of a lesion treated by rotational atherectomy At baseline, there is a long stenosis in tandem involving the proximal and mid left anterior descending coronary artery. (Panel A) The burr *in situ* (Panel B) during rotational atherectomy. Rotational atherectomy alone (Panel C) results in a satisfactory final result.

29% had previously undergone PTCA. Most (64.8%) had multiple vessel disease. Rotational atherectomy was most commonly performed on the left anterior descending coronary artery (48% of lesions), less frequently on the right (29%) or circumflex (19%) coronary arteries. A protected left mainstem lesion was treated in 3% of patients. Most of the lesions had complex characteristics. Sixty-five percent were eccentric, 26% were located at bifurcations, 54% were longer than 10 mm, and 46% had at least moderate calcification. Primary success was defined as a reduction in stenosis severity by at least 20% with a residual stenosis of less than 50% in the absence of major complications (acute myocardial infarction, emergent coronary artery bypass surgery, or in-hospital death). The primary success rate achieved with use of rotational atherectomy alone was 30%. When the residual stenosis was more than 50%, the procedure was completed by adjunctive balloon angioplasty or less frequently with another technic, yielding a final procedural success rate of 95%. The primary success rate was independent of lesion length. Myocardial infarction occurred in 6.4% of patients, Q-wave in 5.4% and non Q-wave in 1%. Emergent coronary artery bypass surgery was undertaken in 2.2% of patients. Death occurred in 0.9% of patients. The complication rate was related to the characteristics of the lesions treated. The complication rate for Type A lesions was 1.3%, for Type B lesions 3.9%, and for Type C lesions 6.2%.

The location of the treated lesions did not have a significant effect on primary success rates. The success rates at lesions that were heavily calcified and at long lesions were similar to the results obtained at other types of lesion. The overall restenosis rate in the 825 patients who underwent angiographic follow-up was 48%. In the patients who were treated by rotational atherectomy alone the restenosis rate was 42% compared to 54% in patients who had undergone adjunctive balloon angioplasty.

Effects of rotational atherectomy: Insights from quantitative angiography

Acute elastic recoil

The use of quantitative coronary angiography has provided invaluable insights into the mechanisms of balloon angioplasty. Immediately after balloon angioplasty, the minimal lumen diameter is invariably less than the diameter of the inflated balloon, due to immediate elastic recoil. In theory, rotational atherectomy, by shaving away atheromatous plaque, might reduce the extent of this immediate recoil. Ideally, the minimal lumen diameter immediately after a rotational atherectomy procedure should be equal to the diameter of the burr used. We systematically investigated the extent of elastic recoil after rotational atherectomy. We compared the diameter of the burr employed with the minimal lumen diameter immediately after the procedure in consecutive patients who were undergoing rotational atherectomy [9]. The measurements were performed on angiograms obtained in the same projections, and after administration of isosorbide dinitrate immediately before and just after the procedure. The coronary arteriograms were analysed with use of the CAESAR system (Computerised Assisted Evaluation of Stenosis And Restenosis). The validation of this system together with the accuracy and reproducibility of measurements obtained under routine clinical conditions have been previously described in detail [10].

The degree of immediate elastic recoil after rotational atherectomy as a function of the size of the most commonly employed burrs is presented in Figure 22.2. The absolute minimal diameter of the residual lumen was significantly less than the diameter of the burr employed. Overall, in 95 consecutive procedures, the lumen diameter after rotational atherectomy alone was 24 ± 21% less than that of the largest burr employed. Thus the

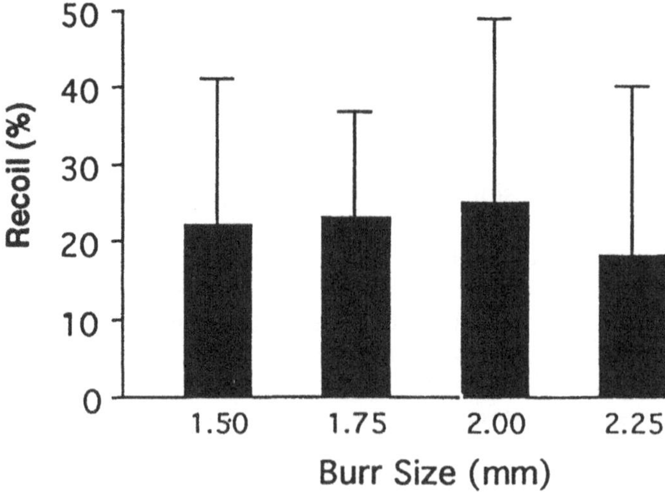

Figure 22.2. The relationship between the size of the burr employed and the minimal lumen diameter at the dilated site immediately after the procedure. The mean minimal lumen diameter after rotational atherectomy was 76% of the burr size.

mean minimal lumen diameter immediately after the procedure was 76 ± 21% of the diameter of the burr used. When the procedure was completed by adjunctive balloon angioplasty, the mean minimal lumen diameter immediately after the procedure was 68 ± 14% of the diameter of the balloon employed, representing a immediate elastic recoil of 32 ± 14%. Of course, the mean percentage residual stenosis after rotational atherectomy cannot be directly compared with that achieved by balloon angioplasty because the maximal burr size that can be used in the coronary circulation is only 2.5 mm. However these results demonstrate that the degree of immediate elastic recoil after rotational atherectomy alone is less than that after rotational atherectomy combined with adjunctive balloon angioplasty, and less than that after balloon angioplasty alone (Figure 22.3) which in a consecutive series of 255 patients was 38 ± 13% (n = 255).

The observation that the luminal diameter immediately after rotational atherectomy is less than the size of the burr employed is consistent with the findings of most other investigators. One recent study has however suggested that the converse is true. In a series of patients studied with intravascular ultrasound immediately after rotational atherectomy, the cross-sectional area of the lumen was significantly greater than that of the largest burr employed. However, in this study there was no consistent relationship between the intravascular ultrasound measurements of lumen diameter and the equivalent values obtained by angiography [11].

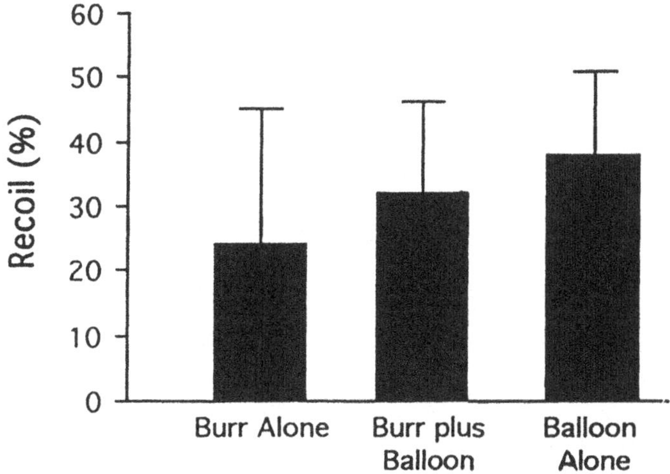

Figure 22.3. The degree of elastic recoil after rotational atherectomy alone (24 ± 21%) was less than that after rotational atherectomy followed by balloon angioplasty (32 ± 14%) or after balloon angioplasty alone (38 ± 13%, ACCORD Study)

Delayed elastic recoil

It has been suggested that a 'delayed' elastic recoil phenomenon may account for some cases of early 'restenosis' after conventional balloon angioplasty. We studied this phenomenon in patients who were enrolled in a multicenter European trial designed to examine the effect of nadroparine (Fraxiparine), a low molecular weight heparin, on the occurrence of restenosis after balloon angioplasty. In this study angiography is performed by protocol 24 hours after initially successful procedures. In the first 123 patients who underwent 24 hour angiography, there was no significant change in mean proximal or distal reference diameters or in mean minimal lumen diameter at 24 hours [12]. Similar results were reported by Foley *et al.* who studied 110 patients before, immediately after, and 24 hours after angioplasty. [13]. They found no change in mean minimal lumen diameter at 24 hours compared to the equivalent value just after the procedure.

To evaluate whether such delayed elastic recoil might occur after rotational atherectomy, we studied early changes in minimal lumen diameter in a group of patients treated by rotational atherectomy alone, and in a group treated by rotational atherectomy with adjunctive balloon angioplasty [14]. The patients were restudied the morning after the procedure. The angiograms were obtained after the intracoronary injection of isosorbide dinitrate. There was no significant difference between the mean minimal lumen diameter immediately after the procedure (1.76 ± 0.48) mm and that at 24 hours (1.77 ± 0.46) in

Table 22.1. Relationship between burr-artery ratio and the occurrence of angiographic or clinical complications in 116 patients.

Burr-artery ratio[a]	Patients	Uncomplicated	Complication	
			Angiographic[b]	Clinical[c]
<0.5	5	4 (80%)	0	1
0.5–0.7	63	49 (78%)	8	4
0.7–0.8	19	15 (79%)	3	1
>0.8	29	16 (55%)	10	3
	116	84 (72%)	21	9

[a] Diameter of burr (mm) divided by the diameter of the reference segment (mm).
[b] Acute reocclusion, coronary dissection or coronary spasm.
[c] Death (0), acute myocardial infarction (Q-wave 3, non-Q-wave 4), emergent coronary artery bypass surgery (2).

the patients treated with rotational atherectomy alone. These results suggest that 'delayed' elastic recoil does not occur after rotational atherectomy.

Reisman *et al.* found that the mean minimal lumen diameter at 24 hours after rotational atherectomy, with or without adjunctive balloon angioplasty, was significantly greater than the equivalent value immediately after the procedure [15]. It is not clear whether in this study, intracoronary nitrates were systematically administered before each angiography. The improvement in luminal diameter reported by Reisman *et al.* at 24 hours which was greater (21%) in the group treated by rotational atherectomy alone than in the group that had adjunctive balloon angioplasty (14%), suggests that a further improvement in lumen diameter may occur in the first 24 hours, perhaps related to changes in vasomotor tone at the dilated site.

Burr size: Relation to procedural outcome

It has been clearly shown that the use of oversized balloons is associated with a high risk of acute complications during balloon angioplasty. Our experience, and that of others, suggests that during rotational atherectomy the relative size of the burr employed is strongly associated with the occurrence of procedural complications. In our initial 116 patients treated with rotational atherectomy, we examined the relationship between the burr/reference diameter ratio (the diameter of the burr divided by that of the adjacent reference diameter) and the occurrence of complications during rotational atherectomy. In this series of patients, the rate of immediate angiographic complications (occlusion, spasm, dissection) when the burr to reference diameter ratio was <0.8 was 22% compared to 45% when the ratio was >0.8. For clinical complications, a similar pattern was observed. When the burr to reference diameter ratio was <0.8 the rate of clinical complications was 6.9% compared to 10.3% when the ratio was >0.8 (Table 22.1).

Based on these two observations, namely that the mean minimal lumen diameter to burr ratio is 0.76 after rotational atherectomy and that the incidence of complications is significantly higher when the burr to reference diameter ratio is >0.8, the mean ratio of minimal lumen diameter to burr size after uncomplicated atherectomy would be 0.61. This corresponds to a residual 39% stenosis after uncomplicated rotational atherectomy.

Treatment strategies with rotablator

Two general treatment strategies have been advocated with Rotablator. Firstly, an attempt to achieve an angiographically satisfactory result with use of rotational atherectomy as a 'stand-alone' procedure. This strategy proposes the use of a single large burr, chosen to approximate the size of the normal vessel, or alternatively, the initial use of a small burr to debulk the lesion followed by stepwise increments in burr size until a satisfactory angiographic result has been achieved. The second general approach proposes the use of a deliberately undersized burr to debulk the lesion with a minimal risk, followed by adjunctive balloon angioplasty, if needed, to obtain an angiographically satisfactory final result.

Rotablator-alone strategy

Several groups have deliberately attempted to achieve successful dilation with use of Rotablator alone. Teirstein *et al.* treated a group of 42 patients who were suboptimal candidates for balloon angioplasty; most had diffuse coronary disease with stenoses >1 cm in length [16]. Adjunctive balloon angioplasty was not performed, except as a salvage procedure in 2 patients. The overall success rate (<50% stenosis without complication) was 76%, 92% at lesions <1 cm in length, 70% at lesions >1 cm in length. One patient died after emergency bypass grafting; 19% had significant enzyme rises without clinical sequelae. Severe coronary spasm occurred during 36% of procedures and often required up to 20 minutes for resolution. Follow-up angiography in 91% of patients showed restenosis in 59% overall, 22% for short lesions and 75% for long lesions. Although the size of the burr relative to the artery was not reported, the largest burr used was 2.0 mm and the reference diameter of the arteries was ≤3 mm. They concluded that rotational atherectomy should not be recommended for patients with long, diffuse coronary stenoses.

Zacca *et al.* reported 31 consecutive patients (36 lesions) in whom they performed rotational atherectomy with single large burrs [17]. Lesion length was <10 mm in 39%, >10 mm in 50%, and >20 mm in 11%. Procedural success was achieved at 97% of lesions. One patient underwent emergent coronary artery bypass surgery. An interesting technical feature was the use of continuous nitroglycerin infusion during burr rotation, and the attempt to limit the number of passes, which they felt accounted for the low incidence of coronary spasm. The restenosis rate was not reported.

Burr-balloon strategy

As reported above, we have found that the initial use of a burr whose size is >80% of the diameter of the reference vessel is associated with a higher incidence of complications. Stertzer *et al.* recently reported their experience in a series of 242 patients in whom 302 rotational atherectomy procedures were performed [18]. They initially used a strategy based on the use of a small burr with stepwise increases in burr size until a satisfactory result was obtained. However, an additional balloon angioplasty was performed in 78% of patients. They classified such additional balloon angioplasty as adjunctive, when it was performed as a salvage procedure due to a complication (dissection, abrupt closure) during rotational atherectomy; they performed adjunctive angioplasty in 6.7% of cases. The remaining balloon angioplasties were described as complementary. This term was used to describe a low pressure inflation with a balloon 'to relieve vasospasm or to smooth a satisfactorily ablated segment'. Of the 302 procedures, rotational atherectomy as a stand-alone procedure was successful in 22.8% of procedures. Adjunctive (6.7% procedures) or complementary (69.5% procedures) was performed in the remaining 77.2% procedures.

Stertzer *et al.* noted that the incidence of complications appeared to be related to the size of the burr employed. They analyzed the factors associated with the 23 (7.6%) acute complications (dissection, severe vasospasm, embolism). In 60% of these cases the initial burr size (1.75–2.00 mm) was relatively large, or alternatively, after an initially small burr, the operator skipped to a large sized burr contrary to their usual policy of using stepwise increments in burr size. After the initial 200 procedures, they attempted to increase the burr/artery ratio to >90% of the lumen diameter of the vessel. However, in several cases this resulted in the formation of pseudoaneurysms. They therefore recommended the use of stepwise increments in burr size, with a final burr/artery ratio of 0.75.

Safian *et al.* reported a series of 116 high-speed mechanical rotational atherectomy procedures in 104 patients with predominantly complex lesion morphology [19]. The mean diameter stenosis decreased from 70 ± 13% to 54 ± 23% after rotational atherectomy alone. Adjunctive balloon angioplasty was performed at 89 (77%) lesions. The final diameter stenosis was 30 ± 20%. Angiographic complications occurred at 39.6% of lesions; this included severe dissection leading to abrupt closure directly related to rotational atherectomy at 13 (11.2%) lesions. The vast majority of these complications (86%) were managed by 'salvage' balloon angioplasty. Clinical sequelae included death (1%), emergent coronary artery bypass surgery (1.9%), and myocardial infarction (7.1%). Angiographic follow-up was performed in 84% of eligible patients. Angiographic restenosis (>50% stenosis) occurred at 50% of primary lesions and 54% of restenosis lesions.

In summary, in the absence of any documented benefit of rotational atherectomy on the occurrence of restenosis, the major advantage of rotational atherectomy lies in its ability to tackle lesions with characteristics unsuited to balloon angioplasty. The available evidence suggests that a burr-balloon strategy, or a strategy that employs successively larger burrs provide the safest approach. We currently employ a burr-balloon strategy, which consists in the initial use of a deliberately undersized burr to 'debulk' the lesion with adjunctive balloon angioplasty, if required, to achieve an angiographically satisfactory result. This appears to produce results similar to the use of sequential increments in burr size, but at considerably less expense.

Angiographic restenosis after rotational atherectomy

No randomized controlled trial has directly compared the restenosis rate after rotational atherectomy alone with the restenosis rate after conventional balloon angioplasty. One inherent difficulty in the design of such a study would be the necessity to include only lesions in arteries which could be treated by both devices as the largest burr size that can be introduced into the coronary circulation is 2.75 mm.

We compared the angiographic rate of restenosis in patients who underwent rotational atherectomy alone with that in patients treated during the same time period who underwent rotational atherectomy completed by adjunctive balloon angioplasty. The patient population consists of patients who underwent rotational atherectomy during our early experience in Lille and who underwent angiographic follow-up. We identified 82 such patients; 45 (55%) of them were treated by rotational atherectomy alone, while the remaining 37 (45%) had an adjunctive balloon angioplasty because the residual stenosis after rotational atherectomy alone was >50%. Follow-up angiography was undertaken at a mean of 4.6, range 3 to 6, months after the procedure. The mean stenosis severity before the procedure was 73.7 ± 11.3% in the group treated by rotational atherectomy alone and 77.4 ± 11.4% in the group treated by rotational atherectomy with adjunctive balloon angioplasty. After the procedure the mean residual stenosis was 42.0 ± 19.2% in the group treated by rotational atherectomy alone and 36.0 ± 17% in the group treated by rotational atherectomy with adjunctive balloon angioplasty. At follow-up angiography, 44.2% of patients treated with rotational atherectomy alone had developed restenosis compared with 41.2% of those who had adjunctive balloon angioplasty. These results are compatible with those reported in the International Registry where the overall restenosis rate in the 825 patients who underwent angiographic follow-up was 48%. In the patients who were treated by rotational atherectomy alone the restenosis rate was 42% compared to 54% in patients who had undergone adjunctive balloon angioplasty.

Present and future role of rotational atherectomy

There are no randomized trials that have directly compared the outcome after rotational atherectomy with that after angioplasty with traditional balloon equipment. A particular problem related to the performance of such a trial relates to the maximum burr size (2.50 mm) that can at present be employed in the coronary circulation. An expandable burr, currently under development, will facilitate the performance of such a study. Based on the results reported to date, and on our personal experience, there are several specific situations where the use of high speed rotational atherectomy appears particularly promising.

Rotational atherectomy as primary therapy

Specific lesion types have been shown, in observational studies, to be associated with a suboptimal outcome when treated with balloon equipment. Such lesions include those that have heavy calcification, those that have moderate or heavy calcification and that are also eccentric, those that are ostial in location, and those that are long (>10 mm but <25 mm) or located in vessels with diffuse atheroma. In our experience, discrete lesions that are heavily calcified, and lesions that are long or in tandem in diffusely diseased vessels respond well to treatment with rotational atherectomy. On-line quantitative coronary angiography is performed before rotational atherectomy and a burr size 70% of the reference diameter is chosen. Adjunctive balloon angioplasty is performed when required, in preference to the use of a larger burr. In diffusely diseased vessels, with long stenoses or stenoses in tandem, adjunctive angioplasty with a long balloon is frequently performed.

Of course such an approach reflects our experience and cannot, at present, be validated scientifically. The extent of calcification, the degree of eccentricity, and the extent of 'diffuse' disease, are with our present technics of quantitation, characteristics that have a high degree of interobserver variability. The advent of intravascular ultrasound will allow a more precise and objective assessment of the extent of calcification, and of the degree of angiographically 'invisible' atherosclerosis, that will enable a more balanced evaluation of the role of different treatment modalities in specific situations.

'Rescue' rotational atherectomy

A second potential role for rotational atherectomy relates to its use as an adjunctive strategy after failed balloon angioplasty. A recent report described the use of rotational atherectomy in a series of 40 patients in whom lesions were encountered that were undilatable with conventional balloon equipment even at high pressures. Brogan *et al.* reported a procedural success rate of 90%, with use of a strategy that consisted in the initial use of rotational atherectomy with additional balloon angioplasty at 88% of lesions [20]. Only 20% of the patients were treated immediately after the initially unsuccessful balloon procedure. This approach to the treatment of balloon failures appears extremely promising; it will be especially useful if it could be performed safely immediately after a failed balloon procedure.

Mintz *et al.* recently described 10 patients with calcified lesions who were successfully treated by rotational atherectomy followed by directional atherectomy. Five of the patients had initially undergone an unsuccessful attempted directional atherectomy [21].

Conclusions

The new devices that have been introduced to overcome the shortcomings of traditional balloon angioplasty do not appear to have any significant impact on the problem of restenosis. The injury produced by the process of dilation, regardless of how the injury is inflicted, provides the stimulus that leads to restenosis. The degree of injury appears to be much more important than the specific technic employed. By contrast, new technics may in specific situations, often with adjunctive balloon angioplasty, produce an adequate primary result where experience with balloon angioplasty alone has been disappointing. Rotational atherectomy, with its unique mechanism of action, appears to fulfil this role for some such lesions. Results to date suggest that rotational atherectomy should be used as a tool to predilate the lesion thus enabling an angiographically satisfactory result to be obtained by subsequent balloon angioplasty. A second potentially promising applicaton is as a treatment for lesions where balloon angioplasty has been attempted without success.

References

1. Gruentzig AR, Senning A, Siegenthaler WE. Nonoperative dilatation of coronary-artery stenosis. Percutaneous transluminal coronary angioplasty. N Engl J Med 1979; 301: 61–8.
2. Holmes DR Jr, Vlietstra RE, Smith HC *et al.* Restenosis after percutaneous transluminal coronary angioplasty (PTCA): a report from the PTCA registry of the National Heart, Lung, and Blood Institute. Am J Cardiol 1984; 53: 77C–81C.
3. Bauters C, Lablanche JM, Mc Fadden EP, Leroy F, Bertrand ME. Clinical characteristics

and angiographic follow-up of patients undergoing early or late repeat dilation for a first restenosis. J Am Coll Cardiol 1992; 20: 845–8.
4. Myler RK, Shaw RE, Stertzer SH *et al.* Lesion morphology and coronary angioplasty: current experience and analysis. J Am Coll Cardiol 1992; 19: 1641–52.
5. Safian RD, Gelbfish JS, Erny RE, Schnitt SJ, Schmidt D, Baim DS. Coronary atherectomy. Clinical, angiographic, and histological findings and observations regarding potential mechanisms. Circulation 1990; 82: 69–79.
6. Sketch MH Jr, Phillips HR. Coronary atherectomy with the TEC device. In Vogel JHK, King SB 3rd (eds): The practice of interventional cardiology, 2nd ed. St. Louis: Mosby-Year Book 1993: 149–55.
7. Fourrier JL, Bertrand ME, Auth DC, Lablanche JM, Gommeaux A, Brunetaud JM. Percutaneous coronary rotational angioplasty in humans: preliminary report. J Am Coll Cardiol 1989; 14: 1278–82.
8. Zotz R, Stahr P, Erbel R, Auth D, Meyer J. Analysis of high-frequency rotational angioplasty-induced echo contrast. Cathet Cardiovasc Diagn 1991; 22: 137–44.
9. Bertrand ME, Lablanche JM, Leroy F *et al.* Percutaneous transluminal coronary rotary ablation with Rotablator (European experience). Am J Cardiol 1992; 69: 470–4.
10. Bertrand ME, Lablanche JM, Bauters C, Leroy F, MacFadden E. Discordant results of visual and quantitative estimates of stenosis severity before and after coronary angioplasty. Cathet Cardiovasc Diagn 1993; 28: 1–6.
11. Mintz GS, Potkin BN, Keren G *et al.* Intravascular ultrasound evaluation of the effect of rotational atherectomy in obstructive atherosclerotic coronary artery disease. Circulation 1992; 86: 1383–93.
12. Lablanche JM. Recoil twenty four hours after coronary angioplasty: a computerized angiographic study [abstract]. J Am Coll Cardiol 1993; 21 (2 Suppl A): 35A.
13. Foley DP, Deckers JW, Serruys PW. There is no elastic recoil in the first 24 hours after PTCA: a quantitative angiographic study [abstract]. Br Heart J 1993; 69 Abstract Suppl: 46A.
14. Bertrand ME, Lablanche JM, Leroy F, Bauters C, McFadden E. Percutaneous transluminal coronary rotary ablation with the Rotablator. In Vogel JHK, King SB 3rd (eds): The practice of interventional cardiology, 2nd ed. St. Louis: Mosby-Year Book 1993: 141–7.
15. Reisman M, Buchbinder M, Bass T, Warth D, Dorros G, Peterson KL. Improvement in coronary dimensions at early 24–hour follow-up after coronary rotational ablation: implications for restenosis [abstract]. Circulation 1992; 86 Suppl I: I332.
16. Teirstein PS, Warth DC, Haq N *et al.* High speed rotational coronary atherectomy for patients with diffuse coronary artery disease. J Am Coll Cardiol 1991; 18: 1694–701.
17. Zacca NM, Kleiman NS, Rodriguez AR *et al.* Rotational ablation of coronary artery lesions using single, large burrs. Cathet Cardiovasc Diagn 1992; 26: 92–7.
18. Stertzer SH, Rosenblum J, Shaw RE *et al.* Coronary rotational ablation: initial experience in 302 procedures. J Am Coll Cardiol 1993; 21: 287–95.
19. Safian RD, Niazi KA, Strzelecki M *et al.* Detailed angiographic analysis of high-speed mechanical rotational atherectomy in human coronary arteries. Circulation 1993; 88: 961–8.
20. Brogan WC 3rd, Popma JJ, Pichard AD *et al.* Rotational coronary atherectomy after unsuccessful coronary balloon angioplasty. Am J Cardiol 1993; 71: 794–8.
21. Mintz GS, Pichard AD, Popma JJ, Kent KM, Satler LF, Leon MB. Preliminary experience with adjunct directional coronary atherectomy after high-speed rotational atherectomy in the treatment of calcific coronary artery disease. Am J Cardiol 1993; 71: 799–804.

PART SIX

'The rivals'

23. Coronary angioscopy – An inner view

JEAN-MARC LABLANCHE, MARTIAL HAMON,
EUGÈNE P. McFADDEN, CHRISTOPHE BAUTERS &
MICHEL E. BERTRAND

Summary

Thanks to recent technical advances, percutaneous coronary angioscopy has become a relatively straightforward technic, applicable in most patients. The angioscope we currently employ (Imagecath, Baxter) is a monorail system incorporating a compliant balloon that when inflated temporarily interrupts blood flow, allowing excellent visualization through its 3000 pixel optic imaging bundle after distal infusion of saline. The device is introduced through a standard guiding catheter, over a 0.014" wire ensuring compatibility with standard balloon dilation equipment. The technic is safe in experienced hands. In our first 200 procedures, performed in 115 vessels before and/or after angioplasty, 2 brief episodes of ventricular fibrillation, 2 localized dissections at the site of balloon inflation, and 2 minor stent displacements occurred early in our experience. None were associated with any detectable clinical consequences.

Angioscopy provides valuable diagnostic information. It is the only method that can provide 'histopathological' data by the percutaneous route. The color of a plaque is strongly associated with the clinical presentation. Unstable plaques are usually yellow and ulcerated,with red or white thrombus. Stable plaques are usually uniformly white or yellow. Restenotic lesions are usually white. Such morphologic information may help to guide therapy. Angioscopy also complements angiography in the assessment of the results of angioplasty, and in defining the need for, and type of, adjunctive therapy. For example, the hazy or irregular angiographic appearance common after coronary angioplasty, is often shown by angioscopy to be due to dissection, and not to thrombus, as previously thought.

Overall, angioscopy allows an evaluation of the degree of instability of a plaque by visualising its color and by defining the presence and age of associated thrombus. The limitations of the procedure include the requirement for an adequate length of proximal vessel to allow inflation of the occlusive cuff, the difficulty encountered in exploring angulated segments, and the inability to visualize the vessel distal to a severe stenosis. Unlike intravascular ultrasound, angioscopy allows lesion visualization from the proximal vessel avoiding the potential trauma associated with crossing a severe lesion.

J.H.C. Reiber and P.W. Serruys (eds): Progress in quantitative coronary arteriography, 369–381.

Introduction

The introduction of coronary angiography was a major milestone in the development of cardiology. It has revolutionized the diagnosis and treatment of coronary disease and has enabled major advances in our understanding of the pathophysiology and the natural history of coronary disease. Angiography provided the conclusive evidence that variant angina was related to intermittent spasm of epicardial vessels [1]. Angiographic studies during the acute phase of myocardial infarction showed that infarction was related to acute thrombosis of an epicardial vessel and rekindled interest in thrombolytic therapy [2].

Angiographic images provide information regarding the size of the internal lumen of an epicardial vessel, and to some extent allow an assessment of the morphological characteristics of epicardial stenoses. This information is obviously critical for clinical decision-making regarding the need for and the preferred method of revascularization. However, pathologic and clinical studies have emphasised some of the shortcomings of angiography. The extent of coronary atherosclerosis on pathological study is much greater that can be appreciated on angiography [3]. Apparently 'normal' segments on angiography may have extensive atherosclerotic involvement; this may not be appreciated on angiography because atherosclerotic arteries undergo compensatory dilation [4]. Thus, to borrow an analogy of Serruys *et al.*, it is important to realise that angiography provides an accurate assessment of size of the 'hole', namely the internal luminal diameter of the vessel, but cannot assess the size of the 'doughnut', namely the thickness of the vessel wall [5]. Another limitation of angiography relates to the inability of angiography to aid in the prediction of future ischemic events. Serial angiographic studies have shown that stenoses responsible for myocardial infarction are not necessarily severe, and that the most severe stenosis, on pre-infarction angiography, is often not the 'culprit' lesion, as assessed by subsequent post-infarction angiography [6]. This is perhaps not surprising, as acute coronary events are most likely related to 'plaque fissuring' with subsequent thrombotic occlusion. Pathologic studies suggest that plaques with specific characteristics, such as those that are rich in lipid, are particularly prone to rupture. Unfortunately, the first clinical manifestation of coronary disease in many individuals is sudden cardiac death, presumably related to arrythmia triggered by sudden coronary occlusion. It is obviously of critical importance to develop accurate clinically applicable methods to assess the characteristics and natural history of atherosclerotic plaques, in order to develop strategies for prevention in high-risk populations.

The era of interventional cardiology has created a new 'limitation' of angiography. Angiography is the only practical method for the assessment of the immediate result after percutaneous transluminal coronary angioplasty. The immediate post-angioplasty angiogram has introduced a new repertoire of angiographic images, the pathophysiological significance of which is incompletely understood. Descriptive terms such as intraluminal 'haziness', intraluminal filling defect, intraluminal and extraluminal dissection have been employed to describe such appearances. However, their pathological and clinical implications have not yet been fully elucidated.

These limitations of coronary angiography have stimulated interest in the development of alternative methods for assessment of epicardial coronary vessels. Two new imaging modalities have been developed, namely coronary angioscopy and intravascular ultrasound imaging. These technics provide information on the morphology of coronary plaques and on the extent of atherosclerosis that complements that obtained by angiography alone.

In this chapter, we describe the initial experience with percutaneous coronary angioscopy in our institution. Initially, we describe the design of the angioscope (ImageCath, Baxter) and the technic of angioscopy. We discuss the potential effects of angioscopy on 'normal' coronary segments exposed to inflation of the angioscopy cuff. Subsequently, we describe the angioscopic appearances encountered and attempt to relate them to the angiographic appearances and to the clinical presentation of the patients. Finally, we discuss the potential role of angioscopy in the future, with particular emphasis on possible applications in conjunction with percutaneous transluminal coronary angioplasty and other new technics for percutaneous revascularization.

Historical background

Although often presented today as a new technic, attempts to visualize intracardiac structures were reported as early as the beginning of the twentieth century [7]. In the early sixties, Carlens and Silander obtained images of the right atrium and right ventricle of the dog with use of a rigid scope introduced through the internal jugular vein [8]. Angioscopy of small vessels, such as the coronary arteries, only became possible in the early 1980's, thanks to the development of ultrathin fibreglass endoscopes. With use of these early, and still somewhat primitive instruments, several groups in Europe, Japan, and the United States began working on the technic of coronary angioscopy in an intraoperative setting and by the percutaneous route [9–11]. Since then, angioscopy has provided a wealth of information that has enhanced our understanding of coronary disease; specific angioscopic appearances have been correlated with particular clinical syndromes and with angiographic findings [12, 13]. Angioscopy after coronary interventions has improved our understanding of the mechanisms of angioplasty, and may have a therapeutic role as an adjunct to such procedures [14, 15].

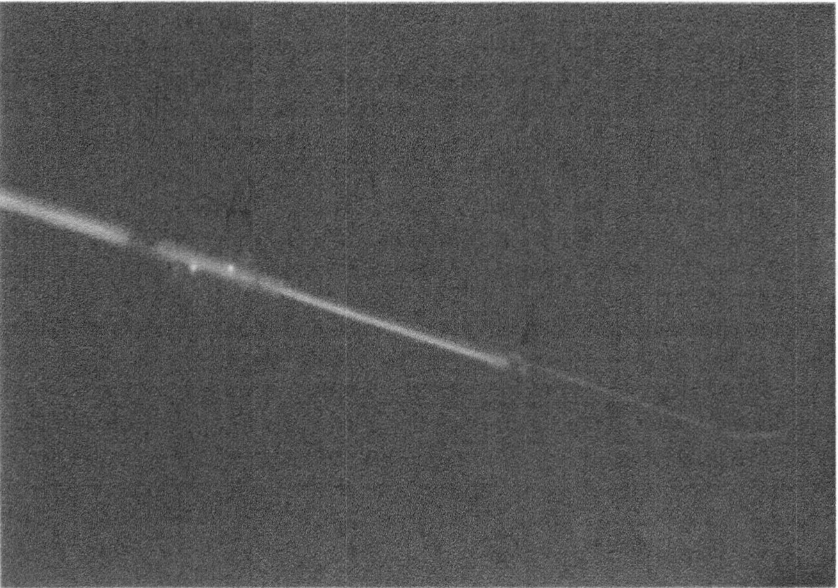

Figure 23.1. The distal end of the angioscope (ImageCath, Baxter). The optical fiber is indicated by a single arrow and the inflated cuff balloon by a double arrow.

The coronary angioscope

A 4.5 French coronary angioscope (Coronary ImageCath, Baxter, Edwards LIS Division, California) was used in all procedures. The 1.5 mm external diameter of the angioscope permits its utilization through a standard 8F guiding catheter. The angioscope consists of a flexible catheter with a distensible occlusion cuff at its distal end (Figure 23.1). The occlusion cuff is inflated to a maximum diameter of 5 mm with a mixture of saline and contrast medium. The optical imaging bundle (0.6 mm, 3000 pixels) passes through the catheter and can explore a 5 cm length of artery distal to the inflated cuff. The optic bundle has a field of view of 55 degrees in air and a depth of field of more than 0.5 mm. The angioscope incorporates a guidewire lumen at the distal end that accomodates a standard 0.014 inch guide wire. Saline perfusion through the catheter when the cuff is inflated allows excellent visualization of the coronary lumen. Saline is injected with use of a standard power injector, initially at a rate of one milliliter per second, that can be reduced to 0.5 milliliters per second when the lumen is blood-free. During the procedure the images are recorded on videotape with an accompanying recorded commentary, for later analysis.

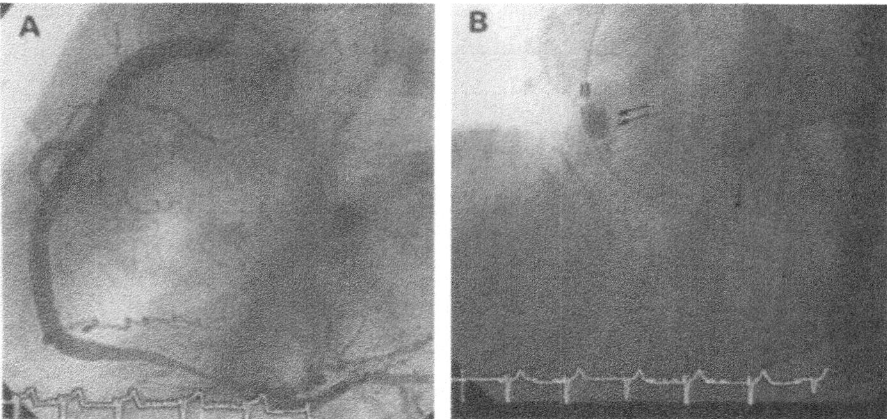

Figure 23.2. Angiogram showing a stenosis in the distal part of the right coronary artery (Panel A). The coronary angioscope in position in the coronary artery (Panel B). The inflated balloon is visible (double arrow) proximal to the stenosis and the optical fiber (single arrow) at the level of the stenosis.

Technique of angioscopy

A standard 8F guiding catheter is introduced into the coronary artery via the percutaneous femoral route. Heparin (10,000 IU) is given intravenously, and a bolus of isosorbide dinitrate is administered into the coronary artery. Baseline angiograms are then performed in at least two projections for the right coronary artery, and three for the left coronary artery.

A standard 0.014 inch guidewire is advanced across the lesion. The angioscope is advanced under fluoroscopic control and the radioopaque marker at the distal end is positioned proximal to the target lesion (Figure 23.2). The occlusive cuff is inflated, and saline is infused through the infusion port of the catheter. The angioscope is then advanced to the lesion and if feasible into the distal vessel. The occlusive cuff is deflated, and electrocardiographic changes, if present, are allowed to resolve. The procedure is then repeated, but this time in the opposite direction. The average duration of a single pass is about 40 seconds. It is important to exercise caution when the angioscope is being withdrawn; on occasion a loop may form in the guidewire; this can be avoided by observing the wire on fluoroscopy, and if necessary, by exerting gentle traction on the wire while withdrawing the angioscope. After withdrawal, the angioscope is carefully flushed with saline. The angioplasty procedure is then performed and the angioscopy procedure repeated afterwards. The average duration of a single angioscopic examination is less than 5 minutes.

Table 23.1. Angiographic and clinical complications encountered during 200 consecutive angioscopy procedures.*

Complication	Frequency (Percent)
Ventricular fibrillation	2 (1%)
Stent displacement	2 (1%)
Localized dissection	2 (1%)
Death, infarction, bypass surgery	0 (0%)

* None of these events had clinical consequences.

Study patients

In general we studied patients who were scheduled for percutaneous transluminal coronary angioplasty. Informed consent was obtained from each patient. Patients were considered for angioscopy if they had a lesion that was situated in a proximal vessel that was not excessively tortuous. The limitation to such lesions is necessary because of the requirement to have a segment proximal to the target lesion of at least 10 millimeters in length, to accommodate the occlusive cuff.

Procedural details and complications

Of the first 200 procedures performed, 113 procedures were performed before an angioplasty procedure, and 87 afterwards (Table 23.1). Several technical complications were encountered, predominantly during our learning phase. On four occasions the optic bundle became caught on the guide wire while it was being retracted; this occurred in highly curved vessel segments. On three occasions the problem was solved by pulling the entire system back into the proximal noncurved segment of the vessel and then retracting the optic bundle.On one occasion, the entire system had to be withdrawn into the guiding catheter. On another occasion, the distensible occlusion cuff failed to deflate; it was withdrawn, while still inflated, into the guiding catheter without angiographically apparent vessel damage. On five occasions the occlusive cuff burst without any clinical or angiographic sequelae.

Angiographic complications occurred in four cases. On two occasions a localized dissection occurred; one was related to inflation of the distensible cuff; the other was produced by the tip of the imaging bundle in a highly curved arterial segment. Neither dissection had clinical consequences. On two other occasions, angioscopy performed immediately after stent placement resulted in slight displacement of the stent by the tip of the imaging bundle.

Chest pain and electrocardiographic changes, more marked than those observed during subsequent balloon angioplasty occurred frequently during angioscopy, presumably related to saline perfusion. On two occasions, ventricular fibrillation occurred that was rapidly cardioverted. These two instances occurred during the first six procedures and were felt to be related to prolonged injection of saline.

Potential adverse effects of angioscopy-induced intimal trauma

Experiments in animals have shown that the trauma induced by balloon inflation in angiographically normal segments may lead to a neointimal proliferative response that is often used as a model of experimental angioplasty. Although the balloon used to occlude the artery during the performance of angioscopy is much more compliant than the balloons used for coronary angioplasty, there is obviously cause for concern that balloon inflation in what are usually angiographically normal arterial segments may have detrimental long-term effects on arterial lumen diameter.

We designed a study to determine whether angioscopy was associated with significant changes in lumen diameter at the site of cuff inflation. We studied 52 consecutive patients undergoing coronary angioscopy. We measured with use of quantitative edge-detection angiography (CAESAR System) the mean and minimal lumen diameters at the site of cuff inflation (localized by filming the inflated cuff) and at control segments before angioscopy, after angioscopy, and at 6 months follow-up. Follow-up angiograms were performed in 37 (71%) patients. At follow-up, the mean (3.22 ± 0.54 mm) and minimal (2.76 ± 0.58 mm) diameters of the segment exposed to the inflated cuff were not significantly different from the equivalent values (3.22 ± 0.58 mm, 2.75 ± 0.61 mm) before angioscopy. No significant changes occurred in the mean or minimal diameters of the control segments over the same period. The late change (follow-up minus pre-angioscopy) in mean lumen diameter at the cuff inflation site (− 0.005 ± 0.18 mm) was not significantly different from that at the control site (0.004 ± 0.20 mm). While it is impossible to determine with certainty whether inflation of the angioscopy cuff causes endothelial denudation in man, these results show that the trauma associated with balloon cuff inflation does not have detectable long-term effects on epicardial lumen diameter [16].

Review of angioscopic findings

Angioscopy provides information that is complementary to that obtained with angiography. Only angiography can provide accurate information regarding the relative anatomic severity of a stenosis. Although some authors have suggested that it is possible to accurately assess the degree of stenosis by angioscopy, the lack of a calibration device and the impossibility of determining the distance between the lens and the stenosis make such determinations extremely subjective [17]. In contrast, only angioscopy allows a

Table 23.2. Lesion color related to clinical presentation in 82 patients before coronary angioplasty.

Clinical presentation	Lesion color			
	Red	Red/Pink	Yellow/Dull	White/Shiny
Recent myocardial infarction	11	8	5	1
Unstable angina	3	4	4	7
Stable angina	0	5	4	7
Restenosis	0	4	4	15

direct view of the color and of surface characteristics of the stenosis and the adjacent, usually angiographically normal, arterial wall (Table 23.2). On angioscopy, the endothelium overlying the normal arterial wall appears white or pink and reflects light, giving a characteristic glistening appearance. Over areas that have luminal irregularities on angiography, or at the site of stenoses, the normal whitish glistening appearance changes to dull-yellow or white.

Detection of intracoronary thrombi: Role of angioscopy

Previous studies have suggested that angioscopy is much more sensitive than angiography for the detection of intracoronary thrombus [11, 12, 18]. Angiographically, the presence of an intraluminal filling defect is regarded as highly specific for the presence of an intracoronary thrombus. Other angiographic appearances that are less specific and less sensitive include an 'irregular' stenosis contour and the presence of intraluminal haziness. On angioscopy, thrombi may appear red and globular protruding into the vessel lumen; they may also be detected as flat red patches adherent to the surface of a yellow or whitish ulcerated plaque. Several authors describe a subdivision of thrombi into red thrombus and white thrombus; red thrombus, containing a predominance of red blood cells has been observed most frequently in the setting of acute myocardial infarction or shortly afterwards, whereas white thrombus occurred most frequently in unstable angina [12].

Angiographic and angioscopic studies have established that acute myocardial infarction is associated with occlusive thrombus formation [2, 12]. Based on the results of such studies, thrombolytic therapy has become the keystone of the modern management of myocardial infarction. Serial angiographic studies demonstrate that the residual stenosis after thrombolytic therapy for acute myocardial infarction often regresses spontaneously. This spontaneous improvement has been attributed to the resolution of associated intracoronary thrombus. However, the extent and time course of changes in the extent of residual thrombus after myocardial infarction remains unclear.

We performed percutaneous coronary angioscopy in 25 patients with semi-recent acute myocardial infarction who had received thrombolytic therapy [19, 20]. Five patients were excluded because the culprit lesion could not be identified (n = 1), or because the angioscopic images were suboptimal (n = 4). The mean time to angioscopy was 15 ± 14 days, range 7 to 60 days in the remaining 20 patients. Most of the infarct-related lesions were located on the left anterior descending artery (n = 11); less often they were found on the left circumflex (n = 4) or right (n = 5) coronary arteries. Three patients with occluded (TIMI Grade 0) infarct-related vessels had red thrombus completely occluding the vessel lumen. Of the remaining 17 patients, thrombi were visualised by angioscopy in 13 patients, whereas only two (12%) had unequivocal evidence of thrombus (in the form of discrete intraluminal filling defects) on angiography.

In seven of the 13 patients who had angioscopically diagnosed thrombus, the thrombus was flat, red in colour, and adherent to the vessel wall. On arteriography, thrombus was suspected in only two of these seven patients; one had an intraluminal filling defect and one had a stenosis with overhanging edges. The other six patients with angioscopically visible thrombi had red thrombus protruding into the vessel lumen. Angiography revealed an intraluminal filling defect in one, a stenosis with hazy arterial borders in one, and stenoses with overhanging edges in three.

Thrombi were less often seen in patients with unstable angina. In 18 consecutive patients with unstable angina, a red globular intraluminal thrombus was seen in three (17%) patients; four (22%) patients had thrombi that were flat or slightly raised and adherent to the stenosis; thrombi were not detected in the remaining 11 (61%) patients.

A somewhat unexpected finding was the not infrequent detection of thrombi in patients with stable angina, or in the nonculprit vessels of these with unstable angina or with recent myocardial infarction. Of 16 'stable' coronary lesions that were examined, thrombi that were invariably small and adherent to the wall were seen at 5 (31%) lesions.

Coronary dissections

Experimental studies in animals, and anecdotal postmortem observations in man suggest that dissection to a greater or lesser extent almost invariably occurs during balloon angioplasty. Angiographically, dissections are seen with moderate frequency after angioplasty; although the presence of visible dissection after angioplasty is not associated with a greater long-term risk of restenosis, it has been associated with an increased risk of acute closure. Angioscopically, dissections may present as thin white wisps of tissue that appear to float in the vessel lumen. Alternatively, there may be longitudinal fissures in the vessel wall with varying degrees of hemorrhage; on occasion, dissections may present as yellow irregular masses apparently floating in the lumen.

In one patient studied after angioplasty, we found a mobile intraluminal mass that corresponded to the typical angiographic description of thrombus. Angioscopy revealed no evidence of thrombus, but rather a yellow mobile flap of tissue floating in the lumen. This led to the decision to perform atherectomy rather than conventional balloon angioplasty. In another patient studied one week after a thrombolysed myocardial infarction, an eccentric stenosis with overhanging edges was seen on angiography in the proximal part of a large right coronary artery. Angioscopy revealed a yellow ulcerated plaque protruding into the vessel lumen with only a small amount of adherent thrombus. Because of the angioscopic findings, we elected to implant an intracoronary stent, which produced a satisfactory acute angiographic result.

Appearance of the restenotic plaque

In our institution, we recommend six-month follow-up angiography to all patients after successful coronary angioplasty. Twenty-three such patients underwent angioscopy of the dilated lesion. The appearance of the stenosis in these patients was remarkably uniform; 15 lesions were white or greyish white in appearance and either completely smooth or only slightly irregular. These appearances, which are similar to those described by White *et al.* presumably are the visual correlate of the fibrous plaque that has been documented histologically in such lesions [21]. Of the remaining eight lesions, four were yellow, and four were reddish-pink.

Potential clinical applications of angioscopy

It is only in recent years that the technic of coronary angioscopy has developed to the extent that it can be performed in the clinical setting. Even now, technical considerations preclude its use as a routine adjunct to coronary angiography. Studies with intraoperative angioscopy, which has been performed now for more than a decade, have suggested a potential role in verifying the integrity of anastomotic sites during coronary bypass surgery, and in inspecting venous grafts for possible damage, and for the presence of incompletely ligated sidebranches, before implantation. Grundfest *et al.* reported that in three cases the angioscopic findings led to a revision of the anastamosis [22].

At the present time, it is too early to predict whether coronary angioscopy will have a role in future clinical practice. Some of the potential indications are listed in Table 23.3. Furthermore, several technical problems remain to be resolved (Table 23.4). However, the additional information provided by

Table 23.3. Potential indications for coronary angioscopy.

Diagnosis of thrombus
Unstable angina
Equivocal angiographic findings
Intraluminal filling defect
'Hazy' angiographic appearances
Evaluation of angioplasty results
Differentiation of dissection/thrombus
Need for adjunctive therapy
Evaluation of new interventional devices

Table 23.4. Limitations of angioscopy.

Limitation	Cause
Extremely proximal segments	Inadequate space for occlusive cuff
Severe angulation	Limited flexibility of optical bundle
Field of view	Tip of optical bundle non-steerable
Viewing time	Ischaemia related to coronary occlusion
Collateral circulation	Saline flush may be insufficient for adequate viewing
No quantification	Lack of calibration device

angioscopy is clearly of benefit in specific situations in deciding the optimal therapeutic approach, as has been shown in anecdotal reports.

The advent of intracoronary stenting has introduced yet another iatrogenic problem for the interventional cardiologist, namely that of early stent occlusion. It is conventionally held that early coronary stent occlusion is exclusively due to the development of stent thrombosis. A recent report described a series of patients in whom early stent occlusion was not due to thrombosis, but was a consequence of obstructive intimal dissection [23]. A dissection was not observed in any of the cases on the immediate post-stenting angiogram.

The major advantage of angioscopy is the ability to detect the presence of intracoronary thrombus. Angioscopy has been clearly shown to be superior to angiography in this respect [11, 12, 18–20]. The availability of newer technologies such as transluminal extraction atherectomy, that appear to be associated with a lower acute complication rate than traditional balloon angioplasty, for the treatment of lesions that have a large burden of thrombus suggest a potential role for angioscopy in preangioplasty assessment, when the angiographic appearances are suspicious. A particular niche for angioscopy may lie in the assessment of patients with recent myocardial infarction. Residual stenosis on angiography in such patients may be due to the presence of a significant underlying atherosclerotic stenosis, but may equally be due to the presence of residual thrombus superimposed on a nonsignificant lesion.

Angioscopic assessment may aid in this distinction and may be useful in deciding the optimal therapeutic approach.

Finally, there are numerous potential research applications for percutaneous angioscopy. The assessment of the results of thrombolytic therapy in unstable angina, the assessment of the post cardiac transplant patient, and the assessment of the immediate results of angioplasty and of newer non-balloon technologies represent only a few of the potential applications [24].

References

1. Maseri A, Pesola A, Marzilli M *et al.* Coronary vasospasm in angina pectoris. Lancet 1977; 1: 713–7.
2. De Wood MA, Spores J, Notske R *et al.* Prevalence of total coronary occlusion during the early hours of transmural myocardial infarction. N Engl J Med 1980; 303: 897–902.
3. Dietz WA, Tobis JM, Isner JM. Failure of angiography to accurately depict the extent of coronary artery narrowing in three fatal cases of percutaneous transluminal coronary angioplasty. J Am Coll Cardiol 1992; 19: 1261–70.
4. Glagov S, Weisenberg E, Zarins CK, Stankunavicius R, Kolettis GJ. Compensatory enlargement of human atherosclerotic coronary arteries. N Engl J Med 1987; 316: 1371–5.
5. Beatt KJ, Serruys PW, Luijten HE *et al.* Restenosis after coronary angioplasty: the paradox of increased lumen diameter and restenosis. J Am Coll Cardiol 1992; 19: 258–66.
6. Little WC, Constantinescu M, Applegate R *et al.* Can coronary angiography predict the site of a subsequent myocardial infarction in patients with mild-to-moderate coronary artery disease? Circulation 1988; 78: 1157–66.
7. Allen D, Graham E. Intracardiac surgery – a new method. J Am Med Assoc 1922; 79: 1028–30.
8. Carlens E, Silander T. Method for direct inspection of the right atrium: experimental investigation in the dog. Surgery 1961; 49: 622–4.
9. Hombach V, Höher M, Hannekum A *et al.* Erste klinische Erfahrungen mit der Koronarendoskopie. Dtsch Med Wochenschr 1986; 111: 1135–40.
10. Uchida Y, Tomaru T, Nakamura F, Furuse A, Fujimori Y, Hasegawa K. Percutaneous coronary angioscopy in patients with ischemic heart disease. Am Heart J 1987; 114: 1216–22.
11. Sherman CT, Litvack F, Grundfest W *et al.* Coronary angioscopy in patients with unstable angina pectoris. N Engl J Med 1986; 315: 913–9.
12. Mizuno K, Satomura K, Miyamoto A *et al.* Angioscopic evaluation of coronary-artery thrombi in acute coronary syndromes. N Engl J Med 1992; 326: 287–91.
13. White CJ, Ramee SR, Collins TJ, Mesa JE, Jain A, Ventura HO. Percutaneous coronary angioscopy: applications in interventional cardiology. J Intervent Cardiol 1993; 6: 61–7.
14. Uchida Y, Hasegawa K, Kawamura K, Shibuya I. Angioscopic observation of the coronary luminal changes induced by percutaneous transluminal coronary angioplasty. Am Heart J 1989; 117: 769–76.
15. Nakamura F, Kvasnicka J, Uchida Y, Geschwind HJ. Percutaneous angioscopic evaluation of luminal changes induced by excimer laser angioplasty. Am Heart J 1992; 124: 1467–72.
16. Hamon M, Lablanche JM, Bauters C, Mc Fadden EP, Quandalle P, Bertrand ME. Effect of balloon inflation in angiographically normal segments during coronary angioscopy; a quantitative angiographic study. Cathet Cardiovascular Diagn. In press.
17. Lee G, Garcia JM, Corso PJ *et al.* Correlation of coronary angioscopic to angiographic findings in coronary artery disease. Am J Cardiol 1986; 58: 238–41.

18. White CJ, Ramee SR, Collins TJ, Mesa JE, Jain A. Percutaneous angioscopy of saphenous vein coronary bypass grafts. J Am Coll Cardiol 1993; 21: 1181–5.
19. Lablanche JM, Hamon M, Mc Fadden EP, Bauters C, Quandalle P, Bertrand ME. Persisting intracoronary thrombus is frequently detected by angioscopy three weeks after thrombolysis for acute myocardial infarction [abstract]. Eur Heart J 1993; 14 Abstract Suppl: 404.
20. Lablanche JM, Hamon M, Mc Fadden EP, Bauters C, Quandalle P, Bertrand ME. Angiographically silent thrombus frequently persists after thrombolytic therapy for acute myocardial infarction: a prospective angioscopic study [abstract]. Circulation 1993; 88 (4 Suppl): I595.
21. White CJ, Ramee SR, Mesa JE, Collins TJ. Percutaneous coronary angioscopy in patients with restenosis after coronary angioplasty. J Am Coll Cardiol 1991; 17 (6 Suppl B): 46B–9B.
22. Grundfest W, Litvack F, Sherman T *et al.* Delineation of peripheral and coronary detail by intraoperative angioscopy. Ann Surg 1985; 202: 394–400.
23. Den Heijer P, Van Dijk RB, Twisk SP, Lie KI. Early stent occlusion is not always caused by thrombosis. Cathet Cardiovasc Diagn 1993; 29: 136–40.
24. Ventura HO, White CJ, Jain SP *et al.* Assessment of intracoronary morphology in cardiac transplant recipients by angioscopy and intravascular ultrasound. Am J Cardiol 1993; 72: 805–9.

24. Intracoronary imaging with ultrasound

ANDONIS G. VIOLARIS, CARLO DI MARIO, PATRICK W. SERRUYS, PIM J. DE FEYTER & JOS R.T.C. ROELANDT

Summary

Although intravascular ultrasound transducers were first developed and tested in the early seventies [1] it wasn't until the advent of catheter based coronary interventional techniques that a major impetus was given to their development. Because intracoronary ultrasound allows direct visualisation of the atherosclerotic plaque [2, 3], it may assist in the choice of intervention, guidance during the procedure and assessment of the results and any complications. Furthermore, direct real time visualisation of arterial wall morphology offers unique opportunities for the *in vivo* assessment of arterial pathophysiology and dynamics on a beat-to-beat basis.

Instrumentation

Two approaches are available for obtaining cross-sectional imaging of the vessel wall. Firstly by mechanical rotation, of either the ultrasound transducer itself, or an acoustic reflector in front of a fixed transducer. The advantage of these systems is high resolution imaging without the presence of a near-field artefact. Realising a driving mechanism while keeping the catheter fully flexible and steerable are, however, challenging problems. Flexibility and steerability are not a major concern with the alternative, multi-element electronic approach, where sixty-four transducer elements are mounted circumferentially in a 360° radial array perpendicular to the long axis of the catheter, but this system is limited by near-field artifact and restricted resolution and dynamic range. The choice of equipment is important as there is evidence to suggest that image quality and interpretation varies between manufacturers.

Image interpretation

Comparison with angiography

A major limitation of contrast angiography is that it provides information predominantly about the vessel lumen. Consequently, morphological changes in the vessel wall are largely inferred from their effect on the lumen, but cannot be directly visualised. Furthermore, there is high inter- and intra-

J.H.C. Reiber and P.W. Serruys (eds): Progress in quantitative coronary arteriography, 383–395.

observer variability in the measurement of coronary stenosis and the commonly used percentage stenosis takes no account of the eccentricity, or otherwise of the stenosis or whether the 'normal' part of the vessel is truly normal. By contrast, ultrasound allows direct visualisation of the vessel wall and hence overcomes many of these inherent limitations of contrast angiography. Because intracoronary ultrasound almost invariably shows greater vessel involvement and/or more severe atherosclerosis, it is likely that new criteria for atherosclerotic severity, based on ultrasound findings will be required.

Nevertheless intracoronary ultrasound cannot image the complete coronary tree; therefore, contrast angiography will remain useful for road mapping, guiding the ultrasound probe to the area of interest. Ultrasound imaging will then provide more detailed information on the area of interest or target lesion. Greater integration of intracoronary ultrasound within angiographic equipment will be required to fully exploit the complimentary information provided, for improved real-time decision making during interventional procedures.

Characteristics of the normal wall

In vitro and *in vivo* studies have shown that muscular arteries can be distinguished from elastic arteries on the basis of their echographic characteristics [4]. Muscular arteries have a hypoechoic smooth muscle component in the media which results in a three-layered appearance, whereas elastic arteries and veins have a more homogeneous appearance to their vessel wall. Intimal atheroma and calcification may, however, induce diffuse attenuation or shadowing preventing the evaluation of the underlying media. Furthermore, in up to 20% of muscular arteries fibrous degeneration of the muscular component of the media results in a homogeneous appearance [5]. A homogeneous appearance is also seen in young people where the intimal layer is thin; some diffuse intimal thickening must be present before the (typical) 3–layered appearance is visualised [6].

Study of the atherosclerotic plaque

In vitro *experience*

In vitro studies have shown that two types of atherosclerotic plaque can be distinguished [4, 5]. 'Hard' plaques, composed of dense fibrous tissue, are seen as bright echoreflective lesions with acoustic shadowing and perhaps duplicate echoes in the presence of calcific deposits. 'Soft' lipid rich plaques are weakly echoreflective (Figure 24.1). Thrombi, plaque rupture and dissection after intervention are also detected with great detail.

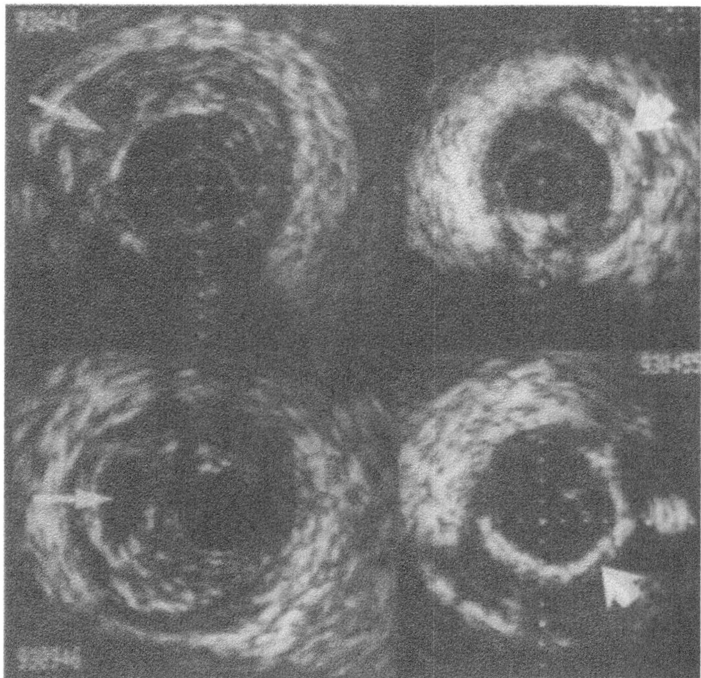

Figure 24.1. Intracoronary ultrasound images from diseased coronary arteries demonstrating: upper left panel. An eccentric, soft, weakly echo reflective plaque (arrow). Lower left panel. An eccentric, soft, weakly echo reflective, plaque with a 'lipid lake' (arrow). Upper right panel. A hard, strongly echogenic, fibrous plaque (arrow) extending from the 12 to the 5 o'clock positions. Lower right panel. A rim of superficial calcification (arrow), extending from the 1 to the 9 o'clock positions. Note the marked acoustic shadowing behind it.

In vivo *experience*

Peripheral vessels

Intravascular imaging of the aorta, iliac and femoral arteries can be obtained easily and the severity of stenosis, type and extent of atherosclerotic plaque and involvement of the medial layer assessed [7, 8]. Quantitative analysis of lumen and plaque area shows a close correlation with digital angiography [9]. Various interventions such as transluminal angioplasty, atherectomy and endovascular stent delivery are accurately monitored [10]. In comparison with angiography, intravascular ultrasound demonstrates a higher sensitivity in depicting presence and extent of dissection, length of intimal tears and characteristics of flow in the true and false lumen. Direct insertion of the ultrasound catheter during surgery can be used to replace more complex angiographic procedures in the evaluation of the efficacy of arterial bypass operation or end-arterectomy in peripheral vessels [11].

Coronary vessels

The limitations of contrast angiography for guidance of coronary interventional procedures has resulted in the development of smaller and more flexible catheters, amenable to coronary insertion. Intravascular ultrasound is able to detect and characterize atherosclerotic changes in what appear to be, angiographically, normal segments and in the presence of edge irregularities or luminal stenoses [12, 13].

Intracoronary imaging has provided direct evidence in support of previous pathology studies showing that coronary arteries undergo a progressive enlargement in relation to increases in plaque area so that a reduction of lumen area is delayed until the atherosclerotic lesion occupies more than 40% of the area circumscribed by the internal elastic lamina [14]. These findings explain why angiographically normal arterial segments show extensive atherosclerotic involvement at surgery. Hermiller and colleagues [15], have demonstrated, in 44 consecutive patients, that when coronary segments with $<30\%$ area stenosis are examined, there is an excellent correlation between internal elastic lamina (IEL) area and plaque area. In these segments the IEL area increased by 2.7 mm^2 for each 1 mm^2 increase in plaque area suggesting that arterial enlargement may overcompensate for early atherosclerotic lesions.

As well as being able to detect and characterize atherosclerotic changes in what appear to be, angiographically, normal segments, intracoronary imaging has also provided additional information in the presence of edge irregularities or luminal stenoses [12, 13]. Furthermore, directional atherectomy in conjunction with intracoronary imaging has confirmed previous *in vitro* studies suggesting that two types of atherosclerotic plaque can be distinguished [4, 5] by demonstrating a higher collagen and calcium content in echogenic 'hard' plaques and increased levels of fibrin, nuclei and lipids in 'soft' plaques [16].

As well as information on atherosclerosis, intracoronary imaging is also providing new insights into the pathogenesis of unstable coronary syndromes and accelerated atherosclerosis in transplant patients [17–23]. In the unstable coronary syndromes, ultrasound imaging has demonstrated more soft lesions and fewer mixed, calcified plaques with fewer intralesional calcium deposits than in stable angina, suggesting that ultrasound morphologic criteria are closely correlated to clinical anginal patterns [18–20]. Whether they correlate with clinical outcome, however, remains unknown.

In cardiac transplant recipients, intracoronary imaging has demonstrated that even angiographically normal vessels show a range of coronary intimal thickening, which includes occasional evidence of focal, early atheromatous lesions [22]. Furthermore, it has also demonstrated a vasoconstrictor response to acetylcholine at 1 year after transplantation suggesting endothelial dysfunction in the epicardial vessels [21] and that the vasodilatory response to nitroglycerin is attenuated during episodes of cardiac rejection, independent of the degree of intimal thickening [23].

Assessment of catheter based interventions

Preliminary evidence suggests that imaging prior to interventions may be helpful for deciding which lesions may be most suitable for which specific treatment modality, and imaging post-intervention may be helpful in delineating which patients are at increased risk of acute occlusion and long-term restenosis.

Prior to intervention ultrasound allows the distinction of 'soft' plaques which are more likely to be dilated by compression, stretching and superficial intimal tears from 'hard' or clearly calcific plaques, which are at increased risk of extensive dissection after balloon angioplasty [24]. Furthermore, the presence of diffuse subendothelial calcification is associated with a lower success rate and higher risk of complications after directional atherectomy [25], indicating that alternative techniques such as rotational or laser atherectomy should be used in this situation. Although echogenic plaques are harder to resect by directional atherectomy than echolucent ones, they are also less likely to restenose [16]. These initial studies confirm previous clinical and pathological studies demonstrating that plaque morphology may affect outcome, and suggest that increased stratification of patients for specific treatment modalities, based on *de novo* plaque morphology, may help in reducing acute occlusion and long-term restenosis post-intervention.

Following intervention, intracoronary ultrasound assessment may be useful in two ways, firstly in assessing and optimising the results and secondly in assessing the risk of acute occlusion and long term restenosis. Since angiography only provides an outline of the vessel lumen, an angiographically successful angioplasty may turn out to be a 'pseudo-success', perhaps because cracks and dissection planes in the vessel wall allow contrast flow, with, in reality, very little increase in the actual luminal area. Subsequent apposition of the split wall layers may result in an angiographic restenosis (a pseudo-restenosis), a lesion being classified as restenosis whereas in fact it was never an actual success. Intracoronary ultrasound by visualising the vessel wall as well as the vessel lumen may have an important role to play in ensuring a good result, with a good luminal cross-sectional area after intervention (Figure 24.2). Furthermore, in the case of stent implantation, the clear imaging of the struts by intracoronary ultrasound ensures that the operator is aware of any incomplete stent expansion and can take appropriate action.

A further important aspect of intracoronary imaging during intervention may be in providing prognostic information regarding the subsequent risk of acute occlusion or restenosis. Angiographic studies have shown that the presence of an intimal flap increases the risk of acute occlusion six-fold. Furthermore, post-mortem studies have shown that extensive medial tears also increase the risk of abrupt closure. As intracoronary ultrasound is very sensitive in detecting the development and characteristics of intimal flaps following interventional procedures [26, 27] it may be able to predict subsequent outcome. Preliminary evidence is supportive of this showing that in-

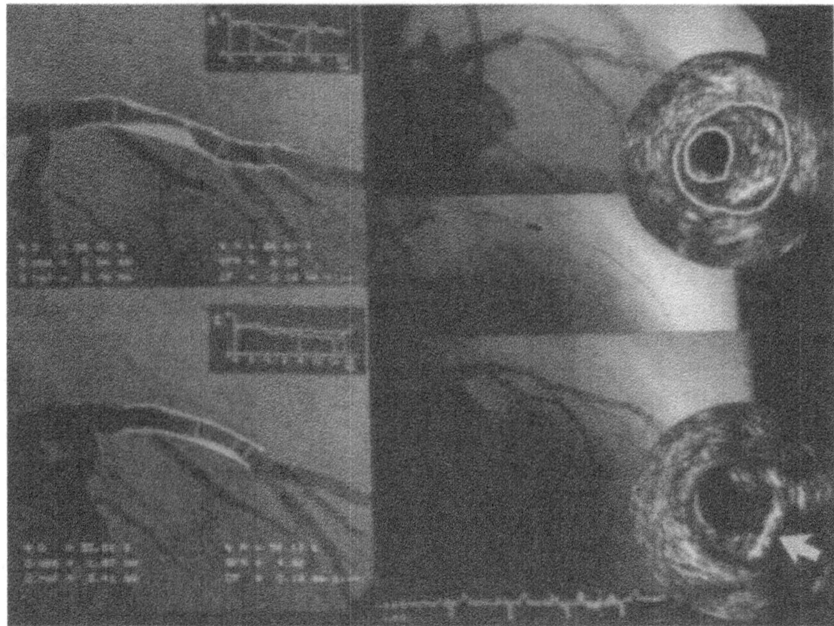

Figure 24.2. Left panels. Quantitative angiographic assessment of an eccentric left anterior descending coronary artery stenosis prior (upper panel), and post (lower panel), successful rotablator therapy. Right panels. Angiograms prior (upper), during (middle) and post (lower) rotablator therapy with ultrasound images prior (upper) and after therapy (lower). Note the eccentric nature of the, mainly fibrous plaque, with deep seated calcification resulting in some acoustic shadowing, at the 5 o'clock position. Following rotablator therapy most of the plaque has been removed apart from the, previously, deep seated, calcification (arrow).

timal tears are twice as common and also more severe in patients who subsequently went on to develop acute occlusion [28]. Preliminary evidence also suggests that intracoronary ultrasound may also be helpful in identifying a subset of patients who have a higher incidence of restenosis [26]. Both of these possibilities now need to be confirmed by the larger ongoing multicenter studies but the preliminary data sited above are already beginning to influence therapy with preliminary data from the ongoing GUIDE (Guidance by Ultrasound Imaging for Decision Endpoints) trial suggesting that the detailed information regarding plaque morphology provided by intracoronary ultrasound leads to a change in therapy in about 50% of cases.

Pathophysiology of intervention and restenosis

Intracoronary ultrasound has made a significant contribution to our understanding of the pathophysiology of coronary interventional procedures and restenosis. Intracoronary ultrasound studies have confirmed previous studies in peripheral vessels showing that luminal enlargement following balloon angioplasty is achieved primarily by arterial wall stretching with lesion volume remaining essentially unchanged [29]. They have also suggested that both vessel stretch and dissection are uncommon after atherectomy [30] thus confirming that plaque removal rather than a 'dotter effect' as the major mechanism for improved lumen area after this procedure.

Intracoronary ultrasound has also brought new understanding to the mechanisms involved in restenosis post-intervention. Our understanding of the mechanisms involved has previously been confined to serial angiographic assessment of the vessel lumen and post-mortem examination of limited histological tissue at specific time points in the disease process. Ultrasound has the potential to differentiate between the nature of the process (elastic recoil, mural thrombosis and intimal hyperplasia) and allow serial assessment of the *in-vivo* vessel wall, hence increasing our understanding of the pathophysiology of restenosis and allowing better targeting of therapeutic agents. These potential advantages have been recently confirmed by preliminary data from Kovach and colleagues, which suggest that chronic arterial recoil may have a far greater influence on late lumen loss and restenosis than previously thought [31].

Safety

The safety of intravascular and in particular intracoronary ultrasound should be a major concern. So far no significant adverse events have been reported when intracoronary ultrasound studies were performed prior to and following interventional procedures, including patients with acute coronary syndromes. Transient coronary spasm has been observed and the catheter can occlude flow when advanced into stenoses or small distal arteries, in which cases prompt withdrawl is clearly necessary. Serial studies in patients have not shown an increase in stenosis of the instrumented vessels when compared to those which were not instrumented making endothelial damage and accelerated atherosclerosis unlikely. These findings are of importance when one considers the use of intracoronary ultrasound in therapeutic trials for the study of regression/progression of atherosclerosis

Potential clinical and research directions

Angiography depicts only a silhouette of the vessel lumen; the extent of atherosclerotic disease and luminal narrowing, particularly in the early pre-stenotic phase, may therefore be misinterpreted. Intravascular ultrasound has the potential for detecting atherosclerotic changes in the pre-stenotic phase and allows accurate measurement of the plaque area as well as the vessel lumen. Furthermore it allows direct evaluation of plaque characteristics. These advantages have important implications for regression studies as dietary and pharmacological interventions are likely to induce regression of the vascular changes in the 'pre-stenotic' rather than the more advanced phases of atherosclerotic disease. Intravascular ultrasound thus has the potential capability to directly visualise these vessel wall abnormalities and may differentiate lipid plaques, potentially amenable to regression from fibrocalcific plaques which are less likely to respond to an intervention. Little progress has been made to date however because of financial costs and major problems in correctly locating the identical imaging position during long-term follow-up.

When a three-layered appearance is present in a muscular artery, the middle hypoechoic layer may be used as a landmark for the detection and quantitation of intimal and medial change [32]. Intravascular ultrasound could thus be useful in assessing changes in medial thickness induced by systemic arterial hypertension and evaluating the effects of long-term anti-hypertensive treatment. Major limitations remain, however, as the plaque has a longitudinal architecture and is complex, requiring true 3–D reconstruction before these potential benefits may be realised.

Work is also in progress in analysis of the backscatter signals to allow a more accurate and quantitative characterisation of plaque components. This may allow better discrimination between soft plaque and thrombus, which have roughly equivalent echogenicity, as well as characterising the lipid content of specific plaques and hence their propensity to rupture and acute occlusion.

Three-dimensional reconstruction

The present imaging field is orthogonal to the catheter and is really only a two-dimensional representation of a complex three-dimensional process. Three-dimensional reconstruction of intracoronary ultrasound images is a major advance since tomographic views are now displayed longitudinally giving a more complete spatial picture of a coronary segment and any associated mural pathology (Figure 24.3). It thus offers an efficient gateway to the quantification of volumetric changes of atherosclerotic plaque, a better understanding of the complex longitudinal patho-anatomy and, when available on-line, would greatly help in guiding interventional techniques and assessing their results. Major problems remain, however, as present algorithms do not take into account catheter shift during withdrawal and lumen curvature, resulting in a straight catheter line reconstruction and hence a three-dimensional image which is not correctly reconstructed spatially.

Forward imaging

All available imaging transducers to date are side facing, requiring advancement of the transducer to the point of interest before images can be acquired.

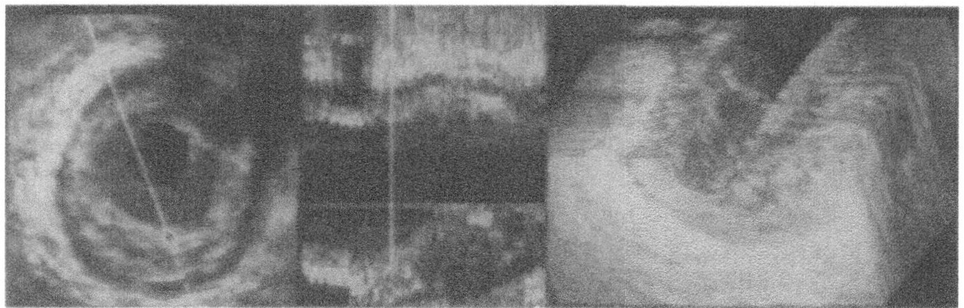

Figure 24.3. Intracoronary ultrasound cross-sectional image (left panel), taken at the level shown (middle panel), with the equivalent three-dimensional reconstruction (right panel). Note the detailed morphology visible on three-dimensional reconstruction.

Forward imaging transducers would allow a more comprehensive assessment of severe stenoses/occlusions and may make the guidance of interventions, such as laser therapy, more feasible.

Combination devices

Therapeutic

A combination device has inherent advantages over dedicated transducers by allowing real time ultrasound imaging during the procedure and obviating the need for repeat catheter exchanges. This would allow direct assessment of the immediate results and any associated elastic recoil. A number of combination devices incorporating balloons [33, 34], laser catheters [35] and atherectomy devices [36] have been developed and preliminary data is encouraging, suggesting that the on line qualitative and quantitative information regarding the vessel wall obtained during the procedure influences operator strategy in over 40% of cases.

Diagnostic

The combination of intracoronary imaging with recording of blood velocity with a Doppler transducer mounted on the same catheter or on a separate guidewire would allow measurement of basal and post-intervention absolute regional coronary flow. In this way the effects of stenoses can be adequately studied by integrating anatomic (stenosis cross-sectional area) and physiologic data (velocity increase at the site of the stenosis, regional flow reserve). The combination of intravascular imaging with simultaneous recording of high-fidelity blood pressure allows arterial compliance to be accurately calculated from the slope of the pressure-dimension relationship [37]. With this method the changes induced by disease or ageing on the arterial wall can be evaluated, and the effects of pharmacological agents monitored.

Problems and limitations

There are important limitations of the present technology which are currently being addressed. Although a marvel of miniaturising technology, imaging transducers are still relatively large precluding the visualisation of clinically significant coronary stenoses prior to intervention or the more distal coronary arteries. Furthermore, the handling characteristics such as trackability, flexibility and steerability of currently available systems are still not optimal. This has important implications, particularly for intracoronary applications, where all the elements of the catheter, including the distal end where the echo-transducer is mounted, must be fully flexible in order to allow safe and successful negotiation of tortuous vessels. Furthermore, increased steerability of the catheters is required to correct for non-coaxial or eccentric intraluminal positions, as the perpendicularity of the ultrasound beam to the vascular wall influences the intensity with which a structure is visualised and partial drop-out occurs above a critical angle [27]. In addition, the 'blooming effect' induced by off-axis positioning of the catheter, results in an overestimation of the vascular lumen and wall.

The present images are not consistently enough adequate for a complete evaluation of vascular dimensions and morphologic changes. Furthermore, relatively long acquisition times limit the study of luminal changes during the cardiac cycle. Shorter acquisition times are desirable for a more precise study of systolic-diastolic changes in luminal dimensions.

These technical problems are currently being addressed with the introduction of even smaller (2.9F), more flexible transducers and with industry talk of imaging guidewires, which would not only allow assessment of severe stenoses, but also serve as a platform for therapeutic devices allowing real time imaging, on-line during the procedure.

Our knowledge of the appearance of normal and diseased vascular walls and the effects of intervention is still in its infancy, however, and the additional diagnostic and prognostic information obtained in small studies to-date must be confirmed in large on-going trials before the expected benefit outweighs the potential costs.

Conclusions

Direct visualisation of the vessel wall by intravascular ultrasound opens up a world of opportunities to us. It may provide prognostic information on atherosclerosis, and allow the assessment of the effects of dietary and pharmacologic interventions in high risk patients. Furthermore, intracoronary ultrasound offers potentially unique information for the selection and guidance of catheter based interventional techniques.

Acknowledgwments

The authors wish to thank Mr J. Tuin for the preparation of the illustrative material.

References

1. Bom N, ten Hoff H, Lancee CT, Gussenhoven WJ, Bosch JG. Early and recent intraluminal ultrasound devices. Int J Card Imaging 1989; 4: 79–88.
2. Roelandt J, Serruys PW. Intraluminal real-time ultrasonic imaging: clinical perspectives. Int J Card Imaging 1989; 4: 89–97.
3. Yock PG, Linker DT. Intravascular ultrasound. Looking below the surface of vascular disease. Circulation 1990; 81: 1715–8.
4. Gussenhoven EJ, Essed CE, Lancee CT *et al.* Arterial wall characteristics determined by intravascular ultrasound imaging: an *in vitro* study. J Am Coll Cardiol 1989; 14: 947–52.
5. Di Mario C, The SH, Madretsma S *et al.* Detection and characterization of vascular lesions by intravascular ultrasound: an *in vitro* study correlated with histology. J Am Soc Echocardiogr 1992; 5: 135–46.
6. Fitzgerald PJ, St. Goar FG, Connolly AJ *et al.* Intravascular ultrasound imaging of coronary arteries. Is three layers the norm? Circulation 1992; 86: 154–8.
7. Nishimura RA, Welch TJ, Stanson AW, Sheedy PF, Holmes DR Jr. Intravascular ultrasound of the distal aorta and iliac vessels: initial feasibility studies. Radiology 1990; 176: 523–5.
8. Gussenhoven EJ, Frietman PA, The SH *et al.* Assessment of medial thinning in atherosclerosis by intravascular ultrasound. Am J Cardiol 1991; 68: 1625–32.
9. Davidson CJ, Sheikh KH, Harrison JK *et al.* Intravascular ultrasonography versus digital subtraction angiography: a human *in vivo* comparison of vessel size and morphology. J Am Coll Cardiol 1990; 16: 633–6.
10. Isner JM, Rosenfield K, Losordo DW *et al.* Percutaneous intravascular US as adjunct to catheter-based interventions: preliminary experience in patients with peripheral vascular disease. Radiology 1990; 175: 61–70.
11. van Urk H, Gussenhoven WJ, Gerritsen GP *et al.* Assessment of arterial disease and arterial reconstructions by intravascular ultrasound. Int J Card Imaging 1991; 6: 157–64.
12. Tobis JM, Mallery J, Mahon D *et al.* Intravascular ultrasound imaging of human coronary arteries *in vivo*. Analysis of tissue characterizations with comparison to *in vitro* histological specimens. Circulation 1991; 83: 913–26.
13. Nissen SE, Gurley JC, Grines CL *et al.* Intravascular ultrasound assessment of lumen size and wall morphology in normal subjects and patients with coronary artery disease. Circulation 1991; 84: 1087–99.
14. Glagov S, Weisenberg E, Zarins CK, Stankunavicius R, Kolettis GJ. Compensatory enlargement of human atherosclerotic coronary arteries. N Engl J Med 1987; 316: 1371–5.
15. Hermiller JB, Tenaglia AN, Kisslo K *et al.* Compensatory enlargement of atherosclerotic coronary arteries: human *in vivo* validation [abstract]. Circulation 1992; 86 (4 Suppl): I-518.
16. Suarez de Lezo J, Romero M, Medina A *et al.* Intracoronary ultrasound assessment of directional coronary atherectomy: immediate and follow-up findings. J Am Coll Cardiol 1993; 21: 298–307.
17. St Goar FG, Pinto FJ, Alderman EL, Fitzgerald PJ, Stadius ML, Popp RL. Intravascular ultrasound imaging of angiographically normal coronary arteries: an *in vivo* comparison with quantitative angiography. J Am Coll Cardiol 1991; 18: 952–8.
18. Hodgson JM, Reddy KG, Suneja R, Nair RN, Lesnefsky EJ, Sheehan HM. Intracoronary ultrasound imaging: correlation of plaque morphology with angiography, clinical syndrome

and procedural results in patients undergoing coronary angioplasty. J Am Coll Cardiol 1993; 21: 35–44.
19. Torre SR, Sharma SK, Israel DH *et al.* Plaque morphology in acute coronary syndromes: new insights from intravascular ultrasound [abstract]. J Am Coll Cardiol 1993; 21(2 SupplA): 194A.
20. de Feyter PJ, Escaned J, Di Mario C *et al.* Combined intracoronary ultrasound and angioscopic imaging in patients with unstable angina: target lesion characteristics [Abstract]. Eur Heart J 1993; 14(Suppl): 25.
21. Mills RM Jr, Billett JM, Nichols WW. Endothelial dysfunction early after heart transplantation. Assessment with intravascular ultrasound and Doppler. Circulation 1992; 86: 1171–4.
22. St. Goar FG, Pinto FJ, Alderman EL *et al.* Detection of coronary atherosclerosis in young adult hearts using intravascular ultrasound. Circulation 1992; 86: 756–63.
23. Pinto FJ, St. Goar FG, Fischell TA *et al.* Nitroglycerin-induced coronary vasodilation in cardiac transplant recipients. Evaluation with *in vivo* intracoronary ultrasound. Circulation 1992; 85: 69–77.
24. Fitzgerald PJ, Ports TA, Yock PG. Contribution of localized calcium deposits to dissection after angioplasty. An observational study using intravascular ultrasound. Circulation 1992; 86: 64–70.
25. Fitzgerald PJ, Muhlberger VA, Moes NY *et al.* Calcium location within plaque as a predictor of atherectomy tissue retrieval: an intravascular ultrasound study [Abstract]. Circulation 1992; 86(4 Suppl): I–516.
26. Honye J, Mahon DJ, Jain A *et al.* Morphological effects of coronary balloon angioplasty *in vivo* assessed by intravascular ultrasound imaging. Circulation 1992; 85: 1012–25.
27. Di Mario C, Madretsma S, Linker D *et al.* The angle of incidence of the ultrasonic beam: a critical factor for the image quality in intravascular ultrasonography. Am Heart J 1993; 125: 442–8.
28. Tenaglia AN, Buller CE, Kisslo KB, Phillips HR, Stack RS, Davidson CJ. Intracoronary ultrasound predictors of adverse outcomes after coronary artery interventions. J Am Coll Cardiol 1992; 20: 1385–90.
29. The SH, Gussenhoven EJ, Zhong Y *et al.* Effect of balloon angioplasty on femoral artery evaluated with intravascular ultrasound imaging. Circulation 1992; 86: 483–93.
30. Tenaglia AN, Buller CE, Kisslo KB, Stack RS, Davidson CJ. Mechanisms of balloon angioplasty and directional coronary atherectomy as assessed by intracoronary ultrasound. J Am Coll Cardiol 1992; 20: 685–91.
31. Kovach JA, Mintz GS, Kent KM *et al.* Serial intravascular ultrasound studies indicate that chronic recoil is an important mechanism of restenosis following transcatheter therapy [abstract]. J Am Coll Cardiol 1993; 21(Suppl A): 484A.
32. Wenguang L, Gussenhoven WJ, Zhong Y *et al.* Validation of quantitative analysis of intravascular ultrasound images. Int J Card Imaging 1991; 6: 247–53.
33. Isner JM, Rosenfield K, Losordo DW *et al.* Combination balloon-ultrasound imaging catheter for percutaneous transluminal angioplasty. Validation of imaging, analysis of recoil, and identification of plaque fracture. Circulation 1991; 84: 739–54.
34. Violaris AG, Linnemeier TJ, Campbell S, Rothbaum DA, Cumberland DC. Intravascular ultrasound imaging combined with coronary angioplasty. Lancet 1992; 339: 1571–2.
35. Aretz HT, Gregory KW, Martinelli MA *et al.* Ultrasound guidance of laser atherectomy. Int J Card Imaging 1991; 6: 231–7.
36. Yock PG, Fitzgerald PJ, Sudhir K, Linker DT, White W, Ports A. Intravascular ultrasound imaging for guidance of atherectomy and other plaque removal techniques. Int J Card Imaging 1991; 6: 179–89.
37. Wilson R, Di Mario C, Krams R *et al.* Changes in large artery compliance measured with intravascular ultrasound [Abstract]. J Am Coll Cardiol 1992; 19 (Suppl A): 140A.

25. Fluorescence spectroscopy for arterial imaging

JOHN R. KRAMER, BRUCE W. LYTLE & MICHAEL S. FELD

Summary

Laser induced autofluorescence offers a new way to image human arterial tissue. Rather than providing a shadow image, intraarterial laser induced autofluorescence allows a subsurface histochemical description of normal and abnormal human artery. This technique may enable the early detection of disease, permit the study of progression of disease, define the early effects of drug therapy, or serve as a real time diagnostic feedback loop for more powerful ablation lasers used to remove atherosclerotic plaque.

Introduction

F. Mason Sones and colleagues at the Cleveland Clinic ushered in modern cardiology with the development of cine coronary arteriography [1]. The ability to visualize coronary atherosclerosis in living patients allowed the physician to tailor therapy to individual patients and led to major advances in the treatment of coronary atherosclerosis including coronary artery bypass grafting and, subsequently, percutaneous transluminal balloon angioplasty. The development of coronary arteriography has rightfully been recognized as "one of the great medical advances of this century" [2].

In turn, the development of newer catheterization laboratory based treatments, such as PTCA, atherectomy, and rotational atherectomy, has stimulated the development of additional intravascular visualization techniques. Coronary angioscopy images vascular structures by allowing the visual assessment of reflected white light collected via a fiberoptic bundle which both delivers and collects light in vessels that have been cleared of blood [3]. Atherosclerotic plaque rupture, thrombus, and intimal dissections can be recognized by this technique. Another technique, intravascular ultrasound, employs a high frequency (20–40 MHz) ultrasound transducer in the tip of an intracoronary catheter which is able to image the vessel in an orientation perpendicular to the axis of the catheter creating a cross-sectional image of the vessel. Arterial wall structures, atherosclerotic plaque, intimal dissections, lipid, fibrous tissue, and calcium can be recognized and luminal diameter and area can be calculated [4].

While angiography, angioscopy, and intravascular ultrasound compliment one another by providing different ways of looking at the shadows of gross

J.H.C. Reiber and P.W. Serruys (eds): Progress in quantitative coronary arteriography, 395–400.

morphologic structures of the vascular system, healthy and diseased, none of these techniques allows a *chemical* evaluation of structures within the vessel wall or lumen. Fluorescence spectroscopy, in contrast, appears to offer an entirely new technique for imaging vascular structures based on a recognition of subsurface histochemical features of normal and abnormal constituents.

Preliminary studies

Kittrell and colleagues [5] were the first to note that normal artery could be differentiated from atherosclerotic plaque using laser induced autofluorescence. By varying the excitation beam wavelength from 300 to 900 nm and collecting induced fluorescence over a 300 to 900 nm range, peaks in the excitation spectrum were found at 350 and 480 nm. Recognizable differences in spectra obtained from normal vessel and vessel containing atherosclerotic plaque were seen when 480 nm excitation was used.

Fitzmaurice and colleagues [6] were able to identify the chromophores responsible for these spectral differences by comparing conventional white light bright-field microscopic images of normal and abnormal coronary arteries to those obtained with an epiillumination fluorescence microscope using an argon ion laser excitation at 476 nm. Normal arteries, as classified by hematoxylin and eosin staining, were found to have intense autofluorescence of the internal and external elastic laminae with much less intense fluorescence in the media from scattered elastin and collagen fibers. There was little variability amongst specimens. Atherosclerotic arteries, also classified by staining with hematoxylin and eosin staining, were described as having intimal fibroplasia, atheromatous plaque, or calcified plaque. In specimens with intimal fibroplasia there was increased autofluorescence of the intima secondary to presence of closely arranged collagen fibers. In specimens with atheromatous plaque, autofluorescence was seen in the fibrous cap, again related to the presence of dense concentrations of collagen, and in the atheroma core related to heterogeneous deposits of extracellular lipids recognized by staining with oil red O. While the internal elastic lamina was detectable by its autofluorescence, it was often disrupted by the atherosclerotic process. Calcified plaques were quite similar to atheromatous plaques except that additional autofluorescence could be observed coming from areas of dense calcification. A good deal of variability was noted in abnormal coronary arteries compared to normal specimens.

Fitzmaurice concluded that normal arteries could be best characterized by the presence of large amounts of the structural proteins elastin and collagen. In abnormal arteries, however, autofluorescence was found to originate from both structural proteins elastin and collagen and from oxidized lipids in the atheroma core and in regions of calcification. While many fluorescent substances may accumulate in the atheroma core, ceroid, a complex of

$$S(\lambda) = kP \frac{\beta sp\ Fce\ (\lambda) + \beta ce\ Fce\ (\lambda)}{Xsp\ Asp\ (\lambda) + XHb\ AHb\ (\lambda)}$$

Figure 25. 1. Equation describing the overall autofluorescent spectra, S (λ), for coronary artery tissue excited by 476 nm light. This signal is a composite of autofluorescence from structural protein (β_{sp}, F_{sp}) and ceroid (β_{ce}, F_{ce}) as altered by the attenuation effects of structural protein (X_{sp}, A_{sp}) and hemoglobin (X_{Hb}, A_{Hb}). In this equation F_{sp} and F_{ce} are fluorescence lineshapes and A_{sp} and A_{Hb} are absorption lineshapes. P is the power of the excitation light, and k is a constant depending on geometry and other factors. In analyzing the spectrum, the parameters β_{sp}, β_{ce} and X_{Hb} are varied to optimize the fit.

oxidized lipoproteins, is a likely candidate for the chromophore of interest in abnormal coronary arteries. Spectral differences between normal and abnormal coronary artery, therefore, could be explained by differences in histomorphological or histochemical characteristics of each tissue.

Richards-Kortum and colleagues subsequently defined a one-layer model of laser-induced fluorescence which allowed the recognition of the relative contribution of chromophores and attenuators to the overall spectra obtained from vascular tissue (Table 25.1, Figure 25.1) [7]. The model assumes tissue to be a single, optically thick layer with a homogeneous distribution of fluorophores and attenuators. Using excitation light at 476 nm and fitting the emission spectra to the equation of Figure 25.1, two diagnostic parameters, β_{sp} and β_{ce}, can be extracted. These model parameters relate to the concentrations of structural proteins and ceroid and allow the diagnosis of arterial tissue as normal or abnormal with a high degree of accuracy. β_{sp} is an abstracted parameter primarily due to the emission from elastic fibers, and β_{ce} is an abstracted parameter indicating the presence of ceroid. Using these two parameters, arterial tissue could be correctly classified as normal, noncalcified plaque, or calcified plaque (Table 25.2). Normal artery was characterized by a high β_{sp} while calcified plaque tended to demonstrate high levels of β_{ce}. *In vitro*, 92% of 82 coronary artery specimens could be correctly classified as normal, non-calcified plaque or calcified plaque using this diagnostic algorithm [8]. Assuming autofluorescent spectral information of this nature could be obtained using catheters constructed of optical fibers, percutaneous, *in vivo*, intraluminal diagnosis of coronary artery disease at almost any stage of development would be feasible.

Richards-Kortum and colleagues [9] have been able to show *in vitro* that a fiberoptic catheter which delivers 476 nm argon ion laser light to arterial tissue can be used to excite laser-induced autofluorescence with intensities low enough to avoid alteration of tissue spectra. The same fiberoptic catheter is able to collect that autofluorescence with a signal to noise ratio comparable to that seen with conventional non-fiberoptic lensed systems as long as the delivery/collection geometry of the fiberoptic catheter is controlled suggest-

Table 25.1. Fluorophores and attenuators of importance in laser induced fluorescence of coronary artery.

Tissue type	Normal	Non-calcified plaque	Calcified plaque
Fluorophores:			
	Collagen	Collagen	Collagen
	Elastin	Elastin	Elastin
	Ceroid	Ceroid	
Attenuators:			
	Collagen	Collagen	Collagen
	Elastin	Elastin	Elastin
	Hemoglobin	Hemoglobin	Hemoglobin

Table 25.2. Average (± SD) β_{sp} and β_{ce} compared to coronary artery histology.

Tissue type	β_{sp}	β_{ce}
Normal	16.95 ± 4.66	0.55 ± 0.91
Non-calcified plaque	6.13 ± 5.79	1.26 ± 1.40
Calcified plaque	5.53 ± 3.77	2.19 ± 2.46

ing that real time, *in vivo*, spectral diagnosis of coronary atherosclerosis in technically feasible.

Clinical studies

Investigators at the Cleveland Clinic, in collaboration with members of the George R. Harrison Spectroscopy Laboratory at the Massachusetts Institute of Technology, are presently testing a prototype portable spectrofluorimeter system (Figure 25.2) to determine the feasibility of real time, *in vivo*, intraarterial diagnosis using laser induced autofluorescence [10]. The system is small and light; compatible with hospital use. The system consists of a N_2-pumped dye laser capable of producing 5 ns, 100 millijoule pulses of 480 nm excitation at approximately 20 Hz. The light is delivered into the vessel via a 200 μm core diameter 0.22 NA fused silica optical fiber contained within a catheter terminating in an optical shield that determines delivery and collection geometry. Laser induced fluorescence is collected by six additional fibers that surround the excitation fiber. The proximal ends of the collection fibers are mounted onto a f/2.5 spectrograph where excitation light is eliminated with a low fluorescence, long pass filter and a photodiode/amplifier system generates and amplifies the electrical signal produced by the incoming autofluorescent light.

During open heart surgery, laser induced fluorescence spectra are obtained by the surgeon while the shield of the catheter is in contact with normal artery (internal thoracic artery) or atherosclerotic plaque (obstructions in the

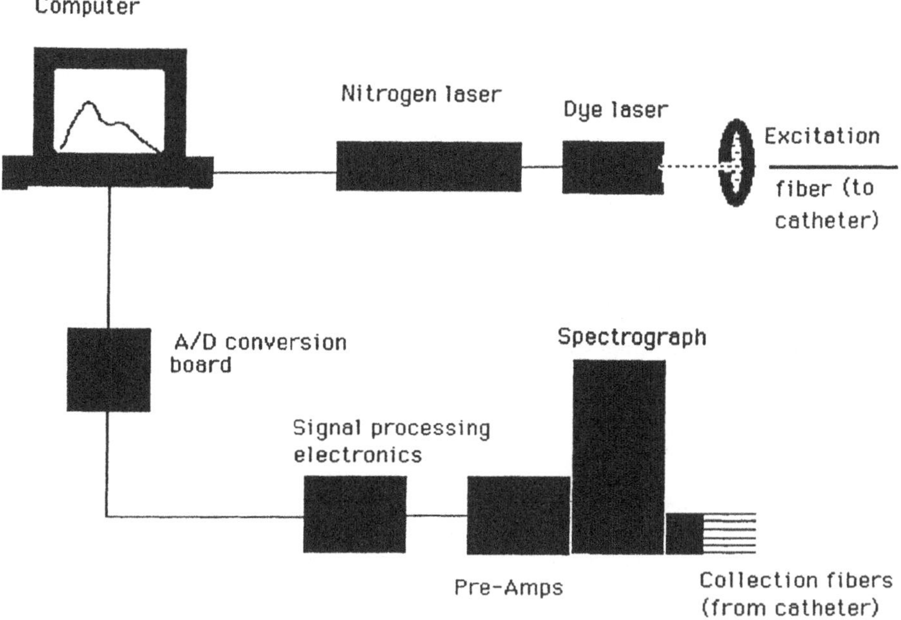

Figure 25.2. Schematic diagram of a portable spectrofluorimeter system used for *in vivo* collection of laser induced autofluorescence.

arteries to be bypassed at the time of operation). Preliminary results show that the system functions efficiently, allowing rapid and safe collection of spectral data at the time of open heart surgery. Initial results suggest that the diagnostic algorithm accurately differentiates normal from abnormal arterial tissue in an *in vivo* setting. Analysis of a large number of these spectra should allow a determination of the sensitivy of this technique for the *in vivo* recognition of abnormal arterial segments.

The future

While the creation of a large laser induced autofluorescence spectral data bank is ongoing, additional experiments utilizing reflectance [11], Raman spectroscopy [12, 13], and multiple fiber delivery/collection catheter systems capable of percutaneous intraarterial mapping [14] are in early stages of implementation.

References

1. Sones FM Jr, Shirey EK. Cine coronary arteriography. Mod Concepts Cardiovasc Dis 1962; 31: 735–8.
2. Hurst JW. A note of appreciation to F. Mason Sones. In Hurst JW (ed): The heart, arteries and veins: update 2: bypass surgery for obstructive coronary disease. New York: McGraw-Hill 1980: 1–2.
3. Ramee SR, White CJ, Collins TJ, Mesa JE, Murgo JP. Percutaneous angioscopy during coronary angioplasty using a steerable microangioscope. J Am Coll Cardio 1991; 17: 100–5.
4. Liebson PR, Klein LW. Intravascular ultrasound in coronary atherosclerosis: a new approach to clinical assessment. Am Heart J 1992; 123: 1643–60.
5. Kittrell C, Willett RL, de los Santos-Pacheo C *et al.* Diagnosis of fibrous arterial atherosclerosis using fluorescence. Appl Optics 1985; 24: 2280–1.
6. Fitzmaurice M, Bordagaray JO, Engelmann GL *et al.* Argon ion laser-excited autofluorescence in normal and atherosclerotic aorta and coronary arteries: morphologic studies. Am Heart J 1989; 118: 1028–38.
7. Richards-Kortum R, Rava RP, Fitzmaurice M *et al.* A one-layer model of laser-induced fluorescence for diagnosis of disease in human tissue: applications to atherosclerosis. IEEE Trans Biomed Eng 1989; 36: 1222–32.
8. Richards-Kortum R, Rava RP, Fitzmaurice M, Kramer JR, Feld MS. 476 nm excited laser-induced fluorescence spectroscopy of human coronary arteries: applications in cardiology. Am Heart J 1991; 122: 1141–50.
9. Richards-Kortum R, Mehta A, Hayes G *et al.* Spectral diagnosis of atherosclerosis using an optical fiber laser catheter. Am Heart J 1989; 118: 381–91.
10. Brennan JF, Zonios GI, Wang TD *et al.* A portable laser spectrofluorimeter system for *in vivo* human tissue fluorescence studies. Applied Spectroscopy. In press.
11. Wu J, Partovi F, Feld MS, Rava RP. Diffuse reflectance from turbid media: an analytical model of photon migration. Appl Optics 1993; 32: 1115–21.
12. Baraga JJ. *In situ* chemical analysis of biological tissue: vibrational Raman spectroscopy of human atherosclerosis [dissertation]. Cambridge, Massachusetts: Massachusetts Institute of Technology, 1992.
13. Manoharan R, Baraga JJ, Feld MS, Rava RP. Quantitative histochemical analysis of human artery using Raman spectroscopy. J Photochem Photobiol B 1992; 16: 211–33.
14. Cothern RM, Hayes GB, Kramer JR, Sacks B, Kittrell C, Feld MS. A multifiber catheter with an optical shield of laser angiosurgery. Lasers Life Sci 1986; 1: 1–12.

26. 3-Dimensional reconstruction of intravascular ultrasound data

MARTIN T. ROTHMAN

Summary

Intravascular ultrasound (IVUS) data is usually represented as 2–dimensional images. By the nature of its acquisition it provides a cross-sectional view of the vessel being examined. This view is not normal for the angiographer who usually tries to view the vessel so as to display its' long axis in silhouette, a view at right angles to that obtained by IVUS imaging. The 2–D view whilst providing instantaneous access to information does not give length perception nor does it provide a feeling for the relationships between structures. Enhancement of the images by reconstruction into a 3-dimensional format may improve comprehension of the data presented and by virtue of adding the length dimension provide a better appreciation of the vessel topography. Digital data processing will speed the reconstruction and may provide as yet unimagined benefits such as on-line 3-dimensional tissue differentiation and 3-dimensional blood flow analysis.

Introduction

The requirement for precise and immediate knowledge during performance of interventional vascular techniques has lead to the development of intravascular ultrasound (IVUS). Resolution of intimal dissections, the detail of the vessel wall and the nature of the material seen as 'stenotic or obstructive' still eludes the operator relying on the X-ray image. Contrast arteriography is the currently accepted method for defining the presence and severity of disease in peripheral and coronary arteries. This technique has limitations: it underestimates the extent and severity of disease [1], it has significant intra-observer and inter-observer error, it may be difficult to assess tortuous segments of vessel, overlying vessels may obscure disease, and it may be difficult to obtain quality images during the performance of interventional procedures [2].

Uses of IVUS during interventional arterio-vascular treatments are varied and exciting:

- selection of appropriate therapeutic technology for treating arterial disease
- definition of the absence of complication and the success of balloon angioplasty

J.H.C. Reiber and P.W. Serruys (eds): Progress in quantitative coronary arteriography, 401–412.

- the positioning of a stent and its appropriate final sizing
- the aiming of a directional atherectomy device and the decision about quantity of tissue to be removed [3]
- the aiming of laser angioplasty devices and assessment of the local tissue effect [4]

Any or all of the above may influence the success rates of these technologies and improve the observed complication and restenosis rates.

The case for ultrasound, rather than direct visualization with fiber optic angioscopy, is made by the understanding that ultrasound can pass through blood and the technique therefore requires no blood replacement strategy during visualization. This may not be very important when considering peripheral vascular disease assessment but is critical when considering detailed prolonged direct visualization in the coronary and cerebral circulation, particularly if frequent instantaneous images are required. Further advantage for ultrasound comes from the fact that sound waves, unlike light waves, can penetrate tissue and so detail may be gleaned about vessel wall structure. Morphological detail can be appreciated and discrimination between elastin and muscular arteries, presence of lipid (hypoechoic), fibromuscular tissue (soft echoes), presence of collagen rich fibrous tissue (bright echoes), and calcified tissue (bright echoes with shadowing behind) can already be achieved [5, 6]. Automated tissue discrimination may be possible using computer assisted tissue characterization algorithms [7, 8, 9].

Ultrasound has other advantages, it is safe and the images readily understood by the operator. It lends itself to incorporation with treatment technologies thereby becoming the 'on-board' diagnostic element of combination devices. A balloon/diagnostic ultrasound combination is already available but todate the images are poor, a prototype directional atherectomy device with ultrasound visualization capability has been demonstrated [3]. IVUS can be combined with Doppler to give flow details and flow field analysis and pictorialisation is already feasible [10].

Background

Intravascular ultrasound systems comprise two basic elements, the CATHETER for intravascular use, and the IMAGE DISPLAY SYSTEM.

Catheter

Understanding the types of catheter design is relevant if the operator is to understand the capabilities and limitations of enhanced image processing techniques that may be applied to the signal. There are a number of different catheter technologies under development for the performance of intravascular ultrasound. These catheters fall into two basic categories, rotational and array-based devices. The general requirements for both types of ultrasound catheter technologies are similar: ultrasound crystals with center frequency between 20–30 MHz, ability to image close to or at the outer wall of the catheter, diameter 1.0–2.5 mm, usable catheter length 135 cm, flexibility especially distally and part or all of the catheter trackable 'over-the-wire' (particularly for coronary application).

Catheters have been developed which have one or more piezoelectric crystals mounted at the distal end. The crystal may be mounted inside the catheter and rotated at high speed, an acoustic mirror rotated instead of the crystal or a number of crystals may be fixed in an array around the circumference of the catheter. The problems related to these catheter designs have been highlighted elsewhere [11]. Whichever catheter technology is used the basic crystal principles are the same. The piezoelectric crystal is caused to resonate at high frequency, 20–30 MHz, by the passage of an electric current. Ultrasound is transmitted out to the tissue interfaces whence it is reflected back to the crystal, causing it to resonate and generate an electric current. The time from outward transmission to return is related to distance and the transmission coefficients of the intervening tissues. In the rotational catheter the crystal is stimulated frequently during the spin cycle so as to build up an image whilst one or more crystals in the array-based catheter are fired sequentially to create the data for the image.

Ring-down time

The main difference to be appreciated between rotational and array-based catheters, other than the obvious design characteristics, is in relation to *ring-down*. A piezoelectric crystal, after it has been electrically stimulated, resonates for a period of time, and this is known as the *ring-down time*. During the period of ring-down returning ultrasound echoes are detected poorly or not at all. In ultrasound physics time relates to distance; the ring-down thus creates a blind spot adjacent to the crystal face. The longer the ring-down time the greater the effective blind spot around the catheter. A device with its' crystals on the surface, like the array-based catheters, will have their blind spot outside the overall dimension of the catheter. The rotational catheter design may have part or all of the blind spot within the catheter body.

The issue of ring-down is thus important and solutions that reduce ring-down time include appropriate selection of the backing and facing layers that are applied to the piezoelectric ultrasound crystal. In addition signal processing algorithm solutions can minimize or remove ring-down from the received signal. The application of the solution may be achieved in hardware or in software and run on a graphic-display work station.

Image display system

The data from the transducer at the distal tip of the ultrasound catheter may be displayed on a relatively simple monochrome analog display screen or be processed to enhance the image. The volume of data involved usually necessitates digitizing of the data before image processing and this may be carried out after analog display or prior to primary presentation of the data. The information returning from the catheter is usually displayed as a cross-sectional slice (B-mode) corresponding to an image perpendicular to the long axis of the vessel. Single crystal catheters can have unsophisticated image display as the data does not have to be processed significantly to produce reasonable cross-sectional slice images. However data from an array-based catheter benefits from image processing to produce a seamless smooth cross-sectional image. Either catheter technology may use more sophisticated systems in which multiple slices may be further processed to allow the construction of a three dimensional colour image [8, 9]. Image reconstruction uses multiple slices of data, data-matching, inter-slice interpolation and allows construction of a smooth 3-dimensional image. It is likely that all image display systems will eventually use sophisticated image processing facilities so that the value of the data may be maximized.

3-Dimensional reconstruction

The method by which multiple cross-sectional slices may be displayed as 3-dimensional images is defined in detail elsewhere [9]. Basically multiple slices are acquired during continuous advancement or more usually pull-back of the catheter. The slices are referenced one to another and the images stacked to create a 3-dimensional image or the signal content of adjacent slices may be interrogated and interpolation algorithms used to create a 3-dimensional reconstruction with a mixture of real data interspersed with computed data.

The quality of a 3-dimensional image after reconstruction relates to a number of factors which will be discussed below. It is important to understand the limitations of an ultrasound system otherwise the operator will reach erroneous conclusions about the B-mode as well as the 3-D image.

Beam characteristics

The ultrasound beam leaves the crystal face and converges before it diverges (Figure 26.1A and 1B). The resolution of the system relates to the beam physics of the ultrasound crystal and it is necessary to define resolution in respect of three co-ordinates; radial (Figure 26.1C), lateral and longitudinal (or axial).

The basic measurement of distance from the crystal face is usually very accurate and thus *radial* resolution for ultrasound is good.

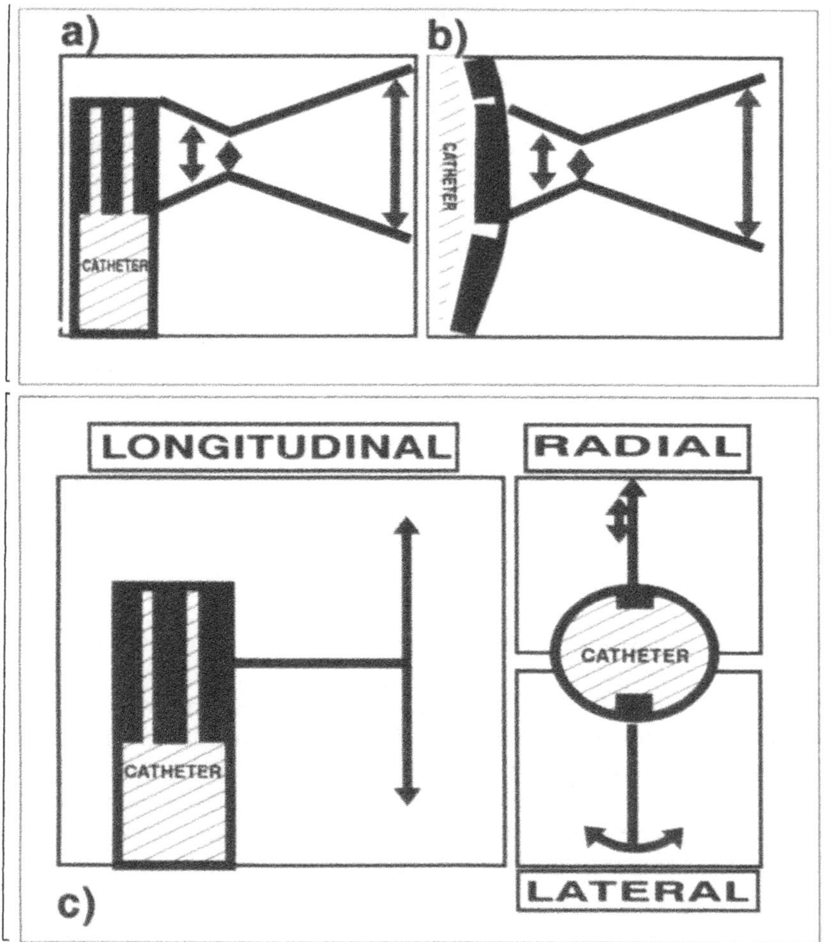

Figure 26.1. Definition of parameters relevant to resolution. (A) Beam plot for long axis of crystal indicating that field from which data acquired is related to length of crystal. (B) Beam plot for width of crystal defining that data from either side of the crystals mid-line is recruited to the image. (C) Resolution is defined in three dimensions; radial, lateral and longitudinally.

The *lateral* resolution of a crystal is usually not as good as radial resolution. This relates to the fact that the beam converges from the crystal face but diverges after the focal point. An object at one or other side of the beams' central line may be detected and displayed as having been detected on the central line. Rotational and array-based catheters may suffer this problem. Array-based catheters connected to a signal-processing facility can use computer algorithms to reduce this artefact. The techniques of data analysis from multiple adjacent crystals to improve the lateral resolution are well known and called 'synthetic aperture' or 'software focus' algorithms.

The longest dimension of the ultrasound crystal is usually along the long axis of the catheter. This adversely effects the beam so that the *longitudinal* resolution is usually poorer than the radial resolution. The thickness of tissue from which data is acquired may be of the order of a millimeter or more. Thus the cross-sectional data that makes up the B-mode image is not infinitely thin and the 'slice thickness' impacts on the reliability of the image.

Image distortion associated with rotational catheters

The external motor to rotate the tip transducer of a rotational catheter is situated some 135 cm away. The intermediate drive shaft is necessarily thin as it is within the body of the catheter. The desired 1:1 rotational relationship between motor and tip may not always be achieved; the tip may lag consistently behind the motor, may intermittently fall behind and catch-up (stick and slip), or may fail to rotate at all, particularly in the thin shafted coronary devices where coronary vessel tortuosity may conspire to trap the drive shaft. These and other image distortions of rotational devices have been discussed elsewhere [11].

B-mode slice thickness and 3-D reconstruction

As previously described the B-mode slice has thickness and this can influence the 3-dimensional reconstruction result. It is important to know the thickness of each acquired B-mode (Figure 26.2) so that multiple representations of the same data are not assembled on the assumption that each were from unique segments. The inter-slice distance between B-mode images needs to be accounted for in the 3-dimensional reconstruction computation.

Catheter tip pull-back technique

There is a vogue for motorized catheter pull-back but unless the 3-dimensional assembly routine takes account of the B-mode slice thickness no real advantage is achieved. Multiple slices may be acquired during motorized pull-back of the catheter but when the acquisition time is very fast many of the slices may effectively be of the same segment of tissue, moreover the data is coming from a relatively thick slice of tissue but represented as if the data were from an infinitely thin one. Thus longitudinal resolution relates to actual tissue slice thickness and for effective 3-dimensional reconstruction it is important to understand this dimension (Figure 26.2).

Understanding of the motion of the catheter tip within the coronary vessel is necessary for proper appreciation of the 3-D reconstructed image. A measured pull-back of the catheter body outside the patient does not necessarily achieve an equal movement within the coronary artery (Figure 26.3). There is the potential for considerable slack within the guide catheter and within the coronary artery itself and so care is essential to ensure that inter-

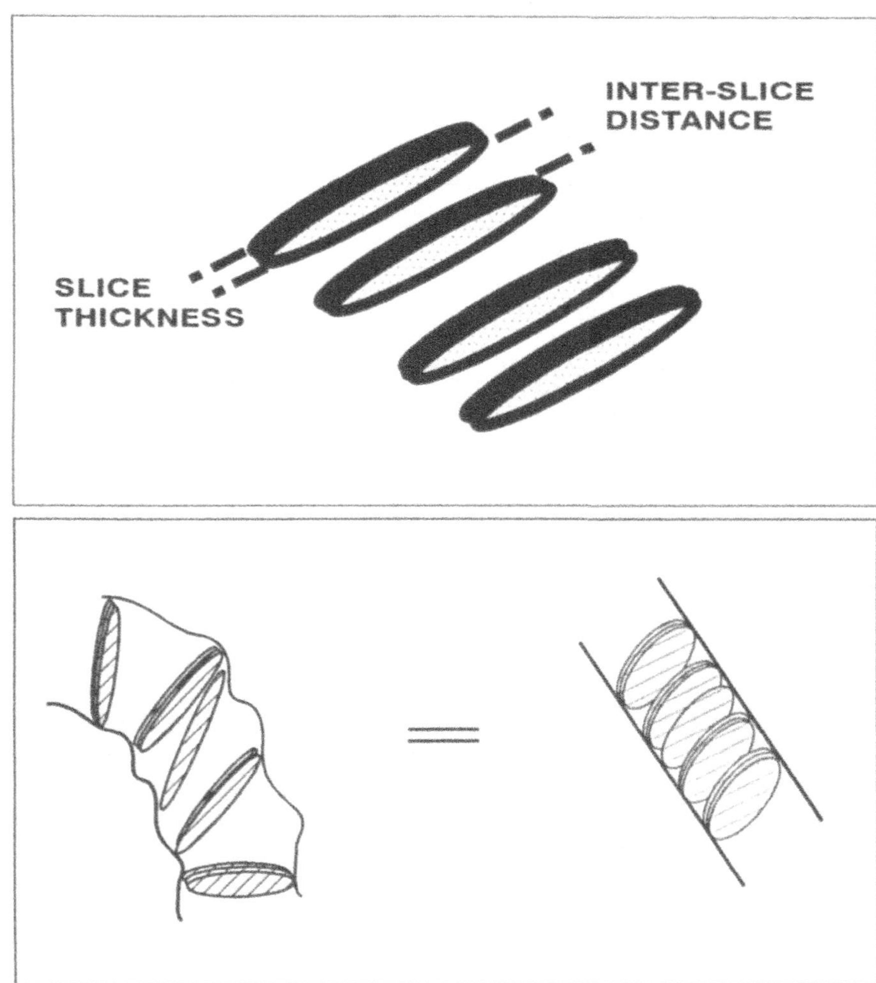

Figure 26.2. Upper panel: all B-mode images comprise data from above and below the mid-line of the crystal and this contributes to the 'slice thickness'. This slice thickness governs the inter-slice interval that should be allowed between B-modes when acquiring for 3–D reconstruction. *Lower panel*: all B-modes are acquired at right axis to the catheter. Although they may not be acquired from parallel planes reconstruction algorithms usually assume they are.

slice distances are correct for the 3-D assembly algorithm and for acquisition of unique B-mode slice (Figure 26.2).

Vessel distortion by 3-D reconstruction

There is no satisfactory method by which B-mode slices may be orientated one to another. All B-mode slices are acquired at right-angles to the catheter

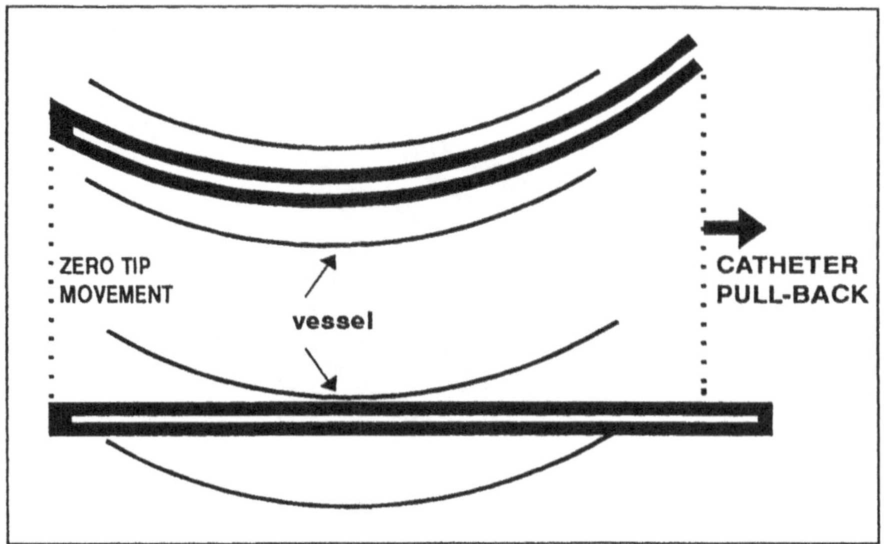

Figure 26.3. Catheter pull-back outside the patient does not necessarily lead to equivalent tip movement within the coronary artery.

body. Any tortuosity of the vessel through which the catheter passes during pull-back is not taken into account during the 3-D reconstruction and so all vessels end up straight (Figure 26.2). Algorithms for manually or automatically acquiring and entering the co-ordinates of the catheter tip position from bi-plane fluoroscopy, so as to orientate the planes of each B-mode slice, are in their infancy.

Value of 3-D reconstruction

Morphology of disease and treatment rationale

The value of 3-D reconstruction for assessment of the topography of the vessel under evaluation depends on the quality of the B-mode data. If this is of good quality then appreciation of length and nature of the disease may be better understood if 3-D reconstruction is used. Balloon size selection may be enhanced by a better appreciation of the bulk of disease present. Eccentric lesions may be better treated by directional atherectomy and it is muted that the presence of circumferential calcification calls for the use of high-speed rotational atherectomy. These opinions require more research before they are substantiated.

The result of intervention may well be reliably assessed by IVUS. The adequacy of dilatation, the quantity of debulking, the positioning of a stent and its completeness of opening may all be better appreciated using IVUS.

The value of 3-D reconstruction may be illustrated by consideration of vessel dissection. If the point of attachment of a flap can be appreciated, its circumferential extent and the degree of spiraling defined, then it may be possible to separate safe from unsafe dissections. In the example (Figure 26.4) a flap of less than 90 degrees is seen, with the flap everted the vessel is not occluded. On tracking this dissection axially over the vessel length it can be seen to be benign as the dissection does not spiral. Alternatively in the same figure is seen a 90 degree arc dissection that spirals through a 180 degree arc of vessel. If this dissection everts it causes a 50% occlusion; more extensive spiraling would lead to greater effective occlusion.

A similar argument is demonstrated in Figure 26.5 where a dissection causing a 50% obstruction at one point can lead to effective total obstruction if the point of attachment of the dissection spirals around the vessel. Appreciation of the risk from this dissection may best be achieved by 3-dimensional reconstruction rather than simple pull-back through the region of interest.

3-D flow-field analysis

The mechanics of coronary blood flow depend in part on the driving pressure and also on the anatomy of the vessel. Insignificant narrowings within a vessel may effect flow depending on their position, the tortuosity of the vessel, their proximity to other narrowings and side-branches. A small stenosis on the inside of a bend may not interfere with flow as it is within the slow flow field; however the same dimension stenosis on the opposite wall, after the bend, may dramatically impair flow. Likewise multiple small stenoses may summate to significantly impair flow, depending on their location.

Basic research on the demonstration of blood-flow fields has been published [10] but rapid on-line analysis of flow fields will most probably require input of the co-ordinates for the tip of the catheter from bi-plane fluoroscopy as well as vessel inlet blood pressure; the development lead time is long but preliminary data is exciting.

Vessel wall characterization

IVUS is the only imaging modality currently available for appreciation of the vessel wall *in-vivo*. Longitudinal studies of disease progression and regression will be enhanced if atheroma and calcification can be reliably identified within vessels. Likewise, if studies confirm that specific interventional treatment modalities are best suited to identifiable abnormalities then IVUS will become adjunctive to the routine performance of interventional treatments.

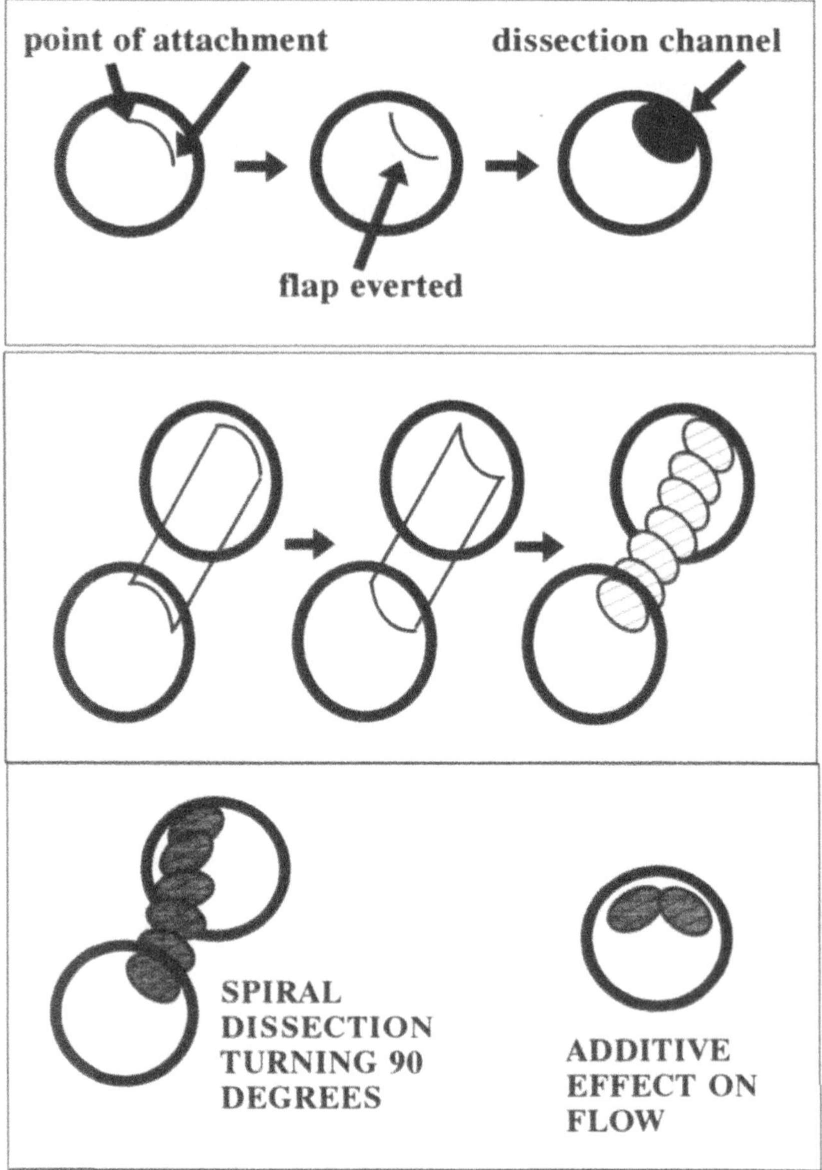

Figure 26.4. Theoretical value for 3–D reconstruction in the appreciation of dissections. *Upper panel*: point of attachment defines the size of the dissection channel. *Middle panel*: no spiral of dissection. *Lower panel*: spiral dissection leads to additional reduction in lumen dimension compared to non-spiral dissection.

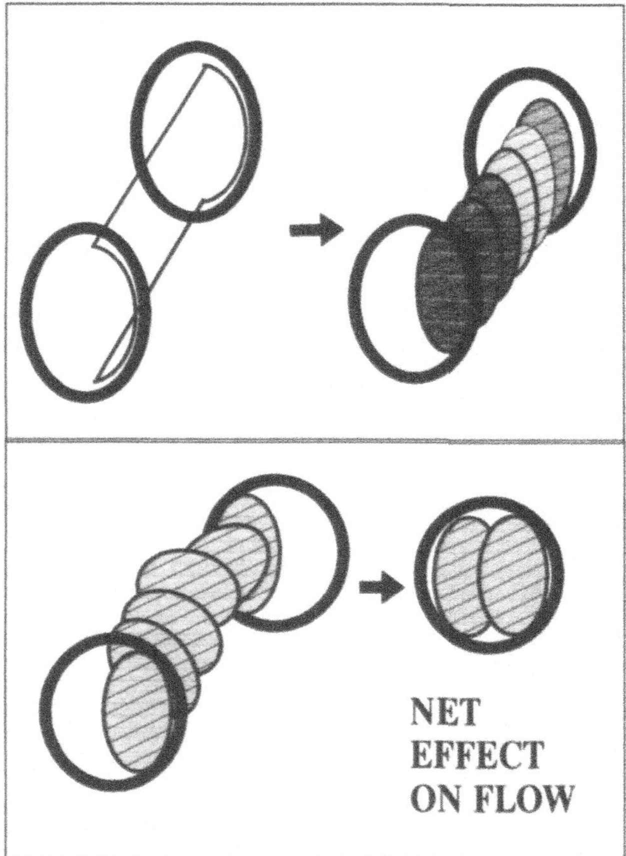

Figure 26.5. Larger dissection channels, if they spiral, lead to relatively more of a flow obstruction. *Upper panel*: limited dissection without spiral leads to moderate flow impairment. *Lower panel*: similar dissection which spirals leads to significant flow impairment.

Published 3-D images of diseased vessels indicate the potential for this enhancement but reliable identification of disease is unproven.

Conclusion

Intravascular, real-time, high resolution ultrasound imaging is an exciting new technology. It produces cross-sectional images of an artery which may be processed to produce 3-dimensional images, allow lumen measurements, and an appreciation of the morphology of a vessel. The potential for new areas of research are legion and practical applications are being appreciated. It is likely to become a major adjunct to interventional vascular procedures assessing the immediate result and perhaps indicating the longer-term outcome.

References

1. Glagov S, Weisenberg EA, Zarins CK *et al.* Compensatory enlargement of human atherosclerotic coronary arteries. N Eng J Med 1987; 316: 1371–5.
2. Fisher LD, Judkins MP, Lespérance J *et al.* Reproducibility of coronary arteriographic reading in the coronary artery surgery study (CASS). Cathet Cardiovasc Diagn 1982; 8: 565–75.
3. Yock PG, Linker DT, White NW *et al.* Clinical applications of intravascular ultrasound imaging in atherectomy. Int J Card Imaging 1989; 4: 117–25.
4. Borst C, Rienks R, Mali WP *et al.* Laser ablation and the need for intra-arterial imaging. Int J Card Imaging 1989; 4: 127–33.
5. Gussenhoven WJ, Essed CE, Frietman P *et al.* Intravascular echographic assessment of vessel wall characteristics: a correlation with histology. Int J Card Imaging 1989; 4: 105–16.
6. Gussenhoven WJ, Essed CE, Lancee CT *et al.* Arterial wall characteristics determined by intravascular ultrasound imaging: an *in vitro* study. J Am Coll Cardiol 1989; 14: 947–52.
7. Kitney RI, Moura L, Straughan K. Three dimensional modelling of arterial structures using ultrasound. Proceedings of the Ninth Annual Conference, IEEE Engineering in Medicine and Biology Society. New York: IEEE 1987; 1: 400–1.
8. Kitney RI, Moura L, Straughan K. 3-D visualisation of arterial structures and Voxel modelling. Int J Card Imaging 1989; 4: 135–43.
9. Burrell CJ, Kitney RI, Rothman MT. Intravascular ultrasound imaging and three dimensional modeling of arteries. Echocardiography 1990; 7: 475–84.
10. Burrell CJ, McDonald AH, Rothman MT, Kitney RI, Straughan K, Moura LD, Giddens DP. 3-D computer visualisation of arteries and blood-flow – *in vitro* and *in vivo*. Comput Cardiol 1990; 122: 41–6.
11. Rothman MT. Intravascular ultrasound: the new dimension. In Labs KH, Jäger KA, Fitzgerald DE, Woodcock JP, Neurenberg-Heusler D (eds): Diagnostic vascular ultrasound. London: Edward Arnold 1992: 312–20.

Index

Developments in Cardiovascular Medicine

50. J. Meyer, R. Erbel and H.J. Rupprecht (eds.): *Improvement of Myocardial Perfusion.* Thrombolysis, Angioplasty, Bypass Surgery. Proceedings of a Symposium, held in Mainz, F.R.G. (1984). 1985 ISBN 0-89838-748-5
51. J.H.C. Reiber, P.W. Serruys and C.J. Slager (eds.): *Quantitative Coronary and Left Ventricular Cineangiography.* Methodology and Clinical Applications. 1986 ISBN 0-89838-760-4
52. R.H. Fagard and I.E. Bekaert (eds.): *Sports Cardiology.* Exercise in Health and Cardiovascular Disease. Proceedings from an International Conference, held in Knokke, Belgium (1985). 1986 ISBN 0-89838-782-5
53. J.H.C. Reiber and P.W. Serruys (eds.): *State of the Art in Quantitative Cornary Arteriography.* 1986 ISBN 0-89838-804-X
54. J. Roelandt (ed.): *Color Doppler Flow Imaging and Other Advances in Doppler Echocardiography.* 1986 ISBN 0-89838-806-6
55. E.E. van der Wall (ed.): *Noninvasive Imaging of Cardiac Metabolism.* Single Photon Scintigraphy, Positron Emission Tomography and Nuclear Magnetic Resonance. 1987 ISBN 0-89838-812-0
56. J. Liebman, R. Plonsey and Y. Rudy (eds.): *Pediatric and Fundamental Electrocardiography.* 1987 ISBN 0-89838-815-5
57. H.H. Hilger, V. Hombach and W.J. Rashkind (eds.), *Invasive Cardiovascular Therapy.* Proceedings of an International Symposium, held in Cologne, F.R.G. (1985). 1987 ISBN 0-89838-818-X
58. P.W. Serruys and G.T. Meester (eds.): *Coronary Angioplasty.* A Controlled Model for Ischemia. 1986 ISBN 0-89838-819-8
59. J.E. Tooke and L.H. Smaje (eds.): *Clinical Investigation of the Microcirculation.* Proceedings of an International Meeting, held in London, U.K. (1985). 1987 ISBN 0-89838-833-3
60. R.Th. van Dam and A. van Oosterom (eds.): *Electrocardiographic Body Surface Mapping.* Proceedings of the 3rd International Symposium on B.S.M., held in Nijmegen, The Netherlands (1985). 1986 ISBN 0-89838-834-1
61. M.P. Spencer (ed.): *Ultrasonic Diagnosis of Cerebrovascular Disease.* Doppler Techniques and Pulse Echo Imaging. 1987 ISBN 0-89838-836-8
62. M.J. Legato (ed.): *The Stressed Heart.* 1987 ISBN 0-89838-849-X
63. M.E. Safar (ed.): *Arterial and Venous Systems in Essential Hypertension.* With Assistance of G.M. London, A.Ch. Simon and Y.A. Weiss. 1987 ISBN 0-89838-857-0
64. J. Roelandt (ed.): *Digital Techniques in Echocardiography.* 1987 ISBN 0-89838-861-9
65. N.S. Dhalla, P.K. Singal and R.E. Beamish (eds.): *Pathology of Heart Disease.* Proceedings of the 8th Annual Meeting of the American Section of the I.S.H.R., held in Winnipeg, Canada, 1986 (Vol. 1). 1987 ISBN 0-89838-864-3
66. N.S. Dhalla, G.N. Pierce and R.E. Beamish (eds.): *Heart Function and Metabolism.* Proceedings of the 8th Annual Meeting of the American Section of the I.S.H.R., held in Winnipeg, Canada, 1986 (Vol. 2). 1987 ISBN 0-89838-865-1
67. N.S. Dhalla, I.R. Innes and R.E. Beamish (eds.): *Myocardial Ischemia.* Proceedings of a Satellite Symposium of the 30th International Physiological Congress, held in Winnipeg, Canada (1986). 1987 ISBN 0-89838-866-X
68. R.E. Beamish, V. Panagia and N.S. Dhalla (eds.): *Pharmacological Aspects of Heart Disease.* Proceedings of an International Symposium, held in Winnipeg, Canada (1986). 1987 ISBN 0-89838-867-8
69. H.E.D.J. ter Keurs and J.V. Tyberg (eds.): *Mechanics of the Circulation.* Proceedings of a Satellite Symposium of the 30th International Physiological Congress, held in Banff, Alberta, Canada (1986). 1987 ISBN 0-89838-870-8
70. S. Sideman and R. Beyar (eds.): *Activation, Metabolism and Perfusion of the Heart.* Simulation and Experimental Models. Proceedings of the 3rd Henry Goldberg Workshop, held in Piscataway, N.J., U.S.A. (1986). 1987 ISBN 0-89838-871-6

71. E. Aliot and R. Lazzara (eds.): *Ventricular Tachycardias*. From Mechanism to Therapy. 1987 ISBN 0-89838-881-3
72. A. Schneeweiss and G. Schettler: *Cardiovascular Drug Therapoy in the Elderly*. 1988 ISBN 0-89838-883-X
73. J.V. Chapman and A. Sgalambro (eds.): *Basic Concepts in Doppler Echocardiography*. Methods of Clinical Applications based on a Multi-modality Doppler Approach. 1987 ISBN 0-89838-888-0
74. S. Chien, J. Dormandy, E. Ernst and A. Matrai (eds.): *Clinical Hemorheology*. Applications in Cardiovascular and Hematological Disease, Diabetes, Surgery and Gynecology. 1987 ISBN 0-89838-807-4
75. J. Morganroth and E.N. Moore (eds.): *Congestive Heart Failure*. Proceedings of the 7th Annual Symposium on New Drugs and Devices, held in Philadelphia, Pa., U.S.A. (1986). 1987 ISBN 0-89838-955-0
76. F.H. Messerli (ed.): *Cardiovascular Disease in the Elderly*. 2nd ed. 1988 ISBN 0-89838-962-3
77. P.H. Heintzen and J.H. Bürsch (eds.): *Progress in Digital Angiocardiography*. 1988 ISBN 0-89838-965-8
78. M.M. Scheinman (ed.): *Catheter Ablation of Cardiac Arrhythmias*. Basic Bioelectrical Effects and Clinical Indications. 1988 ISBN 0-89838-967-4
79. J.A.E. Spaan, A.V.G. Bruschke and A.C. Gittenberger-De Groot (eds.): *Coronary Circulation*. From Basic Mechanisms to Clinical Implications. 1987 ISBN 0-89838-978-X
80. C. Visser, G. Kan and R.S. Meltzer (eds.): *Echocardiography in Coronary Artery Disease*. 1988 ISBN 0-89838-979-8
81. A. Bayés de Luna, A. Betriu and G. Permanyer (eds.): *Therapeutics in Cardiology*. 1988 ISBN 0-89838-981-X
82. D.M. Mirvis (ed.): *Body Surface Electrocardiographic Mapping*. 1988 ISBN 0-89838-983-6
83. M.A. Konstam and J.M. Isner (eds.): *The Right Ventricle*. 1988 ISBN 0-89838-987-9
84. C.T. Kappagoda and P.V. Greenwood (eds.): *Long-term Management of Patients after Myocardial Infarction*. 1988 ISBN 0-89838-352-8
85. W.H. Gaasch and H.J. Levine (eds.): *Chronic Aortic Regurgitation*. 1988 ISBN 0-89838-364-1
86. P.K. Singal (ed.): *Oxygen Radicals in the Pathophysiology of Heart Disease*. 1988 ISBN 0-89838-375-7
87. J.H.C. Reiber and P.W. Serruys (eds.): *New Developments in Quantitative Coronary Arteriography*. 1988 ISBN 0-89838-377-3
88. J. Morganroth and E.N. Moore (eds.): *Silent Myocardial Ischemia*. Proceedings of the 8th Annual Symposium on New Drugs and Devices (1987). 1988 ISBN 0-89838-380-3
89. H.E.D.J. ter Keurs and M.I.M. Noble (eds.): *Starling's Law of the Heart Revisted*. 1988 ISBN 0-89838-382-X
90. N. Sperelakis (ed.): *Physiology and Pathophysiology of the Heart*. Rev. ed. 1988 3rd, revised edition, 1994: see below under Volume 151
91. J.W. de Jong (ed.): *Myocardial Energy Metabolism*. 1988 ISBN 0-89838-394-3
92. V. Hombach, H.H. Hilger and H.L. Kennedy (eds.): *Electrocardiography and Cardiac Drug Therapy*. Proceedings of an International Symposium, held in Cologne, F.R.G. (1987). 1988 ISBN 0-89838-395-1
93. H. Iwata, J.B. Lombardini and T. Segawa (eds.): *Taurine and the Heart*. 1988 ISBN 0-89838-396-X
94. M.R. Rosen and Y. Palti (eds.): *Lethal Arrhythmias Resulting from Myocardial Ischemia and Infarction*. Proceedings of the 2nd Rappaport Symposium, held in Haifa, Israel (1988). 1988 ISBN 0-89838-401-X
95. M. Iwase and I. Sotobata: *Clinical Echocardiography*. With a Foreword by M.P. Spencer. 1989 ISBN 0-7923-0004-1

Developments in Cardiovascular Medicine

96. I. Cikes (ed.): *Echocardiography in Cardiac Interventions.* 1989 ISBN 0-7923-0088-2
97. E. Rapaport (ed.): *Early Interventions in Acute Myocardial Infarction.* 1989 ISBN 0-7923-0175-7
98. M.E. Safar and F. Fouad-Tarazi (eds.): *The Heart in Hypertension.* A Tribute to Robert C. Tarazi (1925-1986). 1989 ISBN 0-7923-0197-8
99. S. Meerbaum and R. Meltzer (eds.): *Myocardial Contrast Two-dimensional Echocardiography.* 1989 ISBN 0-7923-0205-2
100. J. Morganroth and E.N. Moore (eds.): *Risk/Benefit Analysis for the Use and Approval of Thrombolytic, Antiarrhythmic, and Hypolipidemic Agents.* Proceedings of the 9th Annual Symposium on New Drugs and Devices (1988). 1989 ISBN 0-7923-0294-X
101. P.W. Serruys, R. Simon and K.J. Beatt (eds.): *PTCA - An Investigational Tool and a Non-operative Treatment of Acute Ischemia.* 1990 ISBN 0-7923-0346-6
102. I.S. Anand, P.I. Wahi and N.S. Dhalla (eds.): *Pathophysiology and Pharmacology of Heart Disease.* 1989 ISBN 0-7923-0367-9
103. G.S. Abela (ed.): *Lasers in Cardiovascular Medicine and Surgery.* Fundamentals and Technique. 1990 ISBN 0-7923-0440-3
104. H.M. Piper (ed.): *Pathophysiology of Severe Ischemic Myocardial Injury.* 1990 ISBN 0-7923-0459-4
105. S.M. Teague (ed.): *Stress Doppler Echocardiography.* 1990 ISBN 0-7923-0499-3
106. P.R. Saxena, D.I. Wallis, W. Wouters and P. Bevan (eds.): *Cardiovascular Pharmacology of 5-Hydroxytryptamine.* Prospective Therapeutic Applications. 1990 ISBN 0-7923-0502-7
107. A.P. Shepherd and P.A. Öberg (eds.): *Laser-Doppler Blood Flowmetry.* 1990 ISBN 0-7923-0508-6
108. J. Soler-Soler, G. Permanyer-Miralda and J. Sagristà-Sauleda (eds.): *Pericardial Disease.* New Insights and Old Dilemmas. 1990 ISBN 0-7923-0510-8
109. J.P.M. Hamer: *Practical Echocardiography in the Adult.* With Doppler and Color-Doppler Flow Imaging. 1990 ISBN 0-7923-0670-8
110. A. Bayés de Luna, P. Brugada, J. Cosin Aguilar and F. Navarro Lopez (eds.): *Sudden Cardiac Death.* 1991 ISBN 0-7923-0716-X
111. E. Andries and R. Stroobandt (eds.): *Hemodynamics in Daily Practice.* 1991 ISBN 0-7923-0725-9
112. J. Morganroth and E.N. Moore (eds.): *Use and Approval of Antihypertensive Agents and Surrogate Endpoints for the Approval of Drugs affecting Antiarrhythmic Heart Failure and Hypolipidemia.* Proceedings of the 10th Annual Symposium on New Drugs and Devices (1989). 1990 ISBN 0-7923-0756-9
113. S. Iliceto, P. Rizzon and J.R.T.C. Roelandt (eds.): *Ultrasound in Coronary Artery Disease.* Present Role and Future Perspectives. 1990 ISBN 0-7923-0784-4
114. J.V. Chapman and G.R. Sutherland (eds.): *The Noninvasive Evaluation of Hemodynamics in Congenital Heart Disease.* Doppler Ultrasound Applications in the Adult and Pediatric Patient with Congenital Heart Disease. 1990 ISBN 0-7923-0836-0
115. G.T. Meester and F. Pinciroli (eds.): *Databases for Cardiology.* 1991 ISBN 0-7923-0886-7
116. B. Korecky and N.S. Dhalla (eds.): *Subcellular Basis of Contractile Failure.* 1990 ISBN 0-7923-0890-5
117. J.H.C. Reiber and P.W. Serruys (eds.): *Quantitative Coronary Arteriography.* 1991 ISBN 0-7923-0913-8
118. E. van der Wall and A. de Roos (eds.): *Magnetic Resonance Imaging in Coronary Artery Disease.* 1991 ISBN 0-7923-0940-5
119. V. Hombach, M. Kochs and A.J. Camm (eds.): *Interventional Techniques in Cardiovascular Medicine.* 1991 ISBN 0-7923-0956-1
120. R. Vos: *Drugs Looking for Diseases.* Innovative Drug Research and the Development of the Beta Blockers and the Calcium Antagonists. 1991 ISBN 0-7923-0968-5

Developments in Cardiovascular Medicine

121. S. Sideman, R. Beyar and A.G. Kleber (eds.): *Cardiac Electrophysiology, Circulation, and Transport.* Proceedings of the 7th Henry Goldberg Workshop (Berne, Switzerland, 1990). 1991 ISBN 0-7923-1145-0
122. D.M. Bers: *Excitation-Contraction Coupling and Cardiac Contractile Force.* 1991 ISBN 0-7923-1186-8
123. A.-M. Salmasi and A.N. Nicolaides (eds.): *Occult Atherosclerotic Disease.* Diagnosis, Assessment and Management. 1991 ISBN 0-7923-1188-4
124. J.A.E. Spaan: *Coronary Blood Flow.* Mechanics, Distribution, and Control. 1991 ISBN 0-7923-1210-4
125. R.W. Stout (ed.): *Diabetes and Atherosclerosis.* 1991 ISBN 0-7923-1310-0
126. A.G. Herman (ed.): *Antithrombotics.* Pathophysiological Rationale for Pharmacological Interventions. 1991 ISBN 0-7923-1413-1
127. N.H.J. Pijls: *Maximal Myocardial Perfusion as a Measure of the Functional Significance of Coronary Arteriogram.* From a Pathoanatomic to a Pathophysiologic Interpretation of the Coronary Arteriogram. 1991 ISBN 0-7923-1430-1
128. J.H.C. Reiber and E.E. v.d. Wall (eds.): *Cardiovascular Nuclear Medicine and MRI.* Quantitation and Clinical Applications. 1992 ISBN 0-7923-1467-0
129. E. Andries, P. Brugada and R. Stroobrandt (eds.): *How to Face 'the Faces' of Cardiac Pacing.* 1992 ISBN 0-7923-1528-6
130. M. Nagano, S. Mochizuki and N.S. Dhalla (eds.): *Cardiovascular Disease in Diabetes.* 1992 ISBN 0-7923-1554-5
131. P.W. Serruys, B.H. Strauss and S.B. King III (eds.): *Restenosis after Intervention with New Mechanical Devices.* 1992 ISBN 0-7923-1555-3
132. P.J. Walter (ed.): *Quality of Life after Open Heart Surgery.* 1992 ISBN 0-7923-1580-4
133. E.E. van der Wall, H. Sochor, A. Righetti and M.G. Niemeyer (eds.): *What's new in Cardiac Imaging*? SPECT, PET and MRI. 1992 ISBN 0-7923-1615-0
134. P. Hanrath, R. Uebis and W. Krebs (eds.): *Cardiovascular Imaging by Ultrasound.* 1992 ISBN 0-7923-1755-6
135. F.H. Messerli (ed.): *Cardiovascular Disease in the Elderly.* 3rd ed. 1992 ISBN 0-7923-1859-5
136. J. Hess and G.R. Sutherland (eds.): *Congenital Heart Disease in Adolescents and Adults.* 1992 ISBN 0-7923-1862-5
137. J.H.C. Reiber and P.W. Serruys (eds.): *Advances in Quantitative Coronary Arteriography.* 1993 ISBN 0-7923-1863-3
138. A.-M. Salmasi and A.S. Iskandrian (eds.): *Cardiac Output and Regional Flow in Health and Disease.* 1993 ISBN 0-7923-1911-7
139. J.H. Kingma, N.M. van Hemel and K.I. Lie (eds.): *Atrial Fibrillation, a Treatable Disease?* 1992 ISBN 0-7923-2008-5
140. B. Ostadel and N.S. Dhalla (eds.): *Heart Function in Health and Disease.* Proceedings of the Cardiovascular Program (Prague, Czechoslovakia, 1991). 1992 ISBN 0-7923-2052-2
141. D. Noble and Y.E. Earm (eds.): *Ionic Channels and Effect of Taurine on the Heart.* Proceedings of an International Symposium (Seoul, Korea , 1992). 1993 ISBN 0-7923-2199-5
142. H.M. Piper and C.J. Preusse (eds.): *Ischemia-reperfusion in Cardiac Surgery.* 1993 ISBN 0-7923-2241-X
143. J. Roelandt, E.J. Gussenhoven and N. Bom (eds.): *Intravascular Ultrasound.* 1993 ISBN 0-7923-2301-7
144. M.E. Safar and M.F. O'Rourke (eds.): *The Arterial System in Hypertension.* 1993 ISBN 0-7923-2343-2
145. P.W. Serruys, D.P. Foley and P.J. de Feyter (eds.): *Quantitative Coronary Angiography in Clinical Practice.* With a Foreword by Spencer B. King III. 1994 ISBN 0-7923-2368-8

Developments in Cardiovascular Medicine

146. J. Candell-Riera and D. Ortega-Alcalde (eds.): *Nuclear Cardiology in Everyday Practice.* 1994 (in prep.) ISBN 0-7923-2374-2
147. P. Cummins (ed.): *Growth Factors and the Cardiovascular System.* 1993 ISBN 0-7923-2401-3
148. K. Przyklenk, R.A. Kloner and D.M. Yellon (eds.): *Ischemic Preconditioning: The Concept of Endogenous Cardioprotection.* 1993 ISBN 0-7923-2410-2
149. T.H. Marwick: *Stress Echocardiography.* Its Role in the Diagnosis and Evaluation of Coronary Artery Disease. 1994 ISBN 0-7923-2579-6
150. W.H. van Gilst and K.I. Lie (eds.): *Neurohumoral Regulation of Coronary Flow.* Role of the Endothelium. 1993 ISBN 0-7923-2588-5
151. N. Sperelakis (ed.): *Physiology and Pathophysiology of the Heart.* 3rd rev. ed. 1994 ISBN 0-7923-2612-1
152. J.C. Kaski (ed.): *Angina Pectoris with Normal Coronary Arteries: Syndrome X.* 1994 ISBN 0-7923-2651-2
153. D.R. Gross: *Animal Models in Cardiovascular Research.* 2nd rev. ed. 1994 ISBN 0-7923-2712-8
154. A.S. Iskandrian and E.E. van der Wall (eds.): *Myocardial Viability.* Detection and Clinical Relevance. 1994 ISBN 0-7923-2813-2
155. J.H.C. Reiber and P.W. Serruys (eds.): *Progress in Quantitative Coronary Arteriography.* 1994 ISBN 0-7923-2814-0
156. U. Goldbourt, U. de Faire and K. Berg (eds.): *Genetic Factors in Coronary Heart Disease.* 1994 ISBN 0-7923-2752-7
157. G. Leonetti and C. Cuspidi (eds.): *Hypertension in the Elderly.* 1994 ISBN 0-7923-2852-3
158. D. Ardissino, S. Savonitto and L.H. Opie (eds.): *Drug Evaluation in Angina Pectoris.* 1994 ISBN 0-7923-2897-3
159. G. Bkaily (ed.): *Membrane Physiopathology.* 1994 ISBN 0-7923-3062-5
160. R.C. Becker (ed.): *The Modern Era of Coronary Thrombolysis.* 1994 ISBN 0-7923-3063-3

Previous volumes are still available

KLUWER ACADEMIC PUBLISHERS – DORDRECHT / BOSTON / LONDON

The manufacturer's authorised representative in the EU is Springer Nature Customer Service Centre GmbH, Europaplatz 3, 69115 Heidelberg, Germany. If you have any concerns regarding our products, please contact ProductSafety@springernature.com

Printed and bound by CPI Group (UK) Ltd, Croydon, CR0 4YY
23/04/2026
02095607-0004